# Returning to Work in Anaesthesia

## Back on the Circuit

# Returning to Work in Anaesthesia

Back on the Circuit

Edited by

**Emma Plunkett**
Specialist Registrar, Birmingham School of Anaesthesia, UK

**Emily Johnson**
Consultant Anaesthetist, Worcester Acute Hospitals NHS Trust, Worcester, UK

**Anna Pierson**
Specialty Registrar, Birmingham School of Anaesthesia, UK

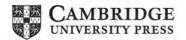
CAMBRIDGE
UNIVERSITY PRESS

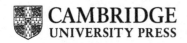

Shaftesbury Road, Cambridge CB2 8EA, United Kingdom

One Liberty Plaza, 20th Floor, New York, NY 10006, USA

477 Williamstown Road, Port Melbourne, VIC 3207, Australia

314–321, 3rd Floor, Plot 3, Splendor Forum, Jasola District Centre, New Delhi – 110025, India

103 Penang Road, #05–06/07, Visioncrest Commercial, Singapore 238467

Cambridge University Press is part of Cambridge University Press & Assessment, a department of the University of Cambridge.

We share the University's mission to contribute to society through the pursuit of education, learning and research at the highest international levels of excellence.

www.cambridge.org
Information on this title: www.cambridge.org/9781107514690

© Cambridge University Press & Assessment 2016

First published 2016

*A catalogue record for this publication is available from the British Library*

*Library of Congress Cataloging-in-Publication data*
Names : Plunkett, Emma V. E., editor. | Johnson, Emily, 1977– , editor. |
Pierson, Anna, 1980– , editor.
Title: Returning to work in anaesthesia : back on the circuit / edited by
Emma Plunkett, Emily Johnson, Anna Pierson.
Description: Cambridge, United Kingdom ; New York : Cambridge University
Press, 2016. | Includes bibliographical references and index.
Identifiers: LCCN 2016006109 | ISBN 9781107514690 (pbk.)
Subjects: | MESH: Anesthesiology – manpower | Return to Work
Classification: LCCR D81 | NLM WO221 | DDC 617.9/6 – dc23
LC record available at http://lccn.loc.gov/2016006109

ISBN    978-1-107-51469-0    Paperback

Additional resources for this publication at www.cambridge.org/returningtowork

· · · · · · · · · · · · · · · · · · · · · · · · · · · · · · · · · · · · · · · · · · · · · · · · · · · · · · · · · · · · · · · · · · · · · · · · · · · · · · · ·

For my husband Adrian and our children; Aubrey, Penelope and Arthur. Three lovely reasons to have had time away from anaesthesia.
*EP*

Dedicated to my son Euan and nephew Alexander.
*EJ*

For the three boys in my life; my husband, Richard, and our sons, George and Henry. Your love and support have made this possible.
*AP*

# Contents

# Section 2: Refreshing Your Knowledge

Nicholas Cowley, Kerry Cullis, Anna Dennis, Hozefa Ebrahim, Ruth Francis, Maria Garside, Sarah Gibb, Emily Johnson, Surrah Leifer, Randeep Mullhi, James Nickells, Anna Nutbeam, Anna Pierson, Jane Pilsbury, Emma Plunkett, Louise Savic, Charlotte Small, Alifia Tameem, Caroline Thomas and Benjamin Walton

# Section 3: Guidelines, Updates and Checklists

# Contributors

**Kathryn Bell**
Consultant Anaesthetist, The Newcastle upon Tyne Hospitals NHS Foundation Trust, UK; Training Programme Director, Northern School of Anaesthesia, UK

**Anna Costello**
Specialty Registrar, Oxford School of Anaesthesia, UK

**Nicholas Cowley**
Consultant in Anaesthesia and Intensive Care Medicine, Worcester Acute Hospitals NHS Trust, UK

**Kerry Cullis**
Consultant Anaesthetist, University Hospitals Birmingham NHS Trust, UK

**Anna Dennis**
Consultant in Anaesthesia and Intensive Care Medicine, Heart of England NHS Foundation Trust, UK

**Hozefa Ebrahim**
Consultant in Anaesthesia and Intensive Care Medicine, Heart of England NHS Foundation Trust, UK

**Carolyn Evans**
Bernard Johnson Advisor LTFT, Royal College of Anaesthetists, UK

**Ruth Francis**
Consultant Anaesthetist, University Hospitals Birmingham NHS Trust, UK

**Laura Fulton**
Specialist Registrar, Barts and the London School of Anaesthesia, UK

**Maria Garside**
Associate Specialist, Bradford Teaching Hospitals NHS Foundation Trust, UK

**Sarah Gibb**
Locum Consultant Anaesthetist, The Newcastle upon Tyne Hospitals NHS Foundation Trust, UK

**Fran Haigh**
Consultant Anaesthetist, Poole Hospital NHS Foundation Trust, UK

**Jill Horn**
Consultant Anaesthetist, Bradford Teaching Hospitals NHS Foundation Trust, UK; Training Programme Director, Leeds/Bradford School of Anaesthesia, UK

**Emily Johnson**
Consultant Anaesthetist, Worcester Acute Hospitals NHS Trust, UK

**Surrah Leifer**
Specialty Registrar, North West School of Anaesthesia, UK

**Katy Miller**
Specialty Registrar, Birmingham School of Anaesthesia, UK

**Randeep Mullhi**
Consultant in Anaesthesia and Intensive Care Medicine, University Hospitals Birmingham NHS Trust, UK

**James Nickells**
Consultant Anaesthetist, North Bristol NHS Trust, UK

**Anna Nutbeam**
Specialty Registrar, South West School of Anaesthesia, UK

**Stephen Phillips**
Specialty Registrar, Wessex School of Anaesthesia, UK

**Anna Pierson**
Specialty Registrar, Birmingham School of Anaesthesia, UK

**Jane Pilsbury**
Specialty Registrar, Birmingham School of Anaesthesia, UK

**Emma Plunkett**
Specialist Registrar, Birmingham School of Anaesthesia, UK

**Nancy Redfern**
Consultant Anaesthetist, The Newcastle upon Tyne Hospitals NHS Foundation Trust, UK; Honorary Membership Secretary, Association of Anaesthetists of Great Britain and Ireland, UK

**Louise Savic**
Consultant Anaesthetist, The Leeds Teaching Hospitals NHS Trust, UK

**Charlotte Small**
Specialty Registrar, Birmingham School of Anaesthesia, UK

**Alifia Tameem**
Consultant in Anaesthesia and Pain Management, The Dudley Group NHS Foundation Trust, UK

**Caroline Thomas**
Specialty Registrar, Leeds/Bradford School of Anaesthesia, UK

**Laura Tulloch**
Consultant in Anaesthesia and Intensive Care Medicine, Worcester Acute Hospitals NHS Trust, UK

**Benjamin Walton**
Consultant in Intensive Care Medicine and Anaesthesia, North Bristol NHS Trust, UK

# Foreword

This is a 'must-have' handbook for any anaesthetist returning to work. It binds the practical-ities, essential knowledge and latest guidance into a friend, companion and guide.

I remember when I first returned to work (I've done it three times- once for sickness and twice for parenthood), there was no clear process; I could not remember which switch was which, or doses for drugs. I was worried and anxious about my performance and patient safety. Since this time, return to work guidance and collaboration from the AAGBI and RCOA, have brought great advances in our safer and phased return to work practice.

And now, at last, *Back on the Circuit*, an anaesthesia return to work book! Written by a highly credible team, who know how we feel as they have returned to work and might again. Emma Plunkett, Emily Johnson and Anna Pierson have worked with drive and dedication, to bring together this unique book, an important milestone for us as a profession and an essential resource for those returning to work.

**Dr Annie Hunningher**
Consultant in Anaesthesia, GASagain course co-lead

# Preface

Doing anything that you've not done for a while can be daunting. People often say, 'It's just like riding a bike', although even for previously experienced cyclists the first time back on the saddle can be uncomfortable and unsteady! For more complex tasks of an unpredictable nature, this 'unsteadiness' is magnified and things that one might have previously done automatically need more deliberate thought. Returning to work in anaesthesia is no different. Anaesthesia is a multifaceted specialty with many different requirements: specialist knowledge, complex clinical skills and timely and effective communication particularly in stressful situations, to name a few. As anaesthetists we are highly trained individuals. Trained in the areas mentioned, but also trained to be aware of our limitations and when we should ask for help.

In anaesthesia, indeed through all the medical specialties, patient safety comes first. We have a duty as doctors to ensure that we are capable and competent. It is therefore important that we acknowledge times when we are a bit 'unsteady' and seek appropriate support. In the past this has not always been easy to do, as extra support when returning from a break has not always been perceived to be required. The service needs of running departments might also at times put pressure on individuals to work outside their comfort zone. In combination this might lead to doctors returning to work being expected to be back up to speed the moment they set foot in the workplace. Anyone who has experienced a significant break will know that this is usually far from how they feel.

Everyone involved in this project has had time away from anaesthesia, for numerous reasons. Many of them also teach on returning to work courses or are responsible for supervising and supporting those returning to work. We have worked together to produce what we hope will be a valuable resource for those preparing to return to anaesthesia after a break. There is a lot of useful information already available; however, it is in many different places and it can feel rather overwhelming working out where to begin.

This book is your starting point. We have thought hard about what we needed when we were in your position. We have a section which gives practical advice, one to help you refresh your knowledge and one that provides all the guidelines and checklists that you might want to look at before you come back or in your first few weeks back.

A commonly quoted problem returning to work is a lack of confidence. We cannot resolve this directly in a book. However, we can help you to feel well prepared for your return and hopefully that will help your confidence to come flooding back. We want this book to be your friend and have worked hard with this goal in mind. We wish it had been available for our returns to work in anaesthesia and hope it is useful for you.

Good luck and please get in touch to let us know how you get on.

# Acknowledgements

This book is the product of hard work from a fantastic team of authors. They have all given their precious time to the project and we appreciate their support and commitment to our shared vision. We think that the strength of the project comes from this collaboration and hope we have created a really useful resource.

As well as this team of authors, we have some other people to thank. Thank you to James Nickells and Ben Walton, lead editors from FRCAQ. They supported the project from the outset and have shared some of their bank of Final FRCA Single Best Answer questions that covered topics in our refresher section. We are incredibly grateful for their contribution.

Thank you to Sara Ormorod for writing the question on the definition of capacity. As a consultant liaison psychiatrist, her expertise is much appreciated. Thank you to Hannah Church, Hari Krovvidi, Nancy Redfern and Amy Walker who have each reviewed chapters for us and provided their wisdom and advice on their areas of expertise.

Thanks to all those individuals and organizations who have granted permission for us to reproduce their images, figures, tables or guideline summaries in this book. Thanks to Sam Salib who took the photo of the epidural set up trolley.

Thanks to Nisha, Jade and Ross from Cambridge University Press. Nisha has been a fantastic support from the inception of the project and throughout the preparation of the manuscript and beyond.

Finally, and most importantly of all, the biggest thank you has to be to our families for their encouragement, patience, understanding and help with childcare. This book really is a team effort and we are so very grateful to have had such a great team.

# Introduction

Emma Plunkett, Emily Johnson and Anna Pierson

If you are reading this book, you are likely to be on a break from working in anaesthesia and may be starting to think about your return. Whatever the reason for your break, the previously familiar beeps from the anaesthetic machine will have faded into a dim and distant memory and you may feel as if you cannot remember how to take an anaesthetic history, let alone give an anaesthetic. You are not alone. The feeling of trepidation returning to work after a break is a common one, shared by many.

People feel apprehensive about different aspects of returning to work. Some agonize over their perceived lack of knowledge, feeling that they have forgotten everything. Others worry about their ability to perform practical procedures. Some may be concerned about human factors: ability to communicate and situational awareness. Plus, there may be factors related to the reason for your leave that cause anxiety, for example worries about health or about leaving a small child or unwell relative. All of these are valid concerns and need to be addressed, but the good news is that many of them can be remedied.

Welcome to your returning to work handbook! This book has been written to help you prepare for your return to anaesthesia, whatever the reason for your break from practice, and whatever your particular concerns are.

## How to use the book

The book is divided into three sections, according to when you might want to use them.

Section 1 considers the more practical aspects of returning to work and so this might be best used when planning a break (if this is possible) or once it is known that you will be taking one. It starts by considering the current state of play regarding management of the return to work process and the potential effects of a break from practice. Next we review the available guidance from the Academy of Medical Royal Colleges (AoMRC), the Royal College of Anaesthetists (RCoA) and Association of Anaesthetists of Great Britain and Ireland (AAGBI), summarizing the important points. After this we discuss ways of preparing for your return to work, with chapters covering topics such as keeping in touch days and phased returns to work. Following the publication of the guidance mentioned above, many regions in the UK have introduced Return to Work Programmes to support those returning to work and guide those supervising them. We have therefore included an example of one such programme, which we have experience of using, which you might want to adapt and use yourself if there is not one already in your hospital or region.

Ways that you can help your return to work are considered next with an important chapter describing how mentoring can help you in your return to work period. This is a period of significant change for you and in the 2013 version of 'Good medical practice', the General Medical Council (GMC) recommends that you 'find and take part in structured support opportunities ... whenever your role changes significantly'. We demystify what mentoring is and give an example situation. To accompany this we also give some anecdotes of people's experiences returning to work and their tips and suggestions. We also consider how you can make technology work to your advantage.

The final chapter in Section 1 discusses how we can support colleagues returning to work – both trainees and consultants.

Section 2 is the knowledge refresher section. In this section we have used the RCoA CPD Matrix as a rough 'syllabus' of important subjects to cover. When considering how to structure this section we felt it was important for it to feel practical and interactive and to be different from reading lists of facts. So we decided to cover each topic using a short scenario, followed by a question or questions, which take a variety of formats. Some of these have been adapted from the FRCAQ.com website as we felt that many of their single best answer questions were appropriately written and covered common clinical topics that you would want to refresh. Please do not consider any of the questions in this section to be a test. They are written this way to engage you and to help you to start thinking like an anaesthetist again! After each scenario and question(s), there follows a concise summary of the topic with references for further reading if you are feeling particularly rusty on that topic. We have gone for breadth of subjects – with 120 topics – rather than detailed discussions. By doing this we hope that we have included many of the common cases that you will encounter on your return to work, as well as the emergency situations that we hope you do not find yourself in, but that you will be better prepared for having refreshed your knowledge! This section might be best used in the few weeks before you return to work.

Section 3 contains important guidelines and checklists. This section is your companion for your first few weeks back at work. The first chapter covers preoperative assessment and includes the relevant National Institute for Health and Care Excellence (NICE) and European Society of Anaesthesiology (ESA) guidelines as well as reminders about what to ask in an anaesthetic history and how to interpret preoperative investigations. Next we cover consent and documentation with a recap of what risks to quote when you see your patients. After this we have included a copy of the World Health Organization (WHO) checklist, which in itself is a good prompt for what you need to consider in your anaesthetic planning, and also a handy drug dose reminder that is probably made superfluous by the many apps available now, but can be useful to carry with you if/when technology is not your thing. We have a chapter on practical procedures, to remind you what you need to lay out on your trolley and a brief refresher on how to use ultrasound. Finally, we have brief summaries of the AAGBI, Difficult Airway Society (DAS), Resuscitation Council, NICE and ICU guidelines and summaries of the National Audit Projects. We don't anticipate that you will commit any/all of this to memory prior to returning to work, but rather that you can dip in and out of this section as necessary during your return to work period (and beyond).

We hope that this structure provides a logical approach to planning, preparing for and accomplishing your return to work in anaesthesia. We are aware that time passes and guidelines are updated and so we have developed an accompanying website to this book which can be updated more frequently than the book itself.

# A break from practice: the current state of play

Carolyn Evans

*In this chapter, Dr Carolyn Evans gives an overview of how the return to work process is managed overseas and what the future holds in the UK.*

If a clinician returns to a different clinical area of practice, agreement about a formal training package with assessment of newly acquired skills and competencies automatically follows. The clinician returning to the same area of practice is assumed to be capable of continuing where they left off, even after a break of years. This return to the front line on day one back at work still continues to be the accepted norm, especially for those returning after maternity leave. Try explaining this approach to a member of the public; they would be, understandably, appalled.

## How is a break from practice managed in other countries?

The Australian and New Zealand College of Anaesthetists (ANZCA) have recommendations on practice re-entry available via their website[1]. The most recent version, PS50 2013, *advises* anaesthetists that after an absence of more than 12 months, they should follow an agreed refreshment of knowledge and skills programme before re-entering independent clinical practice. The timeline suggested is 4 weeks supervision for every year of absence. Their College prospectively approves an individual programme and seeks confirmation that the participant has satisfactorily completed the programme. There is no mention of what happens in the event the individual does not meet the expected standards in the agreed timeline – a further period of supervision would be the most likely way forward. A punitive outcome such as referral for a formal assessment of an anaesthetist's practice by their Medical Board would undermine the current voluntary self-directed return to practice programme.

The American Medical Association (AMA) defines physician re-entry as 'a return to clinical practice in the discipline in which one has been trained or certified following an extended period of clinical inactivity not resulting from discipline or impairment'. There is considerable variation between states around what is expected for physicians re-entering practice. The AMA 2010 Physician Licensure Survey reported 51% of medical boards to have a policy on physician re-entry, with a requirement to complete a re-entry programme after a physician had been out of practice an average of 2.8 years (range 1–10 years)[2]. Information from those running re-entry programmes in 2009 gave a length of time to complete a re-entry programme as between 6 weeks and 12 months, with a minimum cost of $6000. Relocation to attend a programme can increase individual costs, so finance remains a huge barrier to active

---

*Returning to Work in Anaesthesia*, ed. Emma Plunkett, Emily Johnson and Anna Pierson.
Published by Cambridge University Press. © Cambridge University Press 2016.

physician participation in re-entry schemes in the USA. The Re-entry Programme Directors report numbers served by their programmes as extremely small, with an average age of 51 years and predominantly male.

## Are there any predictors of outcome after a break from practice?

Information is limited but the Center for Personalized Education for Physicians (CPEP) in the USA published their retrospective outcome data for 683 physicians who were referred between 2000 and 2010[3], which concluded older physicians were more likely to have unsafe assessment outcomes. However, this cohort of individuals was referred to CPEP for remediation so is a very different entity from the physician looking for 'upgrading' of knowledge and skills after a career break.

A review of 62 physicians participating in the CPEP re-entry programme after a voluntary career break recognized an emerging pattern between years out of practice and increasing physician age as predictors of poorer performance. Reasons for leaving practice were predominantly family and health (60%)[4]. Twenty anaesthetists returning to practice completed a re-entry program which included simulation-based assessment. The outcome data collected from this institution over a 10-year period included identification of two anaesthetists with 'deficits significant enough to preclude likely improvement' but loss of participants to follow up and the small numbers limited any further statistical interpretation[5]. It was concluded that simulation was an effective means of assessing baseline competency in this group returning to clinical practice.

In the UK, a General Medical Council (GMC) 'Skills fade literature review' published in December 2014 confirms the paucity of further evidence around loss of clinical and professional skills following a break from practice[6].

## The way forward

The impetus for change worldwide is clinician shortage, the impact of gender change within the workforce and a greater understanding of the impact of clinical inactivity on patient care and patient safety. The fundamental principles of consistency between state medical licensing boards, quality assurance of all re-entry programmes, programme funding and research to inform re-entry programme development that the AMA is working to are themes we would recognize and support in the UK. The General Practice funded returner scheme was superseded in 2006 by an induction and refresher (I+R) scheme. Primary care organizations expect a general practitioner (GP) returning after a break of 2 years or more to enrol in an I+R scheme. There is no requirement in legislation for this, but it offers some reassurance that these doctors are competent to practise in the NHS. Health Education England and NHS England are due to introduce a new I+R scheme, 3–6 months in duration, recognizing the different needs of those returning from work overseas as compared to those after a formal career break[7]. The I+R scheme will be mandatory for those doctors who have been out of clinical general practice for 5 years and recommended for those returning after a break of 2 to 5 years.

Within secondary care, the principles underpinning the return to work agenda have been embraced by the trainee workforce. This is the generation who will normalize the 'return to work portfolio', making it an expected submission for inclusion within an individual's revalidation package. In the future, it is likely that what is currently voluntary best practice will become an expectation from the regulator.

# References

1. www.anzca.edu.au (accessed 2 January 2016).
2. American Medical Association Physician Re-entry website http://www.ama-assn.org/go/reentry (accessed 2 January 2016).
3. E. S. Grace, E. F. Wenghofer, E. J. Korinek. Predictors of physician performance on competence assessment: findings from CPEP, the Center for Personalized Education for Physicians. *Acad Med* 2014; 89(6): 912–19.
4. E. S. Grace, E. J. Korinek, L. B. Weitzl, D. K. Wentz. Physicians reentering clinical practice: characteristics and clinical abilities. *J Contin Educ Health Prof* 2011; 31(1): 49–55.
5. S. DeMaria Jr, S. T. Samuelson, A. D. Schwartz, A. J. Sim, A. I. Levine. Simulation-based assessment and retraining for the anaesthesiologist seeking re-entry to clinical practice: a case series. *Anaesthesiology* 2013; 119: 206–17.
6. http://www.gmc-uk.org/Skills_fade_literature_review_final_report.pdf_60956354.pdf (accessed 2 January 2016).
7. www.england.nhs.uk/2015/01/26/boost-gp-workforce/ (accessed 2 January 2016).

# Chapter 2

# Returning to work guidance

Emma Plunkett

Ten years ago there was little published guidance on how to manage a return to practice after a break, but the landscape has changed considerably in a decade. In 2008, the Association of Anaesthetists of Great Britain and Ireland (AAGBI) Welfare Resource Pack was published and this contained a section on returning to work. This was the first specialty-specific guidance to be produced and much of what it states remains relevant, although the document has now been archived. This was followed in 2011 by the first version of the Royal College of Anaesthetists (RCoA) Return to Practice guidance, which was then updated in 2012 to account for the Academy of Medical Royal Colleges' (AoMRC) guidance published in the same year. This was the work of a multispecialty working group of experts, including Dr Carolyn Evans from the RCoA, the author of their guidance. In the preface of the AoMRC document, the chair of the group states that there was 'considerable concern and a perceived lack of guidance' on this subject, reflecting the feelings of many.

*In this chapter we highlight the key points in these documents, to help you understand what you should be looking to achieve during the return to work process. All of the guidance stresses the vital importance of patient safety when a doctor is returning to practice after a break and this must be the fundamental principle governing the return to work process.*

## AAGBI guidance[1]

This guidance starts by suggesting that there are three distinct groups of doctors approaching the return to work process and it is useful to consider their needs separately as this affects how the process is managed.

1. Those in whom a rapid return to normal duties is expected, i.e. there is no reason to think they will not be able to return to their previous duties.
2. Those requiring a more prolonged period of supervision to establish whether they will be able to return to normal duties, for example a phased return to work after illness.*
3. Those doctors where capability concerns exist who are likely to require a period of retraining.

\* Please note, there is more information about phased returns to work later in this section.

This guidance and that published subsequently (discussed below) have all recommended that concerns about health, conduct and capability should be addressed before a return to work programme is commenced.

*Returning to Work in Anaesthesia*, ed. Emma Plunkett, Emily Johnson and Anna Pierson.
Published by Cambridge University Press. © Cambridge University Press 2016.

**Table 2.1** Factors to consider when planning a return to work programme

| Individual characteristics and situation | Actions | Methods |
|---|---|---|
| • Learning needs<br>• Learning styles<br>• Job plan<br>• How best to assess outcome<br>• Funding | • Decide what CPD to do<br>• Ensure straightforward cases on initial return<br>• Set aside time for reflection and appraisal | • Observation<br>• Supernumerary time<br>• CPD<br>• Mentoring<br>• Flexible working |

The document then goes on to propose the duties of the department when supporting a member of staff to return to work and the duties of the doctor concerned. Here are some key points:

The department should:

- Involve senior departmental managers
- Agree clear guidelines for the reintroduction period
- Have a named consultant coordinating the process and offer a separate mentor
- Ensure confidentiality and dignity for the doctor and that the process is open, honest and fair.

The doctor should:

- Not attempt to return to work unless they are well
- Have insight regarding the process and recognize that it is stressful
- Set realistic goals and be enthusiastic
- Seek support for the process; at home, at work or both.

# AoMRC guidance[2]

The Academy's guidance has a wide remit and aims to inform all of those involved in the return to work process: doctors, employers, regulators, appraisers (Trust or Local Education and Training Board), locum agencies and those who provide continuing professional development (CPD) for this process. It is aimed at those who have had a break of more than 3 months. Less than 3 months away from the workplace was felt by the working group to be much less significant, although it was recognized that confidence may still be affected.

The group reviewed the evidence regarding what factors are important to consider when doctors take time out from practice. Although there is a lot of anecdotal opinion on the subject, there is relatively little evidence and what there is comes from the USA; this has been discussed in Chapter 1.

As is the case with preparing for anything, it is suggested that proper preparation is the key to success. This should be in the form of an action plan drawn up by the doctor and those responsible for supervising their return together. This should involve consideration of the factors listed in Table 2.1.

The guidance also gives recommendations for how to set up an organizational policy for the return to work process – i.e. for development of a return to work programme. It identifies several stages:

- Preparing for absence (when it is anticipated)
- Preparation for return to plan the reintroduction period, including agreed timelines
- How to assess and agree success.

Checklists of factors to consider at each stage are then included, expanding on the factors mentioned above.

## RCoA guidance[3]

The RCoA guidance is a useful translation of the AoMRC guidance and checklists, making them relevant for anaesthesia. It also suggests that an important factor to consider is the length of time in a post before a period of leave. In terms of length of time away from work (identified in evidence as a key factor) and the likely degree of supervision and speed at which normal duties can be resumed, the following breakdown is proposed:

- 3–6 months: a rapid return
- 6–12 months: some support
- >12 months: a structured process
- 3 years: a significant supervised process with robust assessment.

It then considers the different phases in the return to work process and gives ideas for CPD. The points mentioned in the checklists can then be used to design paperwork to use in Return to Work programmes, as is demonstrated in Chapter 4. We also include the guidance on CPD later in the same chapter.

## BMA guidance[4]

The BMA gives guidance on its website for doctors working in both primary and secondary care. It has identified 'a model process' for those returning to secondary care, which follows an identical structure to the Academy's and RCoA's guidance.

## References

1. http://www.aagbi.org/sites/default/files/welfare_resource_pack_2008_0.pdf (accessed 2 January 2016).
2. http://www.aomrc.org.uk/doc_view/9486-return-to-practice-guidance (accessed 2 January 2016).
3. https://www.rcoa.ac.uk/system/files/PUB-ReturnToWork2012.pdf (accessed 2 January 2016).
4. http://bma.org.uk/developing-your-career/consultant/returning-to-practice-a-model-process (accessed 2 January 2016).

# Chapter 3

# Returning to work experiences

Emily Johnson

*The experience of returning to work in anaesthesia is different for each individual who undertakes the challenge. There is no escaping the fact it can be a daunting time, more so for some than others. In this chapter we include some personal reflections that have kindly been shared with the aim of providing some help and reassurance to those returning to work. We also discuss the results of regional surveys investigating the return to work experience.*

Returning to work for the first day was daunting. It seemed so long since I had been in the role of being an anaesthetist. I had attended an update course, ALS and an airway day to prepare myself as much as possible. The thought of having to complete the practical procedures worried me the most. In reality many of these were like riding a bike – they came back very easily. What I wasn't so prepared for was the feeling of being mentally slower. To this day I don't think that I actually was, but this took me far longer to overcome.

Katy, Anaesthetic StR

For me, I found it much easier to concentrate at work if I was confident in my childcare arrangements. Having a nanny who came to the house was worth its weight in gold. We didn't have to change plans if one of the children was ill or if we'd had a disturbed night and were running late. It cost quite a lot, but it meant the children were happier, they could go to what they wanted in the way of clubs and lessons. I actually had two nannies – one did 4 days a week – about 40–48 hours, and the other did one day a week. Being a good employer, providing a decent car so the children were safe, and doing my best to accommodate what our nanny needed to do, led to a good long-term relationship and therefore good help when things were difficult with children or work.

Another useful learning point was just to be 'good enough'. Prior to being a mum I had rather let work expand into home time, not helped as my husband is a non-medical academic, so was also very busy with grant applications. It was good to be reminded that I am our children's only mum – lots of other people can deal with things at work. Go home on time, and leave work at work.

The same applied to my approach to being a mum. It's about bringing up a child so he or she achieves their potential, not making them do what you want. I've had four children and every one was different, with different needs and enthusiasms. I watch others making their children fit into 'routines' and being told 'no' and 'don't', and suspect that this produces more stress amongst the parents and less happiness in the children. Remember, only people who have children who breast feed for 10 minutes every 4 hours can write books about childcare. The rest of society have

*Returning to Work in Anaesthesia*, ed. Emma Plunkett, Emily Johnson and Anna Pierson.
Published by Cambridge University Press. © Cambridge University Press 2016.

children with different parenting needs and therefore do not write books or spend time on chat lines – we're looking after and enjoying our children.

Nancy, Consultant Anaesthetist

I was concerned about many aspects of returning to work. Particularly being able to do the practical procedures and knowing about any major changes in practice since I had been off. In practice the practical skills returned very quickly but the major hurdle was a reduced level of confidence. This I feel was partly due to returning to work less than full time and actually spending less time at work. Also observing all my peers flourish into confident consultants whilst I was still battling through workplace assessments. I had no objective feedback indicating my perceived reduced confidence was a problem and in fact was described as confident in many a multi-source feedback. I also don't believe it made me any worse at my job, it just made it harder personally. It is for this reason I have chosen to work full time in my consultant role.

Emily, Consultant Anaesthetist

I have taken two periods of maternity leave during my anaesthetic training, and clearly remember how I felt about returning to work. I certainly had mixed emotions about leaving my children; anxiety about leaving them for the first time, logistics of arranging childcare and worrying about whether they were happy seemed consuming at times. I don't think I was alone in feeling the perennial guilt about returning to further my career, rather than become a "stay at home mother". However, I also relished the opportunity to exercise my brain again and to remind myself that I wasn't totally defined by my role as a mother, even though I see it as my most important job.

I felt unprepared for my first return to work. I had tried to keep up to date as much as possible and had taught on an ALS course and on a Primary FRCA revision course. No formal RTW documentation was in place then, and I had an overwhelming sense of not really knowing what I was doing. My main sources of support were the LTFT representative for my school of anaesthesia and a really wonderful job share partner, who guided me through everything, step by step.

Practical procedures were not a problem, drug doses returned quickly. However, my overall 'flow' took a while to return. I felt a need to double check the most minor of details, and generally felt rusty. I think I put an immense amount of pressure on myself to be the best mother I could be, and to be the best I could be at my job, rather than give myself time to adjust. I think it took me several months to feel comfortable at work and enjoy it!

Thankfully, second time around, I was able to manage things very differently. A better sense of perspective, more knowledge of the RTW procedure and experience of managing a family and a busy job made things easier. I used my KIT days, and managed to participate in a number of projects whilst on maternity leave. In addition, a formal RTW process was now established; this forward planning ensured my return to clinical practice was as smooth as possible. Once again, a close support network of fellow LTFT trainees was invaluable to me. I have now used this experience to advise other trainees in my role as LTFT Trainee Representative for my school of Anaesthesia.

Anna, Anaesthetic StR

I have had three returns to work; 2008, 2011 and 2014. Comparing the three, what is most striking is the increase in awareness and support for the return to work process. My first return to work would have involved me starting in a hospital I had never worked in before directly onto night shifts. Thankfully my wonderful LTFT slot-share partner and a seasoned LTFT trainee stepped in to help. I think the first time was more difficult as I was adjusting to being a working mother, whereas the second and third time, this was no longer so new. I definitely worried lots about practical procedures and about having to ask for help in situations where I felt I might have been expected to manage solo. In reality neither of these was an issue. I found that familiarity with practical procedures came back quickly and I reasoned that it was always better to ask for help or just to check something with someone first if I was unsure. I don't recall anyone ever minding that. My second return to work was well supported with a lovely Educational Supervisor who had experience of returning to work herself. I also did the GAS Again course and some keeping in touch days, which helped. My most recent return to work has definitely been the easiest. By the third time I had more faith that I would get back up to speed and I followed a return to work programme so it was more structured. I think what I have found most helpful is support from colleagues who have been in similar situations. Realizing that what I was feeling was completely normal was very reassuring and helped to allay some of the anxiety.

Emma, Anaesthetic SpR

Understanding how others prepared for, and coped with, the transition back into clinical anaesthesia should help those having to return after a career break. However, there are inevitably going to be some elements of the process that come as a surprise and that leave any preparation feeling inadequate. The resulting effect is an undermining of confidence at a time that is already likely to feel daunting. Awareness of the issues one is likely to encounter and preparation tailored to suit individual needs[1] are the only solutions.

To establish the commonly encountered problems in returning to work there have been Return to Work (RTW) Surveys conducted in the West Midlands Local Education and Training Board (LETB)[2]. The first of these was completed for those trainees who returned to work between 2008 and 2012. It established many (>71%) trainees had difficulties on returning to work from a period of >6 months leave and most felt that their RTW could have been improved. Commonly encountered problems included paperwork for less than full time (LTFT) training, pay issues, childcare difficulties and rota issues including inadequate supervision and on-call shifts being allocated too soon. There was a general lack of awareness of keeping in touch (KIT) days and RTW courses. The length of time reported to regain confidence varied from a few days to 6 months. This was noted particularly amongst LTFT trainees. Those returning as full-time trainees reported feeling it took roughly 3 weeks for their confidence to return.

As a result of the shortcomings in the RTW process highlighted by this survey a Return to Work Programme was developed and put into practice in the West Midlands (see Chapter 4). Similar programmes have been established in other LETBs.

Following the introduction of the RTW programme the survey was repeated in 2015 and on this occasion consultants known to have had time off were also surveyed. The results of this second survey indicated some improvements. The trainee responses demonstrated increased awareness and uptake of KIT days; in addition many trainees were using the RTW programme. Overall it appeared that fewer problems were encountered with returning to work and the length of time reported to regain confidence had reduced in variability and length, with the longest estimate being 3 months (compared to the previously reported 6 months).

The consultants' survey indicated some (but poorer overall) uptake of the RTW programme and increased variability in estimated time to return of confidence (days to 6 months). Unsurprisingly common concerns among consultants returning to work highlighted some different areas, which included ability to support trainees and awareness of human factors. It was noted a higher proportion of consultants take career breaks due to sick compared to maternity leave and a concern in this group was having the stamina to work through the day and worries about fatigue. In both trainee and consultant groups less than

50% of individuals had a mentor and the vast majority indicated they would have liked this support.

Other interesting comments included one from a trainee who thought after taking her third period of leave returning to work would become easier when actually she found it was more difficult because of the responsibilities of becoming more senior. One consultant noted that they felt reassured as everything came back very quickly, which they attributed to having been doing it for a long time before they went off.

There are an increasing number of publications providing guidance to smooth individuals' transitions from prolonged periods of leave back into clinical anaesthesia. These aim to make the process as clear and stress free for those returning to work as possible. In the case of RTW programmes this is done by laying out some requirements thereby ensuring some of the responsibility for appropriate reintroduction to the clinical environment lies with the employers. Ultimately, however, the responsibility remains with the individual to prepare for and plan a reintroduction to work. Many of the resources available to help with this are described and illustrated in the following chapters.

## References

1.  L. Jobling. Returning to work – a personal view. *RCOA Bulletin*. 2011; 66: 29–31.
2.  E. V. E. Plunkett, C. L. Baxendale, N. Osborn et al. Returning to work: a survey of recent trainee experience and introduction of a return to work programme. *Anaesthesia* 2013; 68: 991.

# Preparing to return to work

*In this chapter we discuss many of the logistical aspects of returning to work, hopefully answering many of the questions you may have and giving you the knowledge to help you plan a return to work programme that is right for you.*

# RTW programmes

Anna Pierson

As highlighted in Chapter 2, the Academy of Medical Royal Colleges, Royal College of Anaesthetists (RCoA) and Association of Anaesthetists of Great Britain and Ireland (AAGBI) have produced guidance on returning to practice after a break. Returning after an absence for any reason has implications for patient safety, particularly when considering on-calls, the nature of clinical anaesthesia and new locations/equipment, and structured return to work (RTW) programmes can help to mitigate any risks arising from this.

The aim of a formal RTW scheme is therefore to promote patient safety and quality of care, whilst giving the doctor an opportunity to regain their confidence and previously acquired skills in a supported environment. Doctors returning to work must be able to access a scheme that has a comprehensive appraisal of his/her needs to ensure a safe and timely return to practice whether this is full time, less than full time (LTFT) or a phased reintroduction to clinical practice.

The RTW process may be divided into the following phases:

- Pre-Absence Period (planned and unplanned)
- Preparation for Return
- Record of Reintroduction

There are several RTW programmes currently in place in LETBs across the country, with the aim of making the returning process a more formal, structured and better supported process. Examples of well established programmes include those in the Wessex[1] and West Midlands LETBs[2]. However, despite recommendations from the RCoA, there is no national, standardized RTW programme in place, and consequently, trainees may have differing experiences. In addition, the needs of a returning trainee are considerably different from those of a consultant, and a RTW programme should reflect this. We discuss the specifics of each in Chapter 6.

*Returning to Work in Anaesthesia*, ed. Emma Plunkett, Emily Johnson and Anna Pierson.
Published by Cambridge University Press. © Cambridge University Press 2016.

Health Education West Midlands

# RETURN TO TRAINING FLOWSHEET

## ABSENCE PLANNING

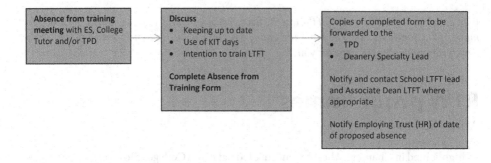

## PREPARATION FOR RETURN

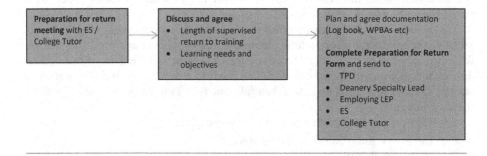

## RECORD OF RE-INTRODUCTION

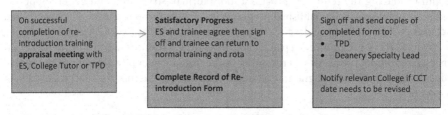

**Figure 4.1** Health Education West Midlands Return to Training Flowsheet.

**Health Education West Midlands**

**Absence from Training Form** **Appendix A**

Details of absence

| Name | | GMC number | |
|---|---|---|---|
| Planned period of leave | From:<br>To: | Reason for leave | |
| Current job title | | | |
| Place of work | | Hours | |
| Time in post | | Educational supervisor | |
| Returning job title | | | |
| Place of return to work | | Hours | |

Preparation for leave from training

| | |
|---|---|
| Is appraisal documentation up to date? | Yes / No |
| Is Hospital Placement Educational Report complete? | Yes / No |
| Any outstanding training needs to be addressed on return? | |
| | |
| Any educational goals planned during period of absence? | |
| | |
| Implications for licence to practice and requirements for revalidation considered? | Yes / No |
| Date of last ARCP | | Date of next ARCP | |

Return to work plan

| | |
|---|---|
| Trainee aware of return to work guidance and re-introduction process? | Yes / No |
| If may wish to change to LTFT training, process for application discussed?<br>http://www.westmidlandsdeanery.nhs.uk/Home/LessThanFullTimeTraining(FlexibleTraining).aspx | Yes / No / N/A |
| Any known updates / guidance to be published during period of leave? | |
| | |
| Planned methods of keeping in touch with work discussed e.g. Keeping in Touch (KIT) days, CPD opportunities, courses. | |
| | |

*Estimated date of next appraisal* (at least 1 month before RTW)

Trainee name:      Educational Supervisor name:

Signature:      Signature:

Date form completed:

**Figure 4.2** Health Education West Midlands Absence from Training Form.

**Preparation for Return Form**

Health Education West Midlands
Appendix B:   Part 1

Details of return

| Name | | GMC number | |
|---|---|---|---|
| Period of leave | From:<br>To: | Reason for absence | |
| Job title | | Length of time in<br>post before leave | |
| Place of work | | | |
| Duties on return | | | |
| Date due to start on calls | | Supervisor | |
| Are there any health issues that need to be considered, and if so has occupational health advice / approval been sought? This should be established before the return to work is planned and if a staged return is necessary, this form may be adapted as required. | | | Yes / No / N/A |

Initial Appraisal                                             Date:

(To be completed a month before returning to work)

| Details of Trainee Preparation for Return to Work<br>e.g.  KIT Days, RTW courses, other relevant CPD activity (please see attached guidance) |
|---|
| |
| Planned hospital / departmental induction (including dates) |
| |

Plan for supervised sessions (10 supervised sessions (1 session = 1 day) are recommended based on current evidence but this will depend on the individual trainee and their circumstances.)

| 1 | | 6 | |
|---|---|---|---|
| 2 | | 7 | |
| 3 | | 8 | |
| 4 | | 9 | |
| 5 | | 10 | |

| Other educational objectives for re-introduction period |
|---|
| |

| Are there any implications on this period of leave for the doctor's licence to practice or revalidation? (For those in a recognised training programme with an annual RITA or ARCP the answer is usually "No") | Yes / No |
|---|---|
| If returning LTFT has the relevant paperwork to secure funding been completed? | Yes / No |

Trainee name:                              Educational supervisor name:

Signature:                                    Signature:

**Figure 4.3**  Health Education West Midlands Preparation for Return Form.

**Record of Re-introduction Form**

**Health Education West Midlands**
**Appendix B: Part 2**

List of supervised sessions

| | Date | Nature of duties | Supervisors signature | Comments |
|---|---|---|---|---|
| | | Hospital induction | | |
| | | Departmental induction | | |
| 1 | | | | |
| 2 | | | | |
| 3 | | | | |
| 4 | | | | |
| 5 | | | | |
| Please contact your educational supervisor at this point if you think you will require additional supervised sessions | | | | |
| 6 | | | | |
| 7 | | | | |
| 8 | | | | |
| 9 | | | | |
| 10 | | | | |

Appraisal after re-introduction                          Date

(To confirm readiness to begin on call duties)

| Induction completed | | Yes / No |
|---|---|---|
| Educational objectives of re-introduction met? | | Yes / No |
| Agreed appropriate to re-commence on call duties? | | Yes / No |
| Appraisal paperwork completed for ongoing education and training plan? | | Yes / No |
| Date of next ARCP | Need to revise CCT date? | Yes / No |
| Any other comments about re-introduction period | | |
| | | |

Trainee name:                                   Educational supervisor name:

Signature:                                      Signature:

**Figure 4.4** Health Education West Midlands Record of Reintroduction Form.

In order to ease the transition back to work, forward planning is essential and there are a number of things you can do to reduce your stress prior to returning. Aiming to complete outstanding projects prior to leave, for example, means you can focus on your time off. Planning your return before your break is also recommended; this is clearly going to be more feasible if the break is planned in advance. Meeting with your educational supervisor/mentor to clarify objectives and formulate a plan for your return will alleviate some of the anxiety. Discussing whether you wish to return full- or less-than-full-time as early as possible gives both you and the LETB/Trust chance to plan ahead. This is discussed in more detail later in this chapter.

Finally, please find in Figures 4.1 to 4.4 an example of the RTW programme that forms part of the Return to Training policy for trainees that is well established in the West Midlands LETB[3]. A flowsheet of the overall process is shown, along with the forms required for completion. Many other LETBs have similar paperwork, and others are in the process of developing them. Increasingly, Trusts are also developing similar programmes for consultants[4]; please see Chapter 6 for more information about this.

# Good medical practice and revalidation

Emma Plunkett

The General Medical Council (GMC) is an independent organization which is responsible for overseeing undergraduate and postgraduate medical education in the UK. It serves to protect patients by setting standards for doctors, ensuring that those standards are met (revalidation) and investigating those doctors who are suspected not to reach those standards of care.

If you are working in the UK, you should be familiar with the latest version of the GMC publication 'Good medical practice'[5], which is split into four domains:

Domain 1: Knowledge, skills and performance
Domain 2: Safety and quality
Domain 3: Communication, partnership and teamwork
Domain 4: Maintaining trust.

For anaesthetists in the UK, all continuing professional development activities can be mapped against these GMC domains. Therefore, when it comes to appraisal and revalidation you will be able to demonstrate that you are achieving the recommended standards. After a break from practice it is worth refreshing your memory of what is written in 'Good medical practice' and the accompanying explanatory notes. The GMC website also has some interactive case studies to help demonstrate good medical practice in action. These can all be found online[6].

## Revalidation

All doctors practising in the UK must hold a licence to practise with the GMC. In order to retain this licence to practice and remain on the GMC register, then it is necessary to revalidate every 5 years[7]. This is done through the annual appraisal process during which doctors demonstrate that they are up to date in their chosen field and able to provide a good level of care. This appraisal is based on the GMC document 'Good medical practice' and should include reflection on serious events, complaints and compliments.

It is not customary to have annual appraisals whilst on leave, but it may be worth arranging one a few months after returning to work, to ensure that your ongoing education and development needs are being met. Although appraisals are time consuming to prepare for, they are an ideal opportunity to review progress, reflect on episodes and to make plans going forward. Participating actively in annual appraisals should mean that revalidation is straightforward, with your responsible officer making a positive recommendation for revalidation.

If you are taking time away from work for any reason, your date for revalidation does not automatically change. However, if you are on leave on your date for revalidation, then your responsible officer will make a request for deferral of the recommendation. This has no effect on your licence to practice and is not published anywhere. It simply means that you have a legitimate reason not to revalidate at that time. (Just for reference, if someone does not demonstrate engagement with the appraisal process then their responsible officer will issue a 'notification of non-engagement' instead.) Your responsible officer can recommend deferring revalidation for up to 12 months. If your time away from anaesthesia has been spent working in a different specialty, this will not affect your revalidation date.

# Statutory and mandatory training
Emma Plunkett

For many people this training feels like a necessity which must be tolerated and endured. I am not sure there is any way to transform these sessions into something more appealing, but perhaps explaining the rationale behind them might at least help you to understand why it is that we must undergo them.

Statutory training, as its name suggests, is training required of staff by law to ensure the safe provision of a service. Mandatory training, on the other hand, is required by organizations to minimize risks to both its users and staff. Examples include manual handling, information governance and fire safety training.

For doctors in the UK, compliance with statutory and mandatory training forms part of the appraisal and revalidation process. For example, keeping up to date with safeguarding and infection control training falls into domain 2: safety and quality; equality and diversity and conflict resolution training will form part of domain 3: communication, teamwork and partnership.

Thankfully, many regions and hospitals deliver much of this training with e-learning via Moodle platforms and there is a move towards trying to standardize this within regions to avoid the need for unnecessary repetition. The e-Learning for Health (e-LfH) Programme[8] covers 10 statutory and mandatory training topics for healthcare staff and Doctors.net[9] also covers some of these areas in its e-learning modules. Please see Table 4.1 for the modules available at the time of writing.

These sessions can sometimes feel unnecessary and patronizing, especially if you are repeating them in a new Trust not that long after having done them elsewhere. However, when you are returning to work after a break, they can actually be a useful reintroduction to the workplace. If you are required to attend face-to-face sessions, even if you feel like you remember the knowledge being presented, use the sessions as an opportunity to meet other members of staff or as a practice run for the logistical aspects of being back at work.

**Table 4.1** Examples of statutory and mandatory training e-learning modules

| Module | e-LfH | Doctors.net |
|---|---|---|
| Conflict Resolution | ✓ | ✓ |
| Equality and Diversity | ✓ | ✓ |
| Fire Safety | ✓ | |
| Health, Safety and Welfare | ✓ | |
| Infection Prevention and Control | ✓ | |
| Information Governance | ✓ | |
| Moving and Handling | ✓ | |
| Resuscitation – Paediatric Basic Life Support | ✓ | |
| Resuscitation – Adult Basic Life Support | ✓ | |
| Safeguarding Adults | ✓ | |
| Safeguarding Children and Young People | ✓ | ✓ |

As with any training or education you undertake these days, make sure you keep a record of it in your portfolio. It is also worth knowing how long the training is valid for and so when you may need to repeat it.

# Returning from sick leave

Emma Plunkett

## Phased returns to work

A phased return to work (RTW) is a supported RTW programme for someone who has been off work owing to illness or injury. It involves gradually increasing the hours of work over a period of weeks or months and introduction of any additional support to the workplace that might be necessary.

According to the government website[10] there is evidence to suggest that people are more likely to get back to work after sick leave if they keep in touch with their employers and plan their RTW. The Association of Anaesthetists of Great Britain and Ireland (AAGBI) guideline, Occupational Health and the Anaesthetist (2014)[11], reports that factors leading to a positive outcome when returning to work after a long-term illness are learning to recognize symptoms of a relapsing illness, having good support and being able to value what can be done, rather than focussing on what cannot. This may not be easy and it is important to be realistic when setting expectations about what can be achieved and the timescale needed. Throwing yourself into work too early or returning too quickly to a previous pattern of work (e.g. full time) can be very detrimental to longer-term health and confidence. Everyone describes being very tired on the first days or weeks.

There is no universally applicable format for a phased RTW programme: it needs to be planned on an individual basis. This planning should involve a consultant occupational health (OH) physician and the Clinical Director from the anaesthetic department, who will need to recommend and make any necessary adjustments to the work environment respectively. Having a good working relationship with an OH physician during a period of illness cannot be underestimated and there are benefits to engaging with OH early. This relationship should be continued throughout the RTW period and beyond for those with ongoing health concerns.

Confidentiality: Doctors returning from illness have a right to expect confidentiality regarding the reason for their absence. Those supervising and supporting that doctor must ensure that this is maintained. The natural curiosity of others in the department can be difficult to manage and it is useful to consider in advance a strategy for doing this. It might be a useful topic to discuss with a mentor or with the consultant OH physician.

Reasonable adjustment: Those supervising and supporting doctors returning from a period of illness have several roles. They have a responsibility to patients to ensure a safe, effective service. Thus they need to know that their staff can provide this. They also have a duty to support the doctor in question and to make reasonable adjustment to the working environment where necessary[12]. Reasonable adjustment can be in the form of changing the way things are done, changing the physical environment or provision of extra aids or service. They do not need to know, and indeed should not ask about the nature of the illness, just about the impact it has on the individual's performance at work.

Support: Supervision and support for the doctor returning is the key to success. Where applicable this might involve consideration of how to manage further unscheduled sickness absences and how to mitigate the chances of recurrence or worsening of symptoms and what to do if this occurs. The supervisor may need to sensitively liaise with other members of the department and this should be done in an inclusive and transparent manner. Putting the doctor returning from illness at the centre of discussions empowers the person and increases their confidence.

# Keeping in touch (KIT) days
Emma Plunkett

Keeping in touch days are an entitlement of employees who are on maternity, paternity, adoption or shared parental leave[13]. They were introduced under legislation in 2007. Prior to this, if an employee were to do any work during their period of leave, this would immediately end their entitlement to the leave. KIT days are designed to facilitate a smooth transition back to work. Here are some useful facts about them:

- A maximum of 10 days can be taken, which do not need to be consecutive.
- They can be taken at any point in the leave period, except in the first 2 weeks of maternity leave, which is compulsory.
- They should be arranged by mutual agreement; neither the employee nor employer can insist on them being taken.
- Taking them does not extend the period of leave.
- Working any part of a day counts as a whole day.
- There is no legal requirement for them to be paid, the level of pay will need to be agreed by both parties.
- They may be spent at work, or undertaking training or other activities which enable the employee to keep in touch with work.

If you would like to take them, then you should discuss a proposed plan for them with your employer and agree whether/how they will be paid. Examples of what could be done on KIT days include shadowing in theatre (getting used to the beeps again!), attending a return to work course, resuscitation course or conference and going to Trust Induction. Other suggestions for courses and other continuing professional development (CPD) for maternity leave can be found on page 21.

# Changing to less than full time (LTFT) working
Anna Pierson

For trainees, the option of being able to work less than full time (LTFT) is available for those who are unable to train full time because of 'well-founded individual reasons' (European Union Council Directive 93/16-/EEC 1993). These reasons can be placed in the following categories:

*Category 1*

>   Disability or ill-health (including those on IVF programmes)
>   Responsibility (men and women) for children
>   Caring for ill/disabled partner, relative or other dependent

*Category 2*

>   Unique opportunities for personal/professional development
>   Service to the wider NHS
>   Other

Normally all Category 1 applicants will be funded. Those in category 2 are assessed individually.

Consultants are able to negotiate working LTFT with their departments. Before making the decision to become LTFT, a number of advantages and disadvantages should be considered.

Pros: Being LTFT reduces working hours, which may enable someone to continue working in circumstances where full-time working would have placed undue pressure on them, possibly resulting in them giving up work. LTFT working offers the flexibility required to balance a busy home and work life or to devote time to maintaining one's health. LTFT training placements may provide fixed weekly sessions and on-calls allowing easy forward planning, e.g. childcare. Trainees may, within reason, work a percentage of full time to suit their needs. This can be adjusted (including a return to full time) provided sufficient notice is given. Consultants may negotiate with their employer to drop a number of programmed activities (PAs). Studies show that LTFT doctors are happier and more enthusiastic than their full-time colleagues. The additional time spent if this is done in training allows more time to achieve continuing professional development (CPD) goals. Being able to postpone your Certificate of Completion of Training (CCT) may also be advantageous. Many LTFT doctors feel that working flexibly provides the best of both worlds; they are able to pursue a career and generate an income, whilst being intellectually stimulated and challenged, yet also have more time to spend at home.

Cons: There are obvious downsides to working LTFT, namely prolonged training and a significant pay cut. Some feel under high pressure to balance work/home and other responsibilities and can experience anxiety at meeting commitments. Doctors who work LTFT can feel that they are perceived differently by full-time colleagues. There is pressure to achieve the same amount of CPD and many find they over-compensate at work to 'prove their worth'. Social life may be affected; this can lead to a feeling of exclusion from other colleagues. Lack of continuity at work can be frustrating and some find practical skills and knowledge are harder to keep up to date; for trainees this may be because not all aspects can be covered within a reduced working week. It can be difficult to attend courses and study days unless your childcare is very flexible and financing these on a reduced budget is challenging.

Finally, although arranging LTFT working can demand time and effort from training programme directors and anaesthetic departments, it works well for many doctors across the country and is a viable, flexible option. There is lots of information about LTFT training on the Royal College of Anaesthetists (RCoA)[14] and Association of Anaesthetists of Great Britain and Ireland (AAGBI)[15]websites and also a section on LTFT consultant careers on the RCoA website[16].

# Continuing professional development (CPD)

Anna Pierson

To ensure your return to work (RTW) runs smoothly, it is strongly suggested in the Royal College of Anaesthetists (RCoA) guidance that you undertake some CPD activity to help you prepare. This may take the form of simulation training, knowledge-based reading or lectures or a resuscitation update. What you choose to do will depend on your level of expertise and your area of practice. All anaesthetists returning to work should read and ensure they meet, as appropriate, the professional attitudes, behaviour and common competencies as listed in the August 2010 CCT in Anaesthesia 'Professionalism in Medical Practice'[17].

There are a wide variety of resources available to help bring you back up to speed. To tailor your CPD activity, the RCoA Matrix (level 1 and 2) gives guidance on which areas to cover in order to support and improve current knowledge and skills[18]. Starting simply, CPD activity may include familiarizing yourself with clinical updates, new guidelines and reading the most recent editions of *BJA Education*.

Under the Essential Knowledge Update, the RCoA has an active educational programme, including regional Core Topic Days, for all levels of anaesthetist. There are a variety of web-based, interactive learning resources, including e-Learning Anaesthesia[19] which covers key concepts and knowledge suitable for trainees. Similarly, the AAGBI also runs regional days of seminars covering essential topics[20] and their e-learning platform[21] contains videos from all recent conferences. Attending meetings, such as the Group of Anaesthetists in Training Annual Scientific Meeting (GAT ASM), can be beneficial from an educational and social perspective. Of note, since 2013, the GAT ASM has a less than full time (LTFT) resource/parent and baby room.

Courses are also a great way to help engage you and prepare for your return. Some schools of anaesthesia, e.g. Wales, Bristol, the West Midlands and the North West, hold specific RTW courses, so it is worth checking availability locally. Other suggestions include resuscitation courses, e.g. ALS or MEPA (Managing Emergencies in Paediatric Anaesthesia). Of particular relevance to anaesthesia are RTW simulation days. They should not be seen as a 'sign off', and require ongoing support from your base hospital. However, they offer an opportunity to gain confidence in a safe environment, in a group with similar anxieties. One example includes the GAS Again courses[22] held in London, Bradford and Bournemouth.

Although this is by no means an exhaustive list of suggestions, we hope this list gives you a starting point for your RTW preparations. More information about online learning can be found in Chapter 5.

# References

1. W. King, F. Haigh, A. Aarvold, D. Hopkins, I. Smith. Returning to work the Wessex Way. *Anaesthesia News* June 2012; 299: 18–19.
2. E. V. E. Plunkett, C. L Baxendale, N. Osborn et al. Returning to work: a survey of recent trainee experience and introduction of a return to work programme. *Anaesthesia* 2013; 68: 991.
3. Health Education West Midlands Return to Training Policy. Available at http://www .westmidlandsdeanery.nhs.uk/LinkClick.aspx?fileticket=3pfIUg2Nc0E%3d&tabid=39& portalid=0&mid=513 (accessed 2 January 2016).
4. H. Church, Z. Nassa. Return to Practice Guidelines for Consultant Anaesthetists. University Hospitals Birmingham NHS Foundation Trust. (For more information about this please contact Dr Hannah Church, Consultant Anaesthetist Hannah.Church@uhb.nhs.uk.)
5. General Medical Council. Good medical practice (2013). Available at http://www.gmc-uk.org/ guidance/good_medical_practice.asp (accessed 2 January 2016).
6. http://www.gmc-uk.org/guidance/case_studies.asp (accessed 28 January 2016).
7. http://www.gmc-uk.org/doctors/revalidation.asp (accessed 2 January 2016).
8. http://www.e-lfh.org.uk/programmes/statutory-and-mandatory-content/ (accessed 2 January 2016).
9. https://www.doctors.net.uk (accessed 2 January 2016).
10. https://www.gov.uk/statutory-sick-pay-employee-fitness-to-work (accessed 2 January 2016).
11. http://www.aagbi.org/sites/default/files/Occupational%20Health%202014%20web_0.pdf (accessed 2 January 2016).
12. https://www.citizensadvice.org.uk/discrimination/what-are-the-different-types-of-discrimination/duty-to-make-reasonable-adjustments-for-disabled-people/ (accessed 2 January 2016).
13. Department for Work and Pensions. Maternity benefits: technical guidance. Updated 26 March 2015. Available at https://www.gov.uk/government/publications/maternity-benefits-technical-guidance/maternity-benefits-technical-guidance (accessed 2 January 2016).
14. http://www.rcoa.ac.uk/training-and-the-training-programme/less-fulltime-training-ltft (accessed 2 January 2016).
15. https://www.aagbi.org/professionals/trainees/training-issues/ltft-training (accessed 2 January 2016).
16. http://www.rcoa.ac.uk/careers-and-training/less-fulltime-consultant-careers (accessed 2 January 2016).
17. Royal College of Anaesthetists. The CCT in Anaesthesia – Professionalism in Medical Practice (Annex A). Edition 2, August 2010. Available at http://www.rcoa.ac.uk/CCT/AnnexA (accessed 23 January 2016).
18. http://www.rcoa.ac.uk/cpd-matrix (accessed 23 January 2016).
19. www.rcoa.ac.uk/e-la (accessed 2 January 2016).
20. http://www.aagbi.org/education/events/core-topics (accessed 2 January 2016).
21. www.learnataagbi.org (accessed 2 January 2016).
22. www.gasagain.com (accessed 2 January 2016).

# Improving your return to work

*In this chapter we consider ways to optimize and improve the return to work (RTW) experience. We discuss the benefits of having a mentor and how embracing technology can help you get back up to speed. We also review human factors and non-technical skills. These are important to get right and, just like knowledge, can need refreshing. We consider some of the perceived limitations or concerns that you may have when returning from a break and think about ways to address these. We give some ideas of where you might go for help and remind you how important it is to ask. Finally we talk about fatigue and burnout and try to give some suggestions of how to avoid them.*

# Should I find a mentor?
## Kathryn Bell and Nancy Redfern

Mentoring is a way of managing change as a professional and doing this in a professional way. It can help an individual put themselves back in charge, and get the best from situations which may feel exciting, daunting or like shifting sand – much like returning to work where both the expectations and risks are high. A mentor might help you review what would be a good balance between work and responsibilities outside and how you can achieve this, or how to get the most from a less than full time job.

Whether you feel skilled and competent or overwhelmed, mentoring is a positive experience: there are very few people who do not do better with mentoring no matter what level they perceive themselves to be at. Nowadays, many senior leaders both in the NHS and in industry use mentors as part of their own professional development. The General Medical Council (GMC) recommend that all doctors should use this sort of structured support whenever we change roles throughout our careers. So the short answer is yes, find a mentor.

## What is mentoring?

Put simply, mentoring is *'Helping without telling'*. The mentor's expertise is in managing the conversation process so the 'mentee' reaches the right decision for them. A more formal definition is:

> Learning relationships which help people to take charge of their own development, to release their potential and to achieve results that they value[1].

*Returning to Work in Anaesthesia*, ed. Emma Plunkett, Emily Johnson and Anna Pierson.
Published by Cambridge University Press. © Cambridge University Press 2016.

The mentoring relationship is confidential, and takes place outside the educational supervision and assessment process. A mentor will encourage and support the mentee, helping the person to challenge their own assumptions and to explore their strengths and weaknesses. The mentor will offer a safe place for reflection, and be an informal audience to try out ideas.

Mentoring is much more successful when it is done by trained mentors. Most mentors also use mentoring for themselves, so are mentees as well as mentors, and have peer support or supervision in their role as mentors. The mentor's skills are in listening carefully to everything the mentee says, encouraging and supporting, empathically challenging blind spots, helping the mentee to develop wider vision about the situation he or she is dealing with, to set goals, develop strategies to achieve these and to plan. When working with a mentee an effective mentor demonstrates a set of core values: respect, empathic understanding and genuine concern, supporting mentees in achieving their full potential, whatever problem or opportunity is being tackled. Different mentees have very different needs and expectations, and a trained mentor should be able to support you whether you need a one-off session to resolve an urgent dilemma or a longer-term relationship.

YOU are the expert on the subject matter (**YOU**) and what you want to do/achieve.

The MENTOR is the expert on the conversation techniques (**PROCESS**).

## How do I find a mentor?

Some hospitals and some Local Education and Training Boards have formal mentoring schemes; find out if anyone you already know is a trained mentor. The Association of Anaesthetists of Great Britain and Ireland (AAGBI) has a team of trained mentors – have a look on their website to see if there is anyone near you. Remember that the mentor does not have to come from the same specialty or background; what matters most is that the mentor is trained and uses frameworks or models to help guide the conversation.

If you want to try mentoring out, the AAGBI offers 'taster' mentoring sessions at all its national meetings: the Annual Congress, Winter Scientific Meeting and Group of Anaesthetists in Training annual scientific meeting. Book a session and discuss a current dilemma or opportunity you have, and find out for yourself whether this is useful.

## Establishing the relationship: working agreements

It is useful to think about some practicalities. Where do you want to meet, how often, for how long and what arrangements do you want if you have to cancel at short notice? Longer-term mentoring relationships seem to work better if people are geographically accessible, either near home or near work. Mentoring can be done via Skype or e-mail, but many people say they get more from having some face-to-face meetings.

The mentor will want to discuss the way you work together, including matters such as confidentiality, regular feedback as to whether mentoring is useful, what you would like more or less of, and that any notes taken belong to you, the mentee. If you are likely to meet your mentor outside the mentoring relationship, for instance during clinical work, you will need to agree whether you would want him or her to acknowledge the mentoring relationship and ask how things are going. Clear role boundaries are useful – your mentor should not normally also be your educational supervisor or clinical director and cannot write a reference for you. At some point you will also need to agree when the mentoring relationship has run its course, and how you want to celebrate what you have achieved at the end.

# What sort of issues/topics do people discuss?

'Typical' dilemmas and opportunities that people bring to mentoring sessions include:

- Improving work–life balance
- CV and career decisions
- Managing work and responsibilities outside work
- Taking on a new project or a new role
- Working relationships
- Handling a difficult situation
- Managing others' expectations (for example, being braver at challenging effectively and making positive suggestions when what others expect is not working for you).

Mentoring is particularly helpful if you are returning to work after a period of illness or have a chronic health condition. The mentor might help you take a longer-term view of the whole situation and identify options that work for you. He or she can help you to test whether you are ready to come back, to pace your RTW, to be realistic and not set unachievable goals. You might think about how to manage others expectations and rehearse ways of handling the natural curiosity of others. Many people feel less confident when coming back to work. Your mentor might encourage you to be braver at challenging effectively, and to make positive suggestions when what is presented is not working. It is easy to feel isolated by a chronic health condition, and a mentoring relationship might facilitate you rediscovering your network, or in getting into new networks, perhaps of people who have faced similar challenges. If your health and performance fluctuate, mentoring and other networks can help you to spot when you are getting ill again. This can be particularly helpful for people with psychological or stress-related illness.

---

**Box 5.1  Example**

Laura decides to have a conversation with a mentor before returning to work after the birth of her first child, now 10 months old. She is considering coming back less than full time [LTFT]. Her long-term career aim is paediatric anaesthesia. Currently in ST3, her next goal is to pass her final FRCA. She has a number of concerns. Will working LTFT compromise her exam preparation and career chances? Will returning to work compromise her family life? Income is also an issue as she is the main wage earner while her partner establishes his business.

The mentor helps Laura to prioritize issues and realize that she should get settled back into work with a weekly timetable that suits her family life before concentrating on exam preparation. She does not have to take the exam immediately as a flexible trainee, and will have a better shot when she feels calmer about childcare and financial issues. She is a bit of a worrier, and her mentor helps her identify that it is important for her core values that her child is happy; if not she will be distracted and will not be able to concentrate on revision.

Matters to do with long-term career are important but not urgent so can be put off to a later date. However, there is some learning about the strengths she brings to her current dilemma and her mentor helps her see how she can draw on this as a part-time consultant paediatric anaesthetist.

Once she is back at work, Laura's mentor helps her to challenge the situation when the rota organizer puts her down for shifts that are very difficult from the childcare perspective. She marshals her resources, particularly in her family life, and is more assertive at bringing in partner as resource and developing plans together. She takes the exam at the end of year 4 and is successful first time.

# Using technology to your advantage

Stephen Phillips and Fran Haigh

Technology has become a fundamental foundation upon which our professional and social lives are organized. The purpose of this chapter is not to serve as an exhaustive list of specialty-specific available technology resources, but to highlight the areas in which technology, including websites and downloadable smartphone applications, can be used to make life more efficient for those returning to anaesthetic practice and act as a starting point for the discovery of further utilities.

## Smartphones and tablets

Following the introduction of the original iPhone® in 2007, the use of smartphones has become increasingly ubiquitous in everyday life. Uptake by anaesthetists has been high[2] and their use has been extended to many aspects of anaesthetic practice. Alongside departmental IT facilities, a modern internet-enabled smartphone or tablet allows rapid and convenient access to the wealth of online resources available, including guidelines, algorithms and journal content[3]. Mobile access to the internet regrettably remains a source of frustration in many departments because of limited Wi-Fi access or cellular reception. Smartphone applications that can be downloaded and retain offline functionality therefore represent a reliable alternative (battery life permitting!) and a continuing area of rapid evolution.

Availability of these apps for specific devices mirrors the dominance in market share of smartphones and tablets based upon the iOS® (e.g. Apple's iPhone and iPad®) and Android™ (including Samsung, Sony and HTC ranges) operating systems. At the present time, availability of apps for those based upon Windows Phone® and BlackBerry OS® unfortunately remains significantly limited.

Most apps are available directly from the inbuilt app stores rather than having to be sourced via an external website, with the majority accessible free of charge. Technical support or the receipt of timely updates remains limited for many, but as the user base of the most popular apps expands these aspects continue to show notable improvement.

## Logbooks

Maintaining an anaesthetic logbook has become an important source of information for appraisal and revalidation purposes. The Royal College of Anaesthetists (RCoA) provides free desktop logbook software (**Anaesthetic Logbook v9**) for both Mac and PC, available for download from the dedicated website www.logbook.org.uk. This website has a wealth of troubleshooting guidance and links to the two published College Bulletins (51 and 79) which confer useful additional information.

Smartphone apps enable a logbook to be maintained away from a desktop PC. Whilst they can be used to export cases into a master desktop logbook, some have the facility to directly generate appropriate summaries or reports and can therefore be used independently. Regular backups are essential in either approach. The **FileMaker Go** (v13) app (*free, iOS only, FileMaker Inc.*) is straightforward and also uses the Logbook v9 college template. Download the app from iTunes then navigate to www.logbook.org.uk for further instructions. A previously popular alternative for iOS was **iGasLog** (*iMobileMedic.com Ltd*) but this has been withdrawn at the time of print owing to incompatibility with the latest version of iOS. The troubleshooting page of the website above offers export instructions to switch to an alternative.

Options for Android include **Log4AS** (*free trial/£17.99, Android only, M-pax*), which is simple to use, can generate reports and receives regular updates. A free but significantly less straightforward alternative is the **Memento Database** (*free, Android only, Luckydroid*) app in conjunction with a template from www.subjective-effect.co.uk.

## E-learning and e-CPD

The award-winning RCoA e-Learning Anaesthesia project (e-LA) is one of the most extensive educational resources available for any medical specialty, with content covering the primary and final FRCA curriculum alongside monthly continuing professional development (CPD) topics and journal articles to support senior practitioners. Access is available to all UK practicing anaesthetists at www.e-lfh.org.uk/programmes/anaesthesia. Activity is automatically logged and certificates can be created for CPD records. No specific app is available but the web interface received a welcome update in 2015 to facilitate more widespread browser support, including touchscreen tablets. Smartphone compatibility is variable and most content is not suited to the smaller screen size.

Access to a vast number of other e-Learning for Healthcare (e-LfH) programmes is available using the same login at www.e-lfh.org.uk, including safeguarding, research and audit tutorials. These can be added by using the Enrolment option within the 'My Account' dropdown menu after signing in to your account.

The RCoA also produces monthly CPD-accredited webcasts with the full catalogue and technical support accessible at www.rcoa.ac.uk/webcasts. Archived webcast content is also available within the e-LA portal but there tends to be a significant delay in the addition of the most recent topics to this interface.

The equally impressive education section of the AAGBI website www.aagbi.org/education contains several distinct resources. Learn@AAGBI is the AAGBI members online learning resource. It contains videos of lectures from all recent AAGBI conferences with opportunity to reflect on these after they are viewed. *Anaesthesia* articles can also be accessed here. Non-members can access other resources via the education pages of the website. The Anaesthesia Tutorial of the Week (ATOTW) archive is here, which can be browsed by category and also there is a link to a new endeavour www.FRCAmindmaps.org, an educational resource for those studying for the final FRCA or who would like a quick refresher in a topic.

To record and reflect upon CPD activities, the RCoA provides an online CPD system that also contains a database of formally approved CPD events. This can be found together with registration instructions at www.cpd.rcoa.ac.uk. Navigating to this website from a smartphone or tablet reveals the mobile option with offline capability, enabling activities and reflection to be added whilst away from a desktop computer.

## Journals

The online presence of the most popular anaesthetic journals has become increasingly extensive. The *BJA* website bja.oxfordjournals.org offers online access to both present and archived journal articles (free with RCoA membership), with a mobile-optimized site accessible from a smartphone browser. *Continuing Education in Anaesthesia Critical Care and Pain* (CEACCP) is also accessible at ceaccp.oxfordjournals.org, from which a certificate of completion for the article MCQ tests can be printed or uploaded into an online CPD diary. As of June

2015, CEACCP was renamed *BJA Education*. Issues from June 2015 onwards are available at bjaed.oxfordjournals.org, with archived content remaining on the CEACCP website.

*Anaesthesia* journal content is available online to AAGBI members via www.aagbi.org/membership/my-account. The well-designed and intuitive apps **BJA Journals** (*free, iOS, Highwire Press inc.*) and **Anaesthesia** (*free, iOS and Android, Wiley Publishing*) offer the additional convenience of offline journal access and are particularly suited to the larger screen of a tablet.

## Reference and guidelines

A trio of useful apps has been created by the National Institute for Health and Care Excellence (NICE) with **NICE Guidance**, **BNF** and **BNFc** (*free with NHS Athens account, iOS and Android, NICE UK*) providing full offline access to the most recent published texts. These benefit from frequent updates although search functions and interface speed can be erratic, particularly with Android versions.

**AAGBI Guidelines** (*free to members, iOS and Android, AAGBI*) includes a large number of complete guidelines and some useful equipment checklists, many of which are highly relevant to the anaesthetist returning to work. Readability on smaller screen sizes can be an issue. The most recent Difficult Airway Society guidelines are available through the **DAS App** (*free, iOS and Android, Subjective Effect Ltd*).

The **Oxford Handbook of Anaesthesia** (*£20.89–£23.99, iOS and Android, Oxford University Press/Medhand Mobile Libraries*) includes all of the content in the most recent paper edition of the handbook in an offline-capable app. Despite an unexpectedly utilitarian interface given the purchase price, the rapidity of navigation throughout the app and the index search function make this an excellent alternative to the original text. It is worthwhile noting, however, that moving to an alternative smartphone platform requires a new purchase.

Currently supported by 42 NHS trusts in the UK, **Microguide** (*free, iOS and Android, Horizon Strategic Partners Ltd*) offers access to trust-specific adult and paediatric antimicrobial prescribing guidelines as a welcome alternative to hunting through hospital intranet portals for the relevant download.

For refamiliarization with both landmark and ultrasound-guided regional anaesthesia techniques, both www.nysora.com and www.neuraxiom.com are excellent free online resources with extensive text, image and video-based descriptive material. The app **SonoAccess** (*free, iOS and Android, FujiFilm SonoSite*) provides offline access to a library of videos and images for a number of common regional blocks, although smartphone screen size can limit the usefulness of this in some instances.

For a more general medical reference resource, **Medscape** (*free after registration, iOS and Android, WebMD LLC*) offers extensive information on a wide range of diseases alongside calculator functions and a formulary (the utility of which is more limited because of the US-centric data). For reliable, highly detailed and scholarly material on most conditions, many trusts now offer employee access to www.uptodate.com from on-site computers, with access also possible with an NHS Athens account.

## Calculator applications

A large number of apps exist to assist with calculations within a number of different fields of anaesthesia. They can be used to double-check drug doses or implement more complex scoring systems.

Calculate by QxMD (*free, iOS and Android, QxMD Medical Software Inc.*) and MedCalc (*free, iOS only, Mathias Tschopp*), whilst not anaesthesia-specific, offer an extensive selection of formulae and scoring systems for treatment guidance, prognostication and perioperative risk assessment. Both are well designed and frequently updated.

More specific apps include Surgical Risk (*free, iOS only, Cardiff Medical Apps Ltd*) or P-POSSUM (*free, Android only, JT Binary*) for P-POSSUM mortality scoring, and the NHS Pre-operative Test checker (*free, iOS and Android, Health Education Thames Valley and Wessex*) for displaying recommended preoperative tests based on the latest UK NICE guidelines.

## Paediatrics

The weight-dependent nature of paediatric anaesthesia and resuscitation lends itself towards easy-access calculators to assist in the management of this patient population. Paediatric Emergency Drugs (*£2.29, iOS only, UBQO Ltd*) is a concise tool that presents resuscitation parameters based upon input age and weight. Both Paeds ED (*£1.49, iOS only, iED Apps*) and Paediatric Emergencies (*£4.99, iOS and Android, ITDCS Ltd*) offer similar reference data and have free trial versions available. A simple, but less comprehensive free Android alternative is Paediatric Anesthesia Calc (*Free, Android only, L.G. Geertshuis*).

# Communication and team working

Emily Johnson

*In this part of the chapter we discuss the non-technical skills that are needed to function effectively at work. We hope that taking the time to consider these now will help to smooth your RTW.*

Communication is fundamental to good team work, increasing efficacy and reducing errors in the workplace. Poor communication was found to be a prime cause in many reported adverse incidents in intensive care units[4]. An individual's communication and team-working behaviours can be shaped and refined by training and their personal awareness and insight.

## Elements of communication

When communicating in a team it is useful to be aware of the elements of communication, which are:

- Sending information concisely and clearly (consider **What** is the information to be communicated, **How** is it to be communicated, **Why** and **Who** to).
- Including the context and content in the information exchange.
- Listening actively and receiving information.
- Identifying and addressing barriers to communication. These include barriers for the individual such as language differences, culture, motivation, prejudices, expectations, past experiences, status, emotions and deafness, and external barriers such as noise level, separation in time or location, lack of visual clues (body language) and interference.

## Models of communication

It is also useful to consider models of communication and use the appropriate model for the situation.

**One-way communication** is the sender directly stating to the receiver what they wish to convey. It is rapid and neat and the sender retains control. However, there is no feedback so it does not permit clarification, which allows potential for the receiver to misinterpret or not listen, and the sender maintains sole responsibility.

**Two-way communication** describes a conversation where the receiver can feedback or clarify. Therefore, it is more reliable and effective, allowing shared responsibility and the opportunity for mutual understanding. However, it takes longer and requires the receiver to communicate in return. Feedback given in two-way communication can be in one of three forms:

1. Informational – objective statement
2. Corrective – challenges to gain clarity
3. Reinforcing – acknowledges receipt and checks understanding.

Making an effort to consider the elements of communication and practice two-way communication, particularly in stressful and emergency situations, is likely to help team working and encourage feedback, involvement and empowerment of all team members. If a team leader actively listens and seeks feedback the team members are likely to become more comfortable communicating and clarifying any queries, leading to an improved situational awareness within the team and reducing the chance of errors. This is a skill that can be practised during simulation sessions and it is worth considering trying to attend one as part of your preparation to return to work.

## Non-verbal communication

Non-verbal communication is also vital and in fact Mehrabian in the 1960s conducted a series of studies concluding that the amount of attention a receiver pays to a sender's message can be broken down as follows[5]:

- Words 7%
- Tone 38%
- Other non-verbal communication (gesture/posture/facial expression) 55%.

Considering this, it follows that the richest communications with most information transfer are likely to be face-to-face interactions allowing for the influence of verbal and non-verbal communication.

## Improving communication

Flin et al.[6] describe four aspects of communication upon which recommendations for improving communication between members of a team are made. These are:

- Explicitness – required for the avoidance of ambiguity. Assumptions must be avoided and an adequate amount of relevant information (sufficient to reduce the chance of errors) should be given without overloading the receiver.

- Timing – the sender should provide information at the most relevant time and be aware of other activities in which the receiver may be engaged.
- Assertiveness – a disposition between passive and aggressive where an individual stands up for themselves without disregarding the other person's opinions. In airline and healthcare industries there is good evidence of status differences affecting communication behaviours and the need for assertive behaviours in more junior team members has been highlighted.
- Active listening – see Table 5.1.

**Table 5.1** Do's and don't's for active listening

| Do | Don't |
|---|---|
| • be patient | • debate your thoughts |
| • ask questions | • change the subject |
| • be supportive | • interrupt |
| • paraphrase | • finish the other person's sentence |
| • make eye contact | • pre-plan |
| • use positive body language | • tune out |
| | • fixate on other tasks |

## Situation awareness

Situational awareness described simply is an understanding of what is going on around you. It can be broken down to three components:

- Information gathering or perception
- Interpreting the information or comprehension
- Anticipating future states or projection.

There are many rapid technological advances and increased interest in computer-based monitoring systems within anaesthesia and many other industries, e.g. aviation. This has led to a re-focus and recognition of the importance of the human operator having a good 'mental model' (picture in their head) representing the task at hand and the surrounding work environment. A lack of this 'mental modelling' or situational awareness is implicated in many incidents within healthcare and other industries. An example within anaesthesia that demonstrated a lack of situational awareness is the Elaine Bromiley tragedy[7]. In this case and others where a loss of situational awareness has occurred there are some common clues:

- Fixation – focussing on one thing to the exclusion of everything else
- Ambiguity – information from different sources does not add up
- Confusion – uncertainty often accompanied by anxiety
- Lack of required information
- Critical tasks not being maintained
- Expected targets or goals being missed
- Discrepancies remain unresolved
- Under-riding feeling of discomfort or that things 'just are not quite right'.

Every individual has a different capacity for picking up new information and maintaining mental awareness of it and this ability can be affected by a number of factors. Fatigue and stress can reduce this cognitive capacity as can distraction, interruption and stimulus over-load as they interfere with working memory, which is vital in maintaining situational aware-ness. Knowing not to distract or interrupt fellow team members involved in tasks retaining information in their working memory is an important element of team working. Points to consider in maintaining good situational awareness are:

- Good briefings – to allow understanding of the nature and risks of a given task.
- Fitness for work – diminished physical or mental fitness will adversely affect the required skills.
- Minimizing distraction and interruption during critical tasks.
- 'Sterile cockpit' rule – from aviation where crew members are prohibited from performing non-essential duties when the aircraft is at a crucial stage of the flight.
- Updating – regularly compare mental model with the real situation.
- Monitoring – remain sensitive to clues of 'zoning out' or fixation or at least be aware of conditions where this may happen.
- Speaking up – encourage speaking up in all team members if there is any uncertainty.
- Time management – use early planning and preparation to resist time pressure.

# Handovers

Many of the communication problems that occur in health care are related to shift handovers and transfer of responsibility. The BMA published an advice booklet Safe Handover, Safe Patients[8] outlining five questions to be asked to help improve the handover process:

1. WHO should be involved? Face-to-face meeting between incoming and outgoing staff with management (e.g. ward managers) present to ensure they are aware of ongoing issues.
2. WHEN should it take place? At a fixed time with a sufficient time allocation to allow necessary information exchange.
3. WHERE should it take place? Close to the work site in a space large enough to allow relevant staff to attend with minimal distractions.
4. HOW should it happen? It should be formal, predictable and follow a consistent format. Leonard et al. (2004) proposed the SBAR situational briefing tool[9]:
   - S – SITUATION – What is wrong with the patient?
   - B – BACKGROUND – What is the clinical background or context?
   - A – ASSESSMENT – What do I think the problem is?
   - R – RECOMMENDATIONS – What would I do to correct the problem?
5. WHAT should be handed over? Written notes or electronic log should be completed by the outgoing personnel and complemented by two-way communication.

# Elements of team working

It is useful to consider the elements of team working as often the role of team leadership and coordination falls to the anaesthetist. These include:

- Supporting other team members including sharing workload, accepting individual responsibility, maintaining good working relationships and establishing openness.

- Conflict resolution, which despite negative connotations can be constructive. West (2004) lists the skills required as[10]:
  1. Fostering useful debate whilst eliminating dysfunctional conflict.
  2. Matching conflict management strategy with source and nature of the conflict.
  3. Using win–win strategies.

- Exchanging information. West (2004) lists skills for team work communication as:
  1. Employing communication that maximizes open flow.
  2. Using open and supportive communication.
  3. Using active listening techniques.
  4. Paying attention to non-verbal messages.
  5. Taking advantage of interpersonal skills and engaging in appropriate small talk.

- Coordination of activities improved by equally distributing activities, monitoring each other's performance and effective information exchange and team members supporting each other.

## The ANTS system

The Anaesthetists' Non-Technical Skills (ANTS) system is a behavioural marker system developed by psychologists and anaesthetists[11]. It describes the main non-technical skills associated with good anaesthetic practice. Non-technical skills are defined as behaviours in the operating theatre environment not directly related to the use of medical expertise, drugs or equipment. They encompass the interpersonal skills and cognitive skills discussed in this chapter. The integration of these skills and technical skills is fundamental to successful task performance and improving safety.

The ANTS system is designed to supply a language for considering and discussing the behavioural aspects of anaesthetists' performance. The components are shown in Figure 5.1

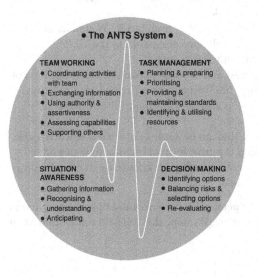

**Figure 5.1** The ANTS system. Reproduced with the kind permission of the University of Aberdeen.

and provide a tool that can be reflected upon to help prepare for a return to the team-working environment.

# Limitations and sources of help

Emma Plunkett

What challenges do people face when returning to work after a break? This is likely to depend on several factors: the reason for leave, the stage the person is at in their career and also the individual.

For those who have been off work because of illness, there is often a degree of uncertainty about how they will be able to cope with the physical and mental demands of being at work. A phased RTW can help here, and seeking advice from an occupational health physician who has experience advising others in similar situations can be reassuring. For those returning from maternity leave, being back at work involves new logistical aspects and a different family dynamic. Days at work and days at home can be very different and it can seem as if they are actually living two different lives. Having robust childcare and a back-up plan for when this does not work is key to being able to leave home at home and concentrate fully on work. Those who are returning from work in another specialty or environment will also have some of the same feelings of unfamiliarity, although perhaps less anxiety about the practical and logistical aspects of being at work.

So what are the potential 'limitations'? What do people worry about when returning? Here are some of the things that have been mentioned in surveys we have done in the West Midlands.

- Practical procedures. From personal experience, I think that the length of time it takes for them to feel familiar again depends upon the level of skill with the procedure beforehand. And actually in reality, these skills usually return very quickly.
- Knowledge. It may feel as if you have forgotten lots, but actually you will be surprised at how much knowledge remains. This can be addressed by CPD to prepare for your RTW and hopefully by reading Section 2 in this book.
- Management of emergencies. This can be addressed by finding a RTW simulation course or another anaesthetic emergency simulation course such as the MEPA (Managing Emergencies in Paediatric Anaesthesia) course.
- Human factors such as situational awareness and decision making or rather, the level of confidence in your own decision making. These can also be addressed on simulation courses. The purpose of a supervised RTW is also to help support the doctor as they refresh these skills.
- Supervision of more junior anaesthetists. This can be a source of anxiety when you are finding your feet again. However, teaching is a great form of revision so with a bit of planning and preparation this can help you to refresh your knowledge. It often becomes apparent that you know more than you think.

Earlier in this section we have included some personal experiences and tips that people who have taken time off work have been willing to share. We hope this will help you to realize that any apprehension you feel is very normal.

So why might people not want to ask for help? I can think of a few reasons, but there are likely to be others. We naturally do not want to bother people. We like to be seen as being able to cope and we do not like to feel as if we are creating work for someone else. This can be compounded by a fear of being judged or a perception that people will think we are wasting their time. In the past I think that asking for help might have been perceived as a weakness, although I hope that this is not the case anymore. Indeed, it should be perceived as a strength to ask for help and as professional colleagues we should strive to support each other for the benefit of our patients.

The first step towards getting the help that you need is to acknowledge that you might need to ask for help in the first place. Be accepting of this and please do not be tempted to see it in a negative light. The next step is knowing what sources of help there are. Suggestions listed below are in addition to the published RTW guidance documents described earlier in this section.

1. Mentoring. This can be a valuable source of support. Mentoring is not for people who are failing. It is for everyone to maximize their potential. Please see the section at the beginning of this chapter for more information. Be sure to use a mentor who has been trained.
2. The AAGBI[12]. The AAGBI has a Support and Wellbeing Committee which aims to provide advice, information and support for anaesthetists and to promote a culture of asking for help. You can email the support and wellbeing committee on wellbeing@aagbi.org.
3. The GAT handbook[13]. This has a section on 'Taking care of yourself', which has lots of helpful advice for trainees (and consultants too!).
4. The BMA[14]. There is lots of information on the BMA website about the practicalities of returning to work.
5. Colleagues. Colleagues who have been through something similar can be an incredible source of support. Sharing your anxieties and concerns with someone who you know can empathize can be therapeutic.
6. Family and friends. Family and friends may not be able to empathize in the same way as colleagues. However, they can listen and reassure and also help to give some perspective to your concerns.

The bottom line is that everybody needs help sometimes. A RTW after a significant period doing something else is a period of change, and it is normal and should be expected that people will need help and support during this time. You should never worry about asking. It is the right thing to do.

---

**Box 5.2  In summary, some helpful tips**

- Set a goal and a plan of how to reach it. Make sure these are realistic.
- Then, take one day at a time.
- Be open and honest with those you are working with.
- Ask for help if you feel you need it.
- Use a mentor for support.

# Avoiding adverse outcomes and what to do if one occurs

Emily Johnson

Adverse incidents affecting patients are something all health professionals strive to avoid. Patient safety is at the forefront of all we do and if this becomes compromised there are numerous consequences that may have knock-on effects on the staff involved. This is particularly pertinent for professionals returning to work after a break for two reasons. Firstly, as mentioned earlier in this section, this is a daunting and stressful time when confidence levels may be low; therefore, an adverse incident will be harder to cope with on an individual level. Secondly, this is a time when individuals may indeed be particularly vulnerable to making an error because of their time out of practice. Appropriate preparation and following RTW programmes should help minimize this but nonetheless an awareness of some of the factors that may help in avoiding adverse outcomes could be beneficial.

James Reason's approach to human error states there are two ways of viewing the problem: the person approach, focussing on the errors of individuals and blaming them, and the system approach, focussing on working conditions and building defences to avert errors and mitigate their effects[15].

Traditionally in medicine the person approach predominates. This approach is more satisfying than targeting institutions. Thankfully, the shortcomings of this approach are increasingly recognized. It is now often appreciated that it is likely to be a counterproductive way of viewing error, and in fact prevents the development of safer healthcare delivery.

High reliability organizations (those with fewer than their fair share of accidents) appreciate human variability is a characteristic that can actually be harnessed in error reduction. Humans are incredibly adaptable and quick to notice changing patterns. Focussing on these characteristics results in efforts being channelled into considering the possibility of failure and how it may be prevented.

Reason's Swiss cheese model of system accidents demonstrates the system approach[15]. There should be defences, safeguards and barriers to protect potential victims against harm (layers of cheese, see Figure 5.2). Ideally these defences would be intact but in reality they

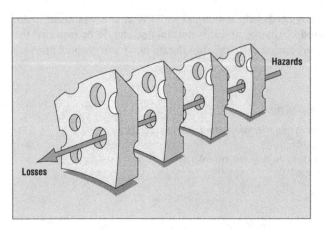

Hazards

Losses

**Figure 5.2** The Swiss cheese model of system accidents. Reproduced with the kind permission of BMJ Publishing Group Ltd.

are like slices of Swiss cheese, having many holes. Although, unlike in the cheese, the holes are always opening, closing and moving. An adverse outcome only happens when the holes momentarily line up to allow a trajectory where hazards can contact victims. This occurs because of either latent conditions or active failures (e.g. mistakes). The active failures can be addressed but will never be eliminated as they are mostly due to human error. It is the latent conditions that can be identified and remedied before an adverse event occurs: this is proactive rather than reactive risk management.

Professor Martin Elliott, a paediatric cardiothoracic surgeon, proposed 10 commandments for preventing error[16]. These are summarized below and are a good focus for doing all you can to avoid and manage adverse outcomes:

1. Adverse events are important – acknowledge adverse events; do all possible to prevent them; tell the truth to create trust.
2. Human error is inevitable – any human can make a mistake (60–70% of an NHS Trust's turnover is spent on staff therefore it is not surprising human error is at the root of most adverse events).
3. Anticipate adverse outcomes – prepare for the worst and in doing this you are doing all you can to mitigate the risks. Ensure you have back-up plans and a get-out strategy.
4. Plan what you are going to do with the whole team – briefings, checklists and discussions are essential (e.g. the World Health Organization (WHO) checklist). Effective communication is essential in achieving this step.
5. Communication – two-way communication is essential – LISTEN and hear what is said. Seek views of others and keep clear records of doing so.
6. Respect the patient – take a time out to remember how important the patient is to others, keep it personal. This aids concentration and reminds everyone of the importance of avoiding error.
7. Check – use the WHO checklist – it is proven to save lives and reduce complications[17]. Engage the team in this process, influence culture.
8. Do it once and do it right – avoid taking short cuts, check with your team.
9. Debrief and learn – identify near misses and share experiences. This allows new processes and protections to evolve. Promote a culture of continuous improvement.
10. Measure, share and improve – put appropriate quality control metrics in place to monitor, present and use as a basis for improvement.

## Coping with an adverse outcome

It is recognized that medical caregivers may experience a number of ill effects following involvement in adverse events. These can be emotions such as shame, guilt, anger, fear, frustration, loneliness and decreased enjoyment of their jobs. They can also be physical signs such as fatigue, sleep disturbance, poor concentration, tachycardia and hypertension. Sufferers of these ill effects are termed the 'second victims'. The frequency and risk factors for becoming a second victim are not clear and whilst most clinicians will experience an adverse event during their career, some do recover with minimal consequence. However, in some, the second victim syndrome can last for an indefinite time period and have far-reaching consequences in their personal and professional lives. Healthcare organizations have a responsibility to look after second victims and this is something that may not currently be done particularly well.

The following are thought to be helpful:

- Formal debriefing
- Talking to a colleague (peer support)
- Psychiatry services.

Peer support has some unique advantages such as:

- Unique insight and empathy
- Credibility of peers
- Immediate access
- Voluntary access
- Confidential
- Emotional 'first aid'.
- Facilitated access to higher level of support (e.g. Employee Assistance Programme).

These are further developed in formal peer support programmes in some centres in the USA and there is an increasing awareness and resources available to support second victims and to develop support programmes[18].

It is important to recognize that emotional stress and the second victim phenomenon is poorly understood. One cannot reliably predict who or how any individual may suffer and it is important to maintain self-awareness and be able to identify the signs in oneself and one's colleagues in order to seek prompt help. The third victim has also been described as a term to identify patients who have suffered suboptimal care as a result of the underperformance of a second victim[19]. Emotional stress is linked to burnout and burnout to increased rates of reported errors, decreased patient satisfaction and prolonged recovery[20-22]. Whilst most anaesthetists recognize their ability may be compromised after an adverse event, the vast majority continue to work, often because of logistical issues and lack of relief. Recognizing these problems, seeking support oneself and providing it for colleagues, preferably in a structured programme within the institution of work, is the first step in preventing unnecessary suffering in patients and professionals.

We mention these subjects here, not to cause undue anxiety, but because it is important to acknowledge that they are likely to happen to you at some point. Perhaps not on your RTW, but at some point during your career, and consideration of what you can do to prevent adverse outcomes and how you will cope with them when they occur is important. Resilience is a term increasingly used in health care. It relates to being adaptable to changing situations. Emotional resilience is a key attribute for doctors (and all healthcare professionals) as we have responsibility for highly changeable and high-stakes situations and we need strategies to cope with these. When you return to work after a break it is conceivable that your resilience may be lower than usual, so it makes sense that you will need to take extra care and access extra support at this time.

# Fatigue and burnout

Emma Plunkett

The risk of fatigue has been reported to cause concern in those preparing to return to work. Working as an anaesthetist is tiring, even in the course of working normal hours, and the effects of shift working add to this considerably. Fatigue is more than just being tired though.

The AAGBI guidance document, Fatigue and Anaesthetists[23], describes fatigue as 'the subjective feeling of the need to sleep, an increased physiological drive to fall asleep and a state of decreased alertness'. For obvious reasons this is of particular concern to those returning from sick leave, but it may also be important for those who are returning from maternity leave, when caring for the new addition to the family also leads to sleep deprivation and fatigue.

So what should you do? Avoidance of sleep deprivation is not an option: all grades of anaesthetists perform out-of-hours work either by working shifts or being on call. Awareness of the implications of lack of sleep and prioritization of good sleep habits are the key to managing sleep deprivation. Most adults need 8 hours sleep per night to enable restorative sleep. Restricted sleep for two or more consecutive nights, leads to development of a sleep debt, which can only be repaid by two 'good night's sleep'. This can be difficult if your home circumstances are such that an interrupted night's sleep is the norm. Recruiting help from your partner, family or friends might be necessary to enable you to get enough sleep to function safely at work. Other good habits to enable you to get the best quality sleep are avoidance of caffeine, heavy meals and exercise too close to bedtime and making sure your bedroom environment is conducive to good quality sleep. Remember that fatigue can be at its worst after overnight on call; it is safer to have a nap than to rush home.

## Burnout

We thought it worth including a few words on burnout here. Burnout is described as emotional exhaustion and it is thought to be due to prolonged levels of occupational stress. Returning to work can be associated with a degree of stress and if this becomes long-standing then it is logical that a risk of burnout follows. Trainees are also thought to be at increased risk. The pressures of examinations, inexperience, and juggling work and young families may all contribute.

There are several inventories described to assess burnout, including one which is available for self-assessment on the Doctors for Doctors section of the BMA website[24]. An article published in *Anaesthesia News* in December 2014 describes the phenomenon of burnout and the results of a survey of East of England trainees[25]: over 35% reported feeling burnt out at least once a week. If you think you may be at risk of developing burnout, it is important to get help. If you are an AAGBI member, you can access a short lecture on burnout by Dr Jon Smith, which gives a personal perspective and some strategies to avoid it. There should be support systems in place in your region, but you can always contact the BMA or AAGBI for help or advice.

## References

1. M. Connor, J. Pokora. *Coaching and Mentoring at Work*. Maidenhead: McGraw Hill, 2007.
2. K. B. Dasari, S. M. White, J. Pateman. Survey of iPhone usage among anaesthetists in England. *Anaesthesia* 2011; 66(7): 630–1.
3. S. D. Burdette, T.E. Herchline, R. Oehler. Surfing the web: practicing medicine in a technological age: using smartphones in clinical practice. *Clin Infect Dis* 2008; 47: 117–22.
4. T. Reader, R. Flin, K. Lauche, B. Cutherbertson. Non-technical skills in the intensive care unit. *Br J Anaesth*. 2006; 96: 551–9.
5. A. Mehrabian, S. R. Ferris. Inference of attitudes from nonverbal communication in two channels. *J Consult Psychol* 1967; 31: 248–52.

6.  R. Flin, P. O'Connor, M. Crichton. *Safety at the Sharp End A Guide to Non-Technical Skills.* Aldershot: Ashgate Publishing Limited, 2008.

7.  Elaine Bromiley case: Coroner's Inquest Verdict http://www.chfg.org/resources/07_qrt04/ Anonymous_Report_Verdict_and_Corrected_Timeline_Oct_07.pdf (accessed 2 January 2016).

8.  BMA Junior Doctors Committee. Safe handover: safe patients. Guidance on clinical handover for clinicians and managers. 2004.

9.  M. Leonard, S. Graham, D. Bonacum. The human factor: the critical importance of teamworking and communication in providing self care. *Qual Saf Health Care.* 2004; 13: i85–90.

10. M. A. West. *Effective Teamwork. Practical Lessons From Organizational Research*, 2nd edn. Leicester: BPS Blackwell, 2004.

11. ANTS System Handbook http://www.abdn.ac.uk/iprc/uploads/files/ANTS%20Handbook %202012.pdf (accessed 2 January 2016).

12. The AAGBI website. http://www.aagbi.org/professionals/welfare (accessed 2 January 2016).

13. The GAT Handbook. http://www.aagbi.org/sites/default/files/GAT%20Handbook%20Web.pdf (accessed 2 January 2016).

14. The BMA. Returning to practice – a model process. Available at http://bma.org.uk/developing-your-career/consultant/returning-to-practice-a-model-process (accessed 2 January 2016).

15. J. Reason. Human error: models and management. *BMJ* 2000; 320: 768–70.

16. M. Elliott. How to avoid adverse outcomes – making it personal: My 10 commandments. *Anaesthesia News* November 2013; 316: 29–30.

17. A. B. Haynes, T. G. Weiser, W. R. Berry, et al.; Safe Surgery Saves Lives Study Group. A surgical safety checklist to reduce morbidity and mortality in a global population. *N Engl J Med* 2009; 360: 491–9.

18. S. D. Pratt, B. R. Jachna. Care of the clinician after an adverse event. *Int J Obstet Anesth* 2015; 24: 54–63.

19. T. W. Martin, R. C. Roy. Cause for pause after perioperative catastrophe: one, two, or three victims? *Anesth Analg* 2012; 114: 485–7.

20. E. S. Williame, L. B. Manwell, T.R. Konrad, W. Linzer. The relationship of organizational culture, stress, satisfaction, and burnout with physician reported error and suboptimal patient care: results from the MEMO study. *Health Care Manage Rev* 2007; 32: 203–12.

21. T. D. Shanafelt, K. A. Bradley, J. E. Wipf, A. L. Back. Burnout and self reported patient care in an internal medicine residency program. *Ann Intern Med* 2002; 136: 358–67.

22. T. D. Shanafelt, C. M. Balch, G. Bechamps et al. Burnout and medical errors among American surgeons. *Ann Surg* 2010; 251: 995–1000.

23. Association of Anaesthetists of Great Britain and Ireland. Fatigue and Anaesthetists. 2014. Available at http://www.aagbi.org/sites/default/files/Fatigue%20Guideline%20web.pdf (accessed 2 January 2016).

24. Doctors for Doctors Burnout questionnaire. Available at https://web2.bma.org.uk/drs4drsburn .nsf/quest?OpenForm (accessed 2 January 2016).

25. B. Fox, E. Stewart. Burnout in anaesthetic trainees. *Anaesthesia News* December 2014; 329: 22–3. Available at http://www.aagbi.org/sites/default/files/ANews_December_web_0.pdf (accessed 2 January 2016).

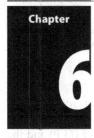

Chapter

6

# Supporting a colleague's return to work

*Support for the return to work process is integral to its success. The principles of support are the same for everyone but there are logistical differences between supporting junior doctors, staff and associate specialist doctors and consultants. We cover each in turn in this chapter.*

# Supporting a trainee: working with Educational Supervisors and College Tutors
Jill Horn

Most consultant anaesthetists will encounter trainees returning to work after a period of absence. It is therefore important that they understand the range of challenges and needs within this group of trainees and what the supervisor's role is.

## Important considerations
### Reason for absence
Trainees may be absent for a variety of reasons which can broadly be divided into those that are planned, chosen absences (e.g. parental leave, out of programme experience) and those which are unplanned or enforced (e.g. illness, suspension). Trainees in the latter group are likely to require a more complex return to work plan.

### Previous experience
Anaesthesia is a practical specialty requiring the mastery of complex skills both technical and non-technical. Many of these become automatic, requiring less cognitive effort the more frequently they are performed. Trainees who have completed only a year or two of anaesthetic practice will have such automatic routines less well embedded[1] and may be virtually 'starting from scratch' when returning to work. Trainees who have prolonged absence during their first or second year of training may well need to repeat their Initial Assessment of Competence (IAC) as part of the return to work process.

*Returning to Work in Anaesthesia*, ed. Emma Plunkett, Emily Johnson and Anna Pierson.
Published by Cambridge University Press. © Cambridge University Press 2016.

## Duration of absence

The duration of absence also affects how easily a trainee resumes their full role; a longer absence requiring a more extended period of supervised practice.

# Responsibilities and roles

One of the biggest challenges for supervisors when supporting a trainee returning to work is the coordination of all the involved parties. Employment arrangements and accountability for health and well-being are shared between the Local Education Provider (LEP) and the Local Education and Training Board (LETB), formerly Deanery.

## Training Programme Directors

The Training Programme Director (TPD)[2] takes overall responsibility for a trainee returning to work and is accountable to the Head of School and the Dean.

In the case of a planned absence, the TPD should have been involved in pre-absence planning, have kept in contact with the trainee during the absence and ensure that initial and review meetings take place. Consideration of training less than full time should be considered.

The TPD is responsible for ensuring that the trainee returns to an appropriate post – usually this will be the post from which the trainee left. Rotating into an unfamiliar post whilst absent from work introduces additional complexity, especially if the trainee has been on prolonged sick leave when support from Human Resources and Occupational Health departments will have been delivered by the LEP. Occasionally, there may be good reasons for placing a trainee into a new post – for example, to achieve specific workplace adjustments such as reducing travel time. In this case the TPD has a key role in the successful transfer of support to the trainee's new post.

Many trainees will choose to synchronize a return with rotation dates. The trainee can then attend the local induction programme and meet their peers. However, trainees who have been absent do have additional needs compared to those who are merely changing post.

The TPD is also responsible for monitoring training. Whilst the trainee is absent, their training 'clock' effectively stops. Resumption of training time occurs whenever the trainee has resumed duties at a level consistent with their stage of training. The Royal College of Anaesthetists (RCoA) and the General Medical Council (GMC) must be informed of any periods of absence since it may be necessary to adjust the trainee's anticipated date of the award of the Certificate of Completion of Training (CCT).

The TPD provides guidance and support to the College Tutor (CT) and Educational Supervisor (ES) to whom the practicalities of the return to work process will usually be delegated.

## College Tutors

The roles and responsibilities of the CT are described by the RCoA (2011)[3] but are less clearly defined than those of the ES and clinical supervisor (CS)[4,5]. However, depending upon local arrangements, the practical task of coordinating a trainee's return to work frequently resides with the CT.

The CT liaises with the trainee, the ES, the TPD, the Departmental Clinical Lead (who has direct managerial responsibility) and CSs as well as other parties including Human

Resources, Occupational Health, the Director of Medical Education (DME) and possibly external parties such as the GMC and the National Clinical Assessment Service (NCAS). Then, in discussion with the trainee and their ES, the CT sets out a return to work plan with a realistic timescale, precise review points, targets and assessments.

Most trainees will begin their return to work under full supervision and without any out-of-hours service commitment. CTs must ensure that those with managerial responsibilities understand the requirements and limitations of the trainee. Occupational health reports are often first sent to the Clinical Lead, rather than the CT or ES, so liaison on these matters is essential. However, information is shared only with the agreement of the trainee, who will usually receive a copy of all relevant correspondence.

It is essential that the trainee receives a departmental and hospital induction to refresh their knowledge of local resources and to inform them of any changes that have occurred since they left work.

Many anaesthetic departments are large and working with a new supervisor every day can be very challenging. Trainees returning to work following sickness or fitness to practise procedures are understandably sensitive regarding what information is given to others about their circumstances. Consequently, it can be useful for the CT to identify a small group of consultants with whom the trainee works. The trainee should be asked what information they wish to share. It is essential that CSs know precisely what level of supervision is required and which areas of practice require focus.

## Educational Supervisors

The ES is the main point of contact for the trainee and is responsible for reviewing and documenting progress. Trainees are used to collecting evidence of their performance; however, in complex cases where confidence is low or when competence is in question, trainees can find formal assessments quite daunting. In the early stages, keeping a reflective diary and obtaining verbal feedback can be reassuring and enable a trainee to see the progress they are making such that they feel more resilient and can request formal assessments. Trainees should use their e-portfolio to collate evidence; a summary will be presented at the Annual Review of Competence Progression using the Educational Supervisor's Structured Report.

Trainees should be encouraged to access local training facilities to refresh skills. Simulation exercises are an opportunity to rehearse non-technical skills and improve confidence in managing emergencies. Practical skills such as central line insertion can be practised on part-task trainers. Trainees need guidance on time management (unfamiliar tasks take longer) and re-establishing a satisfactory work–life balance (especially after maternity leave).

The ES must make clear the boundaries of their role and ensure that the TPD, Clinical Leads and Human Resources personnel are appropriately involved. Some trainees may benefit from support from outside the department, such as counselling or mentoring.

## Documentation

In addition to the use of the e-portfolio as mentioned above, most LETBs have specific documentation[6] for recording a return to work which includes details of meetings: pre-absence, initial review and return review. Occasionally there may be doubt over whether a trainee will make a successful return to work – a decision which will never be taken lightly or in haste. In such cases, accurate documentation to demonstrate that a trainee has received a good level of support is essential.

# Training

An individual CT/ES may only be required to manage a trainee returning to work infrequently. It can therefore be very helpful for the LETB or DME to establish training events to prepare trainers for this occurrence. This can be usefully done using interactive case-based discussions (see Table 6.1).

**Table 6.1** Examples of case-based discussions

| Case summary | Areas for discussion | Main learning points |
|---|---|---|
| ST 5 Trainee returning from 9 months' maternity leave | Post-fellowship so skills well developed<br>Best restart date | Pre-absence planning<br>Use of keep in touch (KIT) days<br>Adjustment to CCT |
| CT2 Trainee returning from 12 months' maternity leave | Limited pre-absence experience so poorly developed automatic skills<br>Considerable training demands ahead | May need to redo IAC<br>May need extension to achieve Basic Level Training Certificate |
| ST 6 Trainee returning after 6 months' sick leave following major shoulder injury | Physical limitations may remain<br>Confidence may be reduced especially regarding emergencies | Workplace adjustments may be required<br>May need phased return<br>Needs to 'test' physical capabilities in safe, supported environment |
| ST 4 Trainee returning after 18 months' sick leave due to mental health problems | Likely low confidence in most areas of practice<br>Ongoing fluctuations in health common | Complex case needing long phased return<br>Must be overseen by experienced TPD with frequent Occupational Health input<br>May need to be supernumerary for prolonged period |

# Conclusion

Trainers who are supporting trainees returning to work must have appropriate training and support. Complex cases require liaison with multiple parties and must be overseen by experienced TPDs.

# Supporting a consultant's return to work

Emma Plunkett

As alluded to in Chapter 1, in many areas of the UK, it has been trainees and those who support them who have driven the development of formal return to work programmes to support the return to work process after maternity leave. However, having a break from anaesthesia is not unique to trainees and it is equally important that consultants, staff grade doctors, and associate specialists are supported when they return to work. Many of the concerns and issues are common to all, although returning as a consultant has unique challenges as it may have been some time since a consultant was supervised by a colleague. However, the consultant is likely to be returning to a working environment and colleagues that they are familiar with, which can be a significant help.

Below we discuss some of the issues pertinent to returning to work as a consultant. The recommendations made reflect those in the Academy of Medical Royal Colleges report

Return to Practice Guidance, April 2012[7], and the Royal College of Anaesthetists guidance Returning to work after a period of absence, May 2012[8], which are discussed previously in Chapter 2. Revalidation is discussed separately in Chapter 4.

## Devising a return to work programme

A consultant should plan their return to work in conjunction with the clinical service lead for their department. The same principles as discussed in Chapter 4 apply to the design of a suitable return to work programme for consultants, i.e. a pre-leave planning meeting should occur for anticipated leave; a preparation to return meeting should be arranged to plan the return to work; all parties should agree what the goals are and how the process will be recorded and assessed. Several trusts now have guidelines covering the return to work process for consultants[9].

The first thing to consider is whether there needs to be any change to their job plan because of the reason for the absence. This may not be known initially, especially if they are returning after illness, so there needs to be a strategy developed to enable this to be assessed. Occupational health advice is key in this situation, but in all cases it is vital that realistic expectations are set.

The clinical service lead is ultimately the person responsible for ensuring a safe and effective reintroduction period, but it is worth considering whether there is someone more suitable to oversee the process as it occurs. This person might vary according to the size of the department and any subspecialty area of practice, and may depend on professional relationships and whom the consultant feels most comfortable working with.

It is important to be transparent about the return to work process. As well as the clinical service lead and group manager, the clinicians/colleagues involved will need to be informed, as will the consultant responsible for the weekly and on-call rotas and the departmental admin team. However, confidentiality must be maintained and the dignity of the doctor ensured. It may be that the consultant prefers to deal with a single member of the admin team for example.

## Supervision

The question of the degree of supervision and by whom does not have a standard answer. It is often appropriate to start with a couple of admin days to help the consultant reacquaint themselves with the department. For those returning from maternity leave these can be KIT days. This time can be used to undertake any mandatory training required by the trust, to reactivate any IT passwords, ID badges, and car park passes. It can also be helpful to meet with the consultant equipment lead and theatre lead to identify any systems or processes that have changed during the leave period, or any new pieces of equipment to get to grips with.

This will progress to directly supervised lists and thereafter lists with distant supervision. The speed at which this occurs is likely to depend upon the length of time off, the reason for the leave and the length of time in post before leave. In a survey of consultants recently returning from either maternity or sick leave in the West Midlands (2013–2015), the number of supervised sessions (half day) ranged from 1 to 22, with a median number of 14 sessions. This is very similar to the 10 supervised days that is commonly used for trainees, although clearly this depends on individual circumstances.

In terms of assessment of progress, suggested tools are the Anaesthetic List Management Assessment Tool (ALMAT)[10] and the Acute Care Assessment Tool (ACAT)[11].

Finally, progression to unsupervised lists will occur and it is worth ensuring (if possible!) that the first few of these are anticipated to be straightforward cases in the first instance.

## How long before on-calls?

Again, this is very much down to the individual situation. However, it is sensible to plan for on-calls to be resumed only at the end of the supervised period and to accept that this may need to change if it is taking longer for the doctor to readjust to working again. For some subspecialty work it may be that a period of doubled-up on-calls is required initially.

Departments are increasingly under-resourced and over-stretched these days. This should not lead to cutting short a planned reintroduction period or phased return to work.

## Potential anxieties

Many of these will be common to all grades of anaesthetist and recognizing limitations and asking for help is discussed in more detail in Chapter 5. Of course everyone is different and will have their own particular worries, which are likely to relate to individual job plans and the circumstances surrounding leave. There may be particular working relationships that add to stress at times of change. These should be identified during the return to work planning meeting and the consultant should be offered a mentor as a source of support and empathetic challenge.

Supervising trainees was mentioned as a source of apprehension in the survey of consultants who had recently returned to work. It makes sense to plan the reintroductory period to allow the consultant time to re-establish confidence in their own practice (which took a median of 3 weeks in the survey), before supervision of trainees is introduced.

## References

1. R. Flin, P. O'Connor, M. Crichton. *Safety at the Sharp End. A Guide to Non-Technical Skills.* Aldershot: Ashgate Publishing Limited, 2008.
2. UK Health Departments. *A Reference Guide for Postgraduate Specialty Training in the UK: The Gold Guide,* 5th edn. UK: UK Health Departments, 2014, p. 19.
3. Royal College of Anaesthetists. *College Tutor – Roles and Responsibilities.* 2011, pp. 1–4.
4. UK Health Departments. *A Reference Guide for Postgraduate Specialty Training in the UK: The Gold Guide,* 5th edn. UK: UK Health Departments 2014, p. 20.
5. General Medical Council. *The Trainee Doctor.* London: GMC, 2011, p. 55.
6. Taylor, P. *Return to Training Scheme.* Leeds: Health Education Yorkshire and the Humber, 2014.
7. http://www.aomrc.org.uk/doc_view/9486-return-to-practice-guidance (accessed 2 January 2016).
8. https://www.rcoa.ac.uk/system/files/PUB-ReturnToWork2012.pdf (accessed 2 January 2016).
9. H. Church, Z. Nassa. Return to Practice Guidelines for Consultant Anaesthetists. University Hospitals Birmingham NHS Foundation Trust. (For more information about this please contact Dr Hannah Church, Consultant Anaesthetist Hannah.Church@uhb.nhs.uk.)
10. Anaesthesia List Management Assessment Tool (ALMAT). Available at www.rcoa.ac.uk/document-store/anaesthesia-list-management-assessment-tool-almat (accessed 2 January 2016).
11. Acute Care Assessment Tool (ACAT). Available at www.ficm.ac.uk/curriculum-and-assessment/assessment-forms (accessed 2 January 2016).

# Refreshing your knowledge

Nicholas Cowley, Kerry Cullis, Anna Dennis,
Hozefa Ebrahim, Ruth Francis, Maria Garside,
Sarah Gibb, Emily Johnson, Surrah Leifer,
Randeep Mullhi, James Nickells, Anna Nutbeam,
Anna Pierson, Jane Pilsbury, Emma Plunkett,
Louise Savic, Charlotte Small, Alifia Tameem,
Caroline Thomas and Benjamin Walton

## Introduction

Following on from the practicalities of planning your return to work, this section is designed to refresh your memory of key topics related to anaesthesia and intensive care medicine, whatever level you may be. The aim is that you may use this as an interactive, informal revision section, rather than a reminder of sitting past or future examinations.

The 120 questions are based on Levels 1, 2 and 3 of the Royal College of Anaesthetists CPD Matrix, and therefore should offer comprehensive cover of most relevant aspects of the anaesthetic syllabus. We have included a variety of question formats to allow you to become focussed on the anaesthetic way of thinking again, to engage you and prompt your memory. The clinical questions in particular will help you to practise your decision-making skills, which can often feel a little rusty when returning to work after a significant break. Each one has been individually written with you in mind. Every author has returned to work after a break and for a variety of reasons; hence we are all too aware of the areas which provoke the most feelings of anxiety, lack of confidence and are often the most difficult to remember. Therefore, the questions aim to focus on specific areas which are often the cause of these concerns, and target issues more relevant to returning from a break from clinical practice.

Each question provides you with a topic summary, referencing relevant and up-to-date guidelines which you should be familiar with. Finally, there are suggestions for your further reading.

Please use the questions as you wish; it may be useful to read them in the run-up to your return to work, or to use them as an aide-memoire to help you once you have returned to clinical practice.

# Scientific principles

*In this chapter, we revisit some of the basic scientific principles fundamental to anaesthesia, from pulmonary compliance to pharmacokinetics. Here, the principles are put into a clinically relevant context as encountered in practice. A variety of question styles are included to help to refresh your decision-making skills.*

## Physiology and biochemistry: pulmonary compliance, resistance and flow-volume loops

You are anaesthetizing a 56-year-old for major lower gastrointestinal cancer surgery who has a history of chronic pulmonary obstructive disease (COPD). You are joined by a very keen CT1 who has a lot of questions about pulmonary function in patients with lung disease.

**What is compliance?**

Compliance is the volume change ($\Delta V$) per unit pressure change ($\Delta P$), and is essentially a measure of the lung's ability to stretch and expand, i.e. their distensibility.

Compliance $= \Delta V/\Delta P (ml/cmH_2O$ or $L/KPa)$, where $\Delta P = \Delta$ transpulmonary pressure.

Since the lungs have a tendency to recoil inwards, inflation requires an increase in transpulmonary pressure (TPP), generated by the respiratory muscles. As TPP increases, lung volume naturally increases. At relatively low lung volumes, the lungs are highly distensible and for a given change in TPP, this results in a relatively large increase in lung volume. However, at high volumes, lungs reach the limit of their distensibility; here there is little change in lung volume for an equivalent change in TPP. Approaching functional residual capacity (FRC), lung compliance is greatest and has a value of approximately 200 ml/cmH$_2$O.

**What factors affect compliance?**

Compliance is reduced by pulmonary oedema; pulmonary fibrosis; extremes of lung volume; restrictive diseases of the chest wall; pregnancy and supine posture. It is increased by old age and emphysema.

---

*Returning to Work in Anaesthesia*, ed. Emma Plunkett, Emily Johnson and Anna Pierson.
Published by Cambridge University Press. © Cambridge University Press 2016.

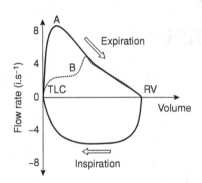

**Figure 7.1** Diagram of normal flow-volume loop. Reproduced with permission from *Physics, Pharmacology and Physiology*, M. Cross and E. Plunkett. Cambridge University Press. 2014 p. 207.

## What is airway resistance and what factors affect it?

This is the resistance of the respiratory tract to gas flow during the respiratory cycle. During laminar gas flow:

Resistance = Driving pressure/gas flow

Factors affecting resistance:

1. Diameter of airways: reduction in diameter increases airway resistance
   - Bronchoconstriction, e.g. asthma, COPD, stimulation of parasympathetic nervous system
   - Reduced elastic recoil, e.g. emphysema
   - Airway inflammation, e.g. asthma, bronchitis
   - Excess mucus, e.g. cystic fibrosis, bronchitis
   - Upper airway obstruction, e.g. foreign body, tracheal stenosis
2. Type of gas flow: during laminar flow there is less resistance than during turbulent flow
   - Low density gases, i.e. helium, are more likely to produce laminar flow
3. Lung volume: at high lung volumes the airways are pulled opened therefore reducing resistance.
4. Anaesthesia: general anaesthesia increases resistance by decreasing FRC.

## What is the appearance of a normal flow-volume loop?

Flow is plotted against volume to produce a diagrammatic representation of spirometric effort. It is a continuous loop of expiration (starting at total lung capacity, TLC) and inspiration (starting at residual volume, RV). The maximal flow rate during expiration is around 8–10 l/s, and during inspiration is 4–6 l/s.

## How would the flow-volume loop change in COPD and other lung pathologies?

### Obstructive lung disease

Peak expiratory flow rate (PEFR) is reduced. There is a scooped out appearance of the expiratory limb and a reduction in flow rates throughout expiration. RV is increased owing to gas trapping.

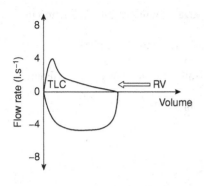

**Figure 7.2** Diagram of flow-volume loop in obstructive lung disease. Reproduced with permission from *Physics, Pharmacology and Physiology*, M. Cross and E. Plunkett. Cambridge University Press. 2014 p. 208.

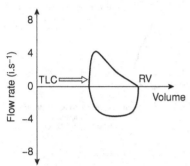

**Figure 7.3** Diagram of flow-volume loop in restrictive lung disease. Reproduced with permission from *Physics, Pharmacology and Physiology*, M. Cross and E. Plunkett. Cambridge University Press. 2014 p. 208.

Restrictive lung disease

The PEFR and total volume expired are reduced. TLC is reduced, shifting the curve to the right.

## Further reading

Appadu B. L., Hanning C. D. Respiratory physiology. In: C. Pinnock, T. Lin, T. Smith, eds. *Fundamentals of Anaesthesia*, 2nd edn. Cambridge: Cambridge University Press, 2006, pp. 402–7.

Cross M. E., Plunkett E. V. E. *Physics, Pharmacology and Physiology for Anaesthetists*. Cambridge: Cambridge University Press, 2008, pp. 119–22, 142.

West J. B. *Respiratory Physiology: The Essentials*, 8th edn. China: Lippincott Williams & Wilkins, 2008.

## Physiology and biochemistry: control of blood pressure

1. Shock can be classified into four different modes; hypovolaemic, cardiogenic, neurogenic and distributive. With regards to this classification, which of the following statements are correct?

    a) Tachypnoea is a relatively early sign in hypovolaemic shock
    b) Tachycardia can be the primary pathology
    c) Capillary refill time is usually low in all forms of shock
    d) Central venous pressure is usually elevated in cardiogenic shock
    e) Skin temperature is not normally changed in obstructive shock

2. With respect to the renal and central nervous control of blood pressure and perfusion, which of the following statements are correct?

a) Hypertension typically results in an increased vagal output causing a reduction in systemic vascular resistance
b) The adrenal medulla is innervated by postganglionic sympathetic fibres
c) The resting autonomic tone is inherently sympathetic
d) Renal blood flow is highly variable, and is controlled by the calibre of the afferent and efferent arterioles
e) Increase in sympathetic outflow increases renal blood flow

Answers: 1. TTFTF; 2. TFTFF

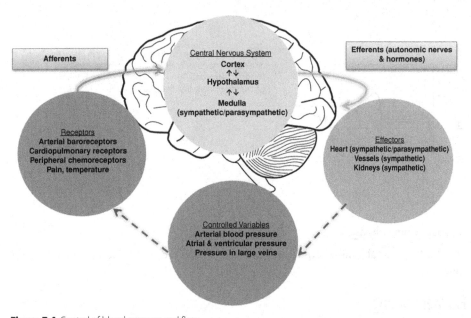

**Figure 7.4** Control of blood pressure and flow.

The control of blood pressure (BP) and blood flow are two distinctly different phenomena, and are central components to the physiology underpinning good anaesthetic practice. This control is via a complex communication between many organ systems.

Figure 7.4 shows the complex communication between the different receptors and effectors, and their connection with the central nervous system. Tachycardia and tachypnoea are both relatively early signs of hypovolaemic shock. However, in the fit, young patient, hypotension may be a late sign of hypovolaemia. Both bradycardia and tachycardia may be a cause of hypotension. As the heart rate (HR) drops, BP will also be reduced. With respect to tachycardia, an extremely high HR will reduce the cardiac filling time in diastole, and hence impact negatively on stroke volume. In most situations, modest tachycardia is a beneficial compensatory mechanism to maintain perfusion pressure.

Table 7.1 shows changes of variables commonly affected by the different types of shock. An understanding of these variables will arm the clinician with the ability to administer the correct treatment in each clinical scenario. The importance of this skill, for example, would be the avoidance of vasopressors in the patient with cardiogenic shock.

**Table 7.1** Classification of shock according to clinical presentation

|  | Hypovolaemic | Obstructive | Cardiogenic | Distributive |
|---|---|---|---|---|
| Blood pressure | ↓ | ↓ | ↓ | ↓ |
| Central venous pressure (preload) | ↓ | ↑ | ↑ | ↓ |
| Capillary refill time | ↑ | ↑ | ↑ | ↓ |
| Skin temperature | ↓ | ↓ | ↓ | ↑ |

Central control of BP is modulated via the autonomic nervous system. The resting tone is inherently sympathetic, and this is evident during a myocardial infarction when all autonomic communication is arrested. In this scenario the HR falls.

The kidney is also involved in maintaining pressure and flow. The afferent and efferent arterioles constrict and dilate in response to changing BP, resulting in a relatively constant renal blood flow. Renal blood flow is reduced by sympathetic nerve activity as part of the arterial baroreceptor response to decreased BP. The macula densa within the kidney is involved in the tubulo-glomerular feedback system. More adenosine is released if the renal perfusion pressure rises. Nitric oxide is a vasodilator and can be produced when the renal perfusion pressure falls.

Therefore, it is important to consider each of the causes of hypotension in turn and systematically determine which is the most likely, thus allowing you to choose the correct treatment.

## Further reading

Bryant H., Bromhead H. Intraoperative hypotension. Anaesthesia Tutorial of the Week 48. 24.8.2009. Royal Hampshire County Hospital, Winchester, UK, 2009. Available at http://www.frca.co.uk (accessed 2 January 2016).

Foex P., Sear J. W. The surgical hypertensive patient. *Contin Educ Anaesth Crit Care Pain* 2004; 4(5): 139–43.

## Physiology and biochemistry: factors affecting ICP

Following a fall down some stairs, a 56-year-old man is promptly admitted to ICU with an isolated head injury. He had a Glasgow Coma Score (GCS) of 5 prior to intubation and has evidence of cerebral contusions on his CT brain scan.

**Immediate management should include maintenance of the following, with the exception of which ONE?**

a) Normocapnia
b) Normoglycaemia
c) Normotension
d) Hypothermia
e) Normoxia

Answer: d)

Head injury is a common presentation to emergency departments, with a significant mortality and morbidity. Eighty-five per cent of patients suffering a severe head injury will be either dead or disabled at 1 year post-injury. It can be classified in a number of ways depending on the mechanism and type of injury, or based on the patient's GCS. The GCS is useful in helping to predict outcome following a significant head injury, with the motor component being particularly useful. Simply speaking, traumatic brain injury (TBI) is graded as mild (GCS 14–15), moderate (GCS 9–13) and severe (GCS ≤ 8).

Intracranial pressure (ICP) depends on the volume of the intracranial contents, which normally comprises 1.4 kg brain, 50–70 ml blood and 50–120 ml cerebrospinal fluid. A normal ICP is 7–17 mmHg (1–2 kPa). An increase in volume of any one of the intracranial components will be counterbalanced by a decrease in the others to a point, after which ICP will exponentially increase, reducing cerebral perfusion and therefore oxygenation (cerebral perfusion pressure (CPP) = mean arterial pressure (MAP) – ICP). Under normal conditions autoregulation maintains a constant blood flow between a MAP 50 mmHg and 150 mmHg. However, in traumatized or ischaemic brains, cerebral blood flow (CBF) may become blood pressure dependent.

Hypercapnia causes vasodilatation, increasing CBF and therefore increasing the intracranial contents and ICP. Hypocapnia ($pCO_2 < 3.3$ kPa) will not cause any further reduction in CBF and offers no advantage. In fact it is detrimental, as it shifts the oxygen dissociation curve to the left, impairing cerebral oxygen delivery. Arterial $pO_2$ has a minimal effect until it falls below 6.7 kPa at which point CBF increases significantly.

This patient has sustained a severe TBI and is at risk of cerebral oedema. He should ideally be managed in a specialist neurosurgical unit with ICP monitoring. He should be discussed with a neurosurgeon, and hopefully arrangement for transfer can be made. While this is happening, it is important to target the prevention of secondary brain injury by addressing the key principles of ongoing management of the head-injured patient on the ICU and maintaining normotension, normoxia, normocapnia, normothermia and normoglycaemia.

There is no evidence that induced hypothermia is beneficial in the immediate management of head injury, but it may be necessary as part of the management of persistently raised ICP.

Please refer to the management algorithm for patients with severe traumatic brain injury in Chapter 31.

## Further reading

Dinsmore J. Traumatic brain injury: an evidence-based review of management. *Contin Educ Anaesth Crit Care Pain* 2013; 13(6): 189–95.

National Institute for Health and Clinical Excellence (NICE). Head injury: triage, assessment, investigation and early management of head injury in infants, children and adults. Clinical Guideline 56. London: NICE, 2007. Available at http://www.nice.org.uk/nicemedia/pdf/CG56NICEGuideline.pdf (accessed 20 April 2012).

Tameem A., Krovvidi H. Cerebral physiology. *Contin Educ Anaesth Crit Care Pain* 2013; 13(4): 113–18.

## Pharmacology and therapeutics: target-controlled infusions (TCI)

A 50-year-old patient presents for elective middle ear surgery. She has a history of postoperative nausea and vomiting and hypertension. You decide to administer a propofol and remifentanil general anaesthetic using a target-controlled infusion (TCI).

With regard to the infusion algorithm model, which of the following would be most appropriate to use for this patient?

a) The Paedfusor model for propofol
b) The Bristol algorithm for propofol
c) The Schnider model for remifentanil
d) The Kataria model for propofol
e) The Minto model for remifentanil

Answer: e)

Propofol and remifentanil are commonly used in combination as part of a total intravenous anaesthesia (TIVA) target-controlled infusion (TCI) general anaesthetic. The advantages of this combination include reduced incidence of post-operative nausea and vomiting and a smooth, easily titratable anaesthetic. It is ideally suited for neurosurgical and longer ENT procedures. These procedures often require a relatively bloodless field for optimal surgical access yet can be highly stimulating in parts with minimal post-operative pain, so the short-acting opioid remifentanil can be increased as required to prevent swings in blood pressure and heart rate.

Most anaesthetic agents are thought to conform to a three-compartment model. The compartment model is used in design of dosing regimens, for example the bolus-elimination-transfer regimen. This refers to a bolus to fill the central compartment (blood) then a constant infusion to match the elimination rate, plus an infusion to compensate for the transfer to peripheral tissues (redistribution), which would be an exponentially decreasing rate.

TCIs aim to target the effect site, which is the site at which the drug exerts its principal effects; for anaesthetics this is the brain. The drug concentration at the effect site ($C_e$) cannot be measured but there are many algorithms for calculating blood and effect site concentrations. The plasma concentration ($C_p$) lags behind the $C_e$ until steady state is achieved.

There are a number of microprocessor-containing infusion devices available with preprogrammed algorithms that can be used for both propofol and remifentanil. The commonest propofol model is the Marsh model, and the commonest remifentanil model is the Minto model. The Marsh model uses total body weight in the calculation, which can result in significant overdose in obese patients if their actual body weights are entered. It is important to calculate ideal body weight based on height in such patients.

The Schnider model is newer and requires age, height and total body weight to be entered. It calculates lean body mass, which it uses for propofol delivery. It is well suited to elderly patients, who may have lower lean body mass. The Paedfusor and Kataria models are used in paediatrics. The Marsh model in TCI administration of propofol has demonstrated overestimation of blood concentrations in children. The Bristol algorithm is the original TIVA method, as used before the introduction of pre-programmed TCI infusion pumps.

## Further reading

Sivasubramaniam S. Target controlled infusions (TCI) in anaesthetic practice. Anaesthesia UK 2007. Available at www.frca.co.uk/article.aspx?articleid=101001 (accessed 9 January 2015).

## Pharmacology and therapeutics: local anaesthetics

You are in theatre anaesthetizing for a day case plastics list. The Plastics SHO is planning to infiltrate the surgical field with local anaesthetic (LA), but is unsure how to calculate the safe maximal dose. The surgical site is infected and the SHO asks you to explain why LA may not work as effectively in this situation.

### What is the mechanism of action of LA?

Local anaesthetics reversibly block sodium channels within the neuronal membrane. They are weak bases and exist in equilibrium between two states: the ionized form and the non-ionized lipophilic form. Equilibrium is dependent on both the $pK_a$ of the LA and the surrounding pH. It is the non-ionized form that passes into the cell down its concentration gradient. Within the cell a new equilibrium is established because of the intracellular pH, and the ionized form then moves into the open sodium channels, blocking them, preventing further neuronal conduction. The 'membrane expansion' theory, where unionized LA dissolves in the cell membrane, disrupting the ion channels, offers an alternative explanation.

### Why is LA less effective when used on infected tissue?

When tissues are infected the extracellular pH is lower than normal, reducing the proportion of LA in the non-ionized lipophilic form, meaning less is available to cross the cell membrane to the site of action. An acidic environment therefore reduces the potency of LA. There may also be higher vascularity within infected tissues, increasing removal of LA from the site.

### Other than pH, what other factors influence the activity of local anaesthetics?

1. Protein binding – increasing the protein binding of LA increases affinity for membrane proteins, therefore prolonging the duration of action.
2. Lipid solubility – increasing lipid solubility increases the potency of LA. It also increases the speed of onset and toxic potential.
3. $pK_a$ – the higher the $pK_a$, the lower the proportion of LA in the non-ionized lipophilic state at any given pH, and therefore the slower the onset of action as less drug is available to cross the cell membrane.

### What are the maximum safe doses of the various local anaesthetics?

**Table 7.2** Maximum safe doses of local anaesthetics

| Local anaesthetic | Maximum safe dose |
| --- | --- |
| Lidocaine | 3 mg/kg |
| Lidocaine with adrenaline | 7 mg/kg |
| Prilocaine | 6 mg/kg |
| Prilocaine with adrenaline | 9 mg/kg |
| Bupivacaine | 2 mg/kg |
| Bupivacaine with adrenaline | 2.5 mg/kg |
| Ropivacaine | 3 mg/kg |

### What other agents can be added to local anaesthetics?

1. Glucose – when dextrose is added to bupivacaine it increases the density of the solution, producing hyperbaric or 'heavy' bupivacaine. When injected intrathecally it therefore sinks within the cerebrospinal fluid because of gravity.

2. Vasoconstrictors – adrenaline and felypressin can be used. Local vasoconstriction reduces the systemic uptake of the LA, therefore reducing toxicity and increasing duration of action.
3. Analgesics – opioids, clonidine and ketamine.
4. Hyaluronidase – used to aid the spread of LA within connective tissue, i.e. after IM or subcutaneous injection.
5. Alkalizing agents – bicarbonate can be added to increase pH, which increases the proportion of LA in the non-ionized lipophilic form, resulting in a quicker onset of action.

## Further reading

Anaesthesia UK. Pharmacology of regional anaesthesia. 2007. Available at http://www.frca.co.uk/article.aspx?articleid=100816 (accessed March 2015).
Peck T. E., Hill S. A., Williams M. *Pharmacology for Anaesthesia and Intensive Care*, 3rd edn. Cambridge: Cambridge University Press, 2008.
Pinnock C., Lin T., Smith T. *Fundamentals of Anaesthesia*, 2nd edn. Cambridge: Cambridge University Press, 2006.

# Pharmacology and therapeutics: reversal of neuromuscular blockade

You are drawing to the close of an urgent laparotomy in a 68-year-old obese patient with an obstructing sigmoid tumour. You have inserted an epidural preoperatively for post-operative pain relief, and are planning to extubate the patient and transfer them to a high dependency bed. The surgeons are closing the abdomen, and request muscle relaxation to facilitate this. You administer a further dose of rocuronium. The surgeons finish operating 10 minutes later.

**Which of the following statements are true or false?**

a) Neostigmine can be administered immediately to effectively reverse rocuronium
b) Sugammadex can be administered immediately to effectively reverse rocuronium
c) Upon return of all four twitches on train of four (TOF) ratio neuromuscular monitoring, the patient may still have up to 70% receptor sites blocked
d) A post-tetanic count of one suggests imminent return of first twitch on TOF monitoring

Answers: FTTF

It is important to ensure adequate reversal of neuromuscular blockade in this patient, both to minimize aspiration risk, and because of risk of airway compromise on extubation secondary to obesity. In view of the recent administration of rocuronium, and additional risk factors, it would actually be reasonable to use sugammadex here to optimize the patient for tracheal extubation. Alternatively, an acetylcholinesterase inhibitor such as neostigmine could be used, along with neuromuscular monitor evidence of suitability for reversal.

A neuromuscular monitor is placed transcutaneously over an accessible peripheral nerve, and used to both assess the patient's suitability for administration of reversal agent, and for residual blockade. The negative (black) electrode is placed distally over the nerve and the positive (red) electrode proximally. The ulnar nerve in the distal forearm is commonly chosen, as it is usually available for visual and tactile assessment of twitch intensity (thumb adduction) and ratio of twitch heights can be assessed. Place the negative electrode over the flexor crease on the palmar surface of the wrist and the positive electrode 2 cm proximally. Peripheral nerve stimulation is delivered for 0.2 ms using a supramaximal electrical stimulus to the nerve (generally > 60 mA for transcutaneous nerve stimulation). (An alternative site is the facial nerve: place the distal (negative) electrode parallel with the tragus of the ear and the proximal electrode at the outer canthus of the eye and look for eyebrow twitching.)

Suitability for use of a traditional acetylcholinesterase inhibitor can be established in the presence of at least three twitches using the 'train of four' (TOF) ratio. Even in this situation, up to 70% of receptor sites remain blocked. It is unusual to have to use tetany and post-tetanic counts with relatively short-acting modern neuromuscular blockers, but if a large dose has just been administered, a post-tetanic count can be made to estimate time to return of single twitch on TOF. A single twitch on TOF should return within 15–20 minutes after emergence of the first twitch post-tetanic count. Following administration of the chosen reversal agent, either TOF or double burst stimulation ratios may be used to assess adequacy of reversal. Both require a first to last twitch ratio of >90% to ensure adequacy of reversal. Double burst stimulation is generally preferable if no objective equipment is available to measure the ratio of twitch size, as it is easier to make a visual assessment with just two twitches.

## Further reading

McGrath C. D., Hunter J. M. Monitoring of neuromuscular block. *Contin Educ Anaesth Crit Care Pain* 2006; 6(1): 7–12.

## Physics and clinical measurement: capnography

Capnography makes a valuable contribution to our standard monitoring during anaesthesia. Recognition of the capnography waveform is a vital skill.

1.  **Match the following themes to the traces in Figure 7.5.**

    a) Normal capnograph
    b) Hyperventilation
    c) Cardiac oscillations
    d) Inadequate paralysis
    e) Rebreathing
    f) Hypoventilation
    g) Malignant hyperpyrexia
    h) Cardiac arrest
    i) System disconnection
    j) Chronic obstructive pulmonary disease (COPD)

2.  **Which of the following statements regarding capnography are true?**

    a) Capnography monitoring is mandatory whilst giving an anaesthetic
    b) A rapid fall in end-tidal $CO_2$ ($EtCO_2$) is a sensitive marker of an air embolism
    c) There are no absolute contraindications to the use of capnography in patients undergoing a general anaesthetic

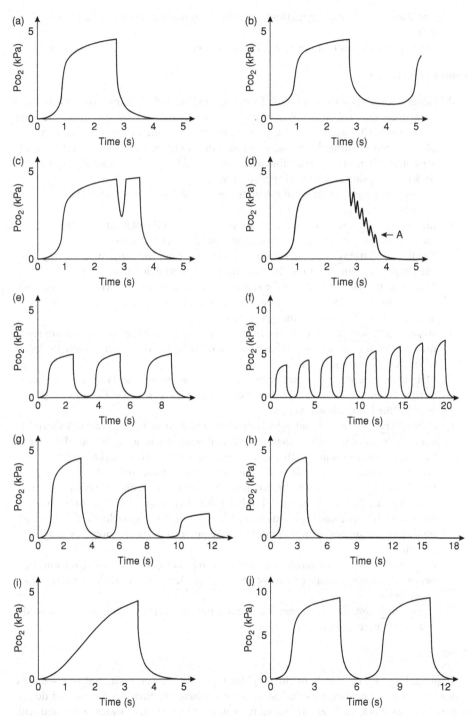

**Figure 7.5** Normal and abnormal capnography traces. Reproduced with permission from *Physics, Pharmacology and Physiology*, M. Cross and E. Plunkett. Cambridge University Press. 2014 pp. 112–16.

d) The side-stream sampling method can produce unreliable results in very small infants
e) Capnography helps to differentiate between tracheal and bronchial intubation

Answers: Question 1:

A. Normal trace: the $CO_2$ level starts from zero, as it initially measures the $CO_2$ content of the fresh gas flow (which is devoid of any $CO_2$). There is subsequently a sharp rise in measured $CO_2$ as the alveolar gas exits the lungs during expiration. The trace plateaus, representing the constant outward flow of more alveolar gas. At the end of expiration, there is a steep decline in the measured $CO_2$ as the inspired gas passes back over the side-stream port (end-tidal value).
B. Rebreathing: baseline does not return to zero, implying there is $CO_2$ in the circulating fresh gas flow.
C. Inadequate paralysis: there is a cleft towards the end of the plateau. This represents the patient's attempt to inspire, and draw fresh gas over the sensor.
D. Cardiac oscillations: note the length of the breath. After the entire tidal volume has been expelled from the lungs, the subsequent inspiration has not occurred. Therefore, the gas flowing over the sensor is increasingly diluted with fresh gas, and the measured concentration slowly drops to zero. However, each heartbeat causes artefacts within the trace as the gas vibrates.
E. Hyperventilation: the shape of the trace remains normal, but owing to the increased minute volume, more $CO_2$ is eliminated from the body. As a result, the $EtCO_2$ level adjusts to a lower equilibrium.
F. Malignant hyperpyrexia: a rare occurrence! Because of increased $CO_2$ production during this adverse reaction, there is a continuous increase in $EtCO_2$ with every breath. This is a medical emergency.
G. Cardiac arrest: this is physiological opposite to malignant hyperpyrexia. A sharp decrease that occurs with cardiac arrest is demonstrated by a continuous decrease in the $EtCO_2$ level. This makes the assumption that the patient is mechanically ventilated. Clearly, this would not occur in a self-ventilating patient!
H. System disconnection: after a breath, there is a sudden and complete disappearance of any further $CO_2$ measurement, implying that there is a circuit disconnection. Alternatively, this could represent an accidental switch from mechanical ventilation mode to spontaneous breathing mode, where no breaths are attempted by the patient.
I. COPD: here, the deep alveolar gases are slow to be completely eliminated from the depths of the lungs because of airway narrowing. Hence, the trace does not reach a true plateau.
J. Hypoventilation: the shape remains normal, but the decreased minute volume leads to a stably increased $EtCO_2$.

Question 2: TTTTF

Capnography monitoring is mandatory during general anaesthesia, and is a sensitive indicator of many complications, including air embolism or other acute causes of deterioration in cardiac output. There are no complications or contraindications associated with its use. In most modern anaesthetic machines, a sample of gas is withdrawn from the breathing system via a side-stream. This flow is usually in the order of 50 ml/h, which can lead to unreliable results in very small infants when the tidal volumes are low, and the relative dead spaces high.

## Further reading

Butterworth J. F., Mackey D. C., Wasnick J. D. *Morgan and Mikhail's Clinical Anaesthesiology*, 5th edn. New York: Lange, 2013, pp. 125–9.

Cross M., Plunkett E. *Physics, Pharmacology and Physiology for Anaesthetists – Key Concepts for the FRCA.* Cambridge: Cambridge University Press, 2008.

Dolenska S. *Basic Science for Anaesthetists.* Cambridge: Cambridge University Press, 2006.

## Physics and clinical measurement: pulse oximetry

1. Consider whether the following statements are true or false regarding the pulse oximeter.

    a) It is used to measure the oxygen carrying capacity of pulsating blood
    b) Pulse oximeters operate on the principle of infrared light absorption through tissue, following the Beer–Lambert Law
    c) A photodetector is used to detect light at a wavelength of 660 nm because deoxyhaemoglobin cannot emit light of this wavelength
    d) Pulse oximeters are superior to the experienced eye in detecting hypoxia in most clinical settings

2. Which of the following can cause an abnormal trace or reading?

    a) Nail varnish or pigment
    b) Bright lights shining on the probe
    c) Patient movement
    d) Poor perfusion
    e) Carbon monoxide poisoning

Answers: 1. FTFT; 2. TTTTT

A pulse oximeter is an instrument designed to measure the oxygen saturation of haemoglobin in whole blood. Rather than measuring the oxygen carrying capacity of pulsating blood, it measures the fraction of saturated blood over the total oxygen carrying capacity. It operates on the principle of infrared light absorption through tissue, following the Beer–Lambert law.

The photodetector cannot distinguish between different wavelengths, i.e. it assumes all the light detected is coming from the light-emitting diode. Hence, there are three settings – 660 nm, 940 nm and off. The photodetector will still receive ambient light in the off position. This is subtracted from the other two readings to produce a reference point.

Light emitted from the diode traverses the finger. It has to pass through pulsatile blood (asterial), non-pulsatile blood (venous) and other tissues. Non-pulsatile components are excluded, leaving the pulsatile to be analysed. Accuracy is to within $+/-$ 2% but is less accurate below saturations of 85% (based on studies in volunteers breathing low oxygen concentrations). Values below 70% are extrapolated and may be grossly inaccurate.

Clinical observation alone has been shown to be notoriously poor at detecting hypoxia. However, pulse oximetry reveals nothing about adequacy of ventilation (e.g. rising $PaCO_2$) or oxygen content (profound anaemia).

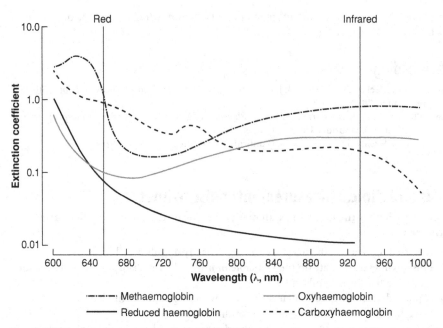

**Figure 7.6** Absorption characteristics of haemoglobin. Reproduced with permission from Elsevier. Jayaprakash J. Patil, Dedan G. Maloney, *Anaesthesia and Intensive Care Medicine*, November 2014.

The trace and reading may be affected by a number of factors. All of the factors mentioned above are possible, but the list is by no means exclusive. Both nail varnish as well as henna pigmentation can cause a clear trace but poor reading, therefore vigilance is required. Movement can affect the trace – a common artefact encountered in recovery includes shivering. Normal light conditions should not affect the accuracy of the reading. However, bright sunlight or close proximity to theatre lights can have a significant effect. Cold-induced vasoconstriction, hypovolaemia and venous engorgement increase the response time. Atrial fibrillation may also cause measurement errors.

Some components within pulsatile blood may affect the measured reading. Pulse oximetry fails to detect the presence of carbon monoxide – it overestimates oxyhaemoglobin and therefore the saturations will be falsely high. Readings should be interpreted with caution in heavy smokers.

## Further reading

Patil J. J., Maloney D. G. Measurement of pulse oximetry, capnography and pH. *Anaesth Intensive Care Med* 2014; 15(11): 522–5.

## Physics and clinical measurement: breathing circuits

You have induced anaesthesia in an 80 kg man for knee arthroscopy.

**Which one of the following statements regarding ventilation is incorrect?**

a) Using a Lack circuit, a fresh gas flow (FGF) of at least 15 l/min will be required for IPPV to prevent rebreathing of carbon dioxide

b) Using a Bain circuit, an FGF of 6 l/min will be inadequate to prevent rebreathing during IPPV
c) Using a Mapleson D circuit, an FGF of at least 12 l/min will be needed to prevent rebreathing during spontaneous ventilation
d) Using a Mapleson A circuit, an FGF of 6 l/min will be adequate to prevent rebreathing during spontaneous ventilation
e) The patient's estimated minute ventilation (MV) is less than 10 l/min at rest

Answer: b)

With the advent of circle systems and increasingly complex anaesthetic machines, the older breathing systems are seen less and less. However, they are still present, especially in anaesthetic rooms and it is worth a quick recap of their characteristics to remind you how to use them.

Breathing systems can be classified as open, semi-open and semi-closed or closed. Mapleson systems used today are in the semi-open category. Semi-closed and closed use a carbon dioxide absorber, allowing gases to recirculate; they include the circle system. Mapleson systems are illustrated in Figure 7.7.

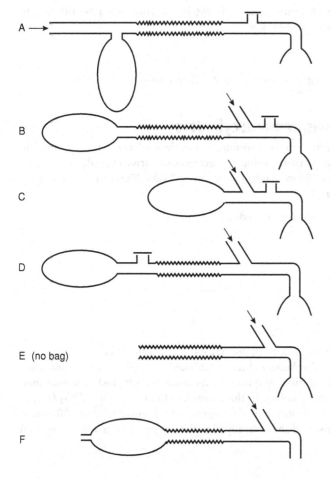

**Figure 7.7** The Mapleson classification. Reproduced with permission from Adrian Cox, 'Introduction to breathing circuits', *Anaesthesia UK*, 2009.

A

B

C

D

E (no bag)

F

**Table 7.3** Mapleson circuits and gas flow

| Mapleson | Systems | FGF for SV (if 80 kg) | FGF for IPPV |
|---|---|---|---|
| A – used for SV | Magill; Lack | 70–100 ml/kg/min (5.6–8 l/min) | Minimum 3 × MV |
| B – not in use today | | | |
| C – used for hand ventilation and resuscitation | | | Min 15 l/min |
| D – used for SV and IPPV | Bain | 150–200 ml/kg/min (12–16 l/min) | 70–100 ml/kg/min (5.6–8 l/min) |
| E – very uncommon today | Ayres T piece | | |
| F – used in paediatrics < 20 kg | Jackson Rees | 2–3 × MV; minimum 4 l/min | |

Lack is a type of Mapleson A circuit, which is typically efficient for spontaneous venti-lation but relatively inefficient for IPPV. The reverse is true of Mapleson D or Bain circuits. Table 7.3 below shows the gas flows required to prevent rebreathing.

To calculate minute ventilation (MV) we need to know the tidal volume (TV) and breaths/min. Tidal volume can be estimated using the formula TV = 10 ml/kg. This is proba-bly an overestimation, and typically a TV of around 500 ml is used to simplify most equations to represent a standard adult patient. But if we stick with the formula here, a TV of 800 ml (10 ml × 80 kg) multiplied by 12 breaths/min = MV 9.6 l/min. Therefore, it is fairly safe to say that this patient's MV is less than 10 l/min.

## Further reading

Anaesthesia UK Introduction to breathing circuits. 2009. Available at www.frca.co.uk/article.aspx? articleid=100136 (accessed 8 April 2015).

## Physics and clinical measurement: cylinders

A patient needs to be transferred from your hospital to a tertiary referral centre for ongoing treatment. He is intubated and ventilated using an electronically driven ventilator. It is cur-rently set with a tidal volume of 500 ml, a respiratory rate of 20 and $FiO_2$ of 1.0. The journey will take approximately 1 hour.

**What is the minimum amount of oxygen needed for transfer?**

a) 600 litres
b) 2400 litres
c) 300 litres
d) 1200 litres
e) 1000 litres

Answer: d)

Oxygen requirement for transfer is an important issue. It is calculated by working out the minute ventilation (MV; tidal volume, in litres, multiplied by respiratory rate) and mul-tiplying that by the $FiO_2$ (as a fraction) and transfer duration (in minutes). It should then be doubled to allow for unexpected delays. In this example: MV (0.5 × 20) × $FiO_2$ (1.0) × minutes (60) × 2 = 1200 l. The publication of *Comprehensive Critical Care* in 2000 made planning for interhospital transfer of the critically ill patient mandatory at a local, regional

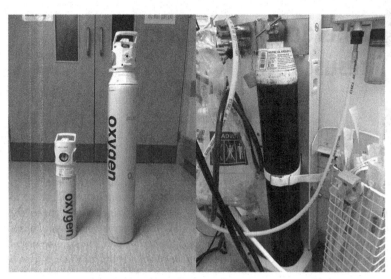

**Figure 7.8** Photograph of cylinders. Common cylinders in use: size CD, 460 l transport cylinder (far left); size HX, 2300 l large transport cylinder for trolley (middle); Size E, 680 l cylinder with standard valve (Pin index) attached to reverse of anaesthetic machine (far right).

and national level. Hospitals should have designated transport teams consisting of identifiable, appropriately trained staff, with appropriate equipment and resources. They should use the same protocols and meet the same standards as other transport teams within the Critical Care Network.

Preparation for transfer is of paramount importance. Equipment should be thoroughly checked and careful consideration given to the amount of drugs and oxygen that will be needed during transfer. A redundancy element must be factored into the calculation to account for delays in transfer such as traffic jams or breakdown.

Oxygen requirements are calculated as described above. The doubling of patient requirements, or carrying at least a 1-hour supply for short journeys, is recommended to allow for unexpected delays. If the ventilator is gas-driven this must also be factored into the calculation (the amount used per minute as a driving gas can be found in the ventilator manual, but it is frequently approximately 1 l/min).

Standard UK oxygen cylinders come in various sizes. D size contain 340 l, CD 460 l, E size 680 l and F size 1360 l. Ambulances commonly carry two F size cylinders connected to a Schrader outlet connection mounted on the wall. They may also carry a number of D size cylinders. It is imperative to establish how much oxygen the ambulance is carrying and check that connections are compatible with the ventilator.

## Further reading

Association of Anaesthetists of Great Britain and Ireland (AAGBI). AAGBI Safety Guideline: Interhospital Transfer. London: AAGBI, 2009.
Intensive Care Society (ICS). Guidelines for the transport of the critically ill adult. London: ICS, 2002.

Chapter

# 8 Emergency management and resuscitation

*As anaesthetists, we are trained to lead and guide resuscitation attempts and to become experts at dealing with the unexpected. Thankfully emergencies are not encountered regularly, so to manage them effectively we need to regularly refresh our knowledge. This chapter covers the recognition and management of the most commonly occurring emergency conditions and problems in anaesthesia, from anaphylaxis to paediatric resuscitation. It also includes some useful further reading options, with links to essential guidelines to help you prepare for when you need to act quickly.*

## Anaphylaxis

You are asked to anaesthetize a 56-year-old woman for a laparoscopic cholecystectomy. She is hypertensive, taking ramipril, and has mild asthma. There is no history of drug allergy, and she has undergone general anaesthesia previously without problems.

You pre-oxygenate, and then induce anaesthesia with fentanyl 100 mcg, propofol 180 mg, and atracurium 40 mg. Shortly after securing her airway with an oral endotracheal tube you administer co-amoxiclav 1.2 g.

Two minutes later the patient becomes blotchy and pale, and the NIBP machine does not read. The radial pulse is impalpable, and the ECG demonstrates a sinus tachycardia of 155 bpm. Simultaneously, the ventilator alarm signals high airway pressures, and you find she is difficult to hand ventilate. The pulse oximeter is no longer reading. The chest is quiet, with no obvious wheeze.

You suspect anaphylaxis, and in an attempt to immediately improve venous return to the heart, you raise her legs in the air. You administer 50 mcg aliquots of adrenaline to a total of 800 mcg, and a litre of crystalloid through a peripheral cannula.

Consider the following questions before turning to the discussion below:

1. **What is the differential diagnosis?**
2. **What further clinical management does she require?**
3. **Would you continue with the case?**
4. **What blood tests and follow-up will she require? Whose responsibility is this to organize?**

1. **Differential diagnoses include:**

   - Exaggerated physiological response to induction, in a hypertensive patient taking an ACE inhibitor

*Returning to Work in Anaesthesia*, ed. Emma Plunkett, Emily Johnson and Anna Pierson.
Published by Cambridge University Press. © Cambridge University Press 2016.

- Myocardial ischaemia
- Bronchospasm following airway manipulation in an asthmatic patient, with subsequent cardiovascular compromise from high intrathoracic pressures
- Equipment failure

2. **A standard ABC approach is needed.**

- Call for help!
- The **early use of adrenaline** is critical. Adrenaline stabilizes mast cells, in addition to its positive inotropy, vasopressor, and bronchodilator effects. An infusion may be required for ongoing maintenance of blood pressure.
- Hydrocortisone 200 mg and chlorphenamine 10 mg are required, to help reduce the severity and duration of the reaction.

3. **Would you continue with the case?**

An elective case such as this should be postponed. For emergency work, the risks of postponing surgery must be weighed against the risk of continuing in the face of suspected anaphylaxis to an unknown agent.

4. **What blood tests and follow-up will she require?**

Serial mast cell tryptase measurements are required, looking for a peak rise. It is the anaesthetist's responsibility to arrange follow-up.

The term 'anaphylaxis' describes the signs and symptoms resulting from widespread mast cell degranulation and histamine release. Degranulation can occur due to cross linking of specific IgE antibodies, or to non-specific, direct degranulation. The former is known as allergic anaphylaxis, the latter as non-allergic anaphylaxis (previously called 'anaphylactoid'). The two cannot reliably be distinguished on clinical grounds alone. However, it is imperative for patient safety to establish the exact cause, in case a specific drug needs to be avoided in future by the patient.

Signs and symptoms of anaphylaxis include:

- Major, unexplained hypotension
- Tachycardia or bradycardia (the latter a more worrying feature associated with severe cases)
- Major, unexplained respiratory compromise
- Angioedema
- Urticaria
- Widespread rash
- Severe itch.

Patients suffering **any** of these require referral to a specialist clinic for follow-up investigation. The referral paperwork is on the Association of Anaesthetists of Great Britain and Ireland (AAGBI) website. Serial mast cell tryptase levels should be taken **immediately**, at **1–2 hours**, and at **24 hours**. 'Peak' levels are at 1–2 hours, but may still be high at up to 6 hours from the event so can be taken up to this point. The 24-hour sample confirms a normal baseline tryptase; persistently raised levels may indicate the presence of a mastocytosis.

Neuromuscular blocking agents remain the most frequent cause of anaphylaxis, followed by antibiotics. However chlorhexidine, ubiquitous both in and out of theatres, has recently emerged as a frequent cause of anaphylaxis and often causes delayed and severe reactions.

Quoted incidence of proven anaphylaxis ranges from 1:1300 to 1:10 000, but incidence of adverse events meeting the AAGBI criteria for referral may be significantly higher. Under-reporting may reflect uncertainty about the referral pathway and blood tests required. To aid the anaesthetist, many hospitals have now developed 'Suspected Anaesthetic Allergy Follow-Up Packs', containing referral paperwork, blood bottles and template letters for the GP and patient. In areas where such packs have been introduced, the number and quality of referrals has increased, improving the likelihood of making a conclusive diagnosis at clinic.

## Further reading

Association of Anaesthetists of Great Britain and Ireland. Management of a Patient with Suspected Anaphylaxis during Anaesthesia Safety Drill. 2009. Available at http://www.aagbi.org/sites/default/files/ana_web_laminate_final.pdf (accessed 18 March 2015).

Association of Anaesthetists of Great Britain and Ireland. Allergies referral form. Available at http://www.aagbi.org/safety/allergies-and-anaphylaxis (accessed 18 March 2015).

Savic L., Garside M., Savic S., Hopkins P. M. Anaphylaxis follow up – making it simple, making it better. *Royal College of Anaesthetists Bulletin* 2014; 87: 33–4.

Savic L., Wood P. M., Savic S. Anaphylaxis associated with general anaesthesia: challenges and recent advances. *Trends Anaesth Crit Care* 2012; 2: 258–63.

# Management of can't intubate can't ventilate

A 20-year-old female is being anaesthetized for an appendicectomy. She is known to suffer from suxamethonium apnoea and so rapid sequence induction was performed using rocuronium 1.2 mg/kg. Her airway had not been predicted to be difficult; however, you are unable to intubate or ventilate her. You have tried an alternative blade, bougie and external laryngeal manipulation. The patient is becoming increasingly hypoxaemic.

**What would be the next most appropriate step in managing this patient?**

a) Perform an emergency needle cricothyroidotomy
b) Administer sugammadex in a dose of 16 mg/kg
c) Attempt intubation using a fibre-optic laryngoscope
d) Insert an oral airway and attempt facemask ventilation with 100% oxygen
e) Reduce cricoid pressure and reattempt intubation

Answer: d)

In this scenario the urgency of surgery is not immediate and the patient should be woken up.

This is an airway emergency as the patient is becoming increasingly hypoxaemic. The priority is to oxygenate the patient. This has already failed using facemask ventilation alone and so the next most appropriate step is to use an oral airway and attempt ventilation with 100% oxygen. If this fails the next step is to attempt insertion of a laryngeal mask airway and ventilate with 100% oxygen. If this fails a surgical cricothyroidotomy will be necessary to allow oxygenation of the patient. Fibre-optic intubation does not have a role in the scenario where a patient is becoming rapidly hypoxaemic.

Sugammadex is a selective relaxant binding agent which is given in a dose of 16 mg/kg to reverse the effects of a 1.2 mg/kg dose of rocuronium. A median time of 1.5 minutes to recovery of the T4/T1 ratio to 0.9 is expected. Sugammadex can be administered; however, the priority here is to oxygenate the patient first.

For further details regarding the management of the difficult airway, see Section 3, Chapter 33.

## Further reading

Difficult Airway Society guidelines flowchart 2015. Available at http://www.das.uk.com/guidelines/das_intubation_guidelines (accessed 9 January 2016).

## Adaptation to basic life support in special circumstances

1. You receive a cardiac arrest call for the antenatal ward in the maternity unit. As you make your way there, you consider the following questions:

   a) **What are the adaptations to standard basic life support needed in a pregnant patient?**
   b) **What are the possible causes of cardiac arrest specific to pregnancy?**

The basic principles of basic and advanced life support are the same in a pregnant as a non-pregnant patient. Some additional points to remember:

- Summon expert help immediately – senior obstetrician and, if fetus viable, neonatologist. Also request the anaesthetic consultant on call attends.
- Aortocaval compression. If more than 20 weeks' gestation then the pregnant uterus presses on the aorta and inferior vena cava, which can impede venous return to the heart, reducing cardiac output and, ultimately, uterine perfusion. It is essential to displace the uterus to the left to reduce aortocaval compression. If the patient is not on an operating table (i.e. a tilting table,) then the most effective way to do this is to manually displace the uterus.
- Effective chest compressions are key to successful resuscitation; therefore, it is important that the patient is supported on a firm surface, e.g. a spinal board or operating table. Using soft pillows to tilt the patient is no longer acceptable (see point above regarding manual displacement of the uterus).
- Increased risk of aspiration; consider early intubation.
- If there is no return of spontaneous circulation within 4 minutes then the obstetrician should perform a perimortem section to deliver the baby by 5 minutes. This can take place anywhere and requires only a scalpel. The patient should be transferred to theatre following return of spontaneous circulation for completion of surgery.

Causes of cardiac arrest to consider in a pregnant patient include:

- Pulmonary embolism
- Sepsis
- Hypertensive disorders of pregnancy
- Haemorrhage
- Placental abruption
- Amniotic fluid embolism
- Cardiac disease

2. A 5-year-old boy collapses on the ward where you are seeing a patient for a preoperative check.

**How would you initially assess and manage this situation?**

- Shout for **help**. Try and get a quick history from the nursing staff/relatives.
- **Confirm cardiac arrest.** Check for breathing, pulse and signs of life. Pulse palpation can be difficult in children, so if there is no breathing/signs of life after 10 seconds begin resuscitation. Ask a nurse to put out a cardiac arrest call.
- Open the airway with head tilt, chin lift and **give five rescue breaths.** In children the cause of cardiac arrest is more commonly respiratory in origin rather than cardiac, so effective breaths are vital.
- **Begin cardiac compressions** and use a rate of 15 compressions to 2 breaths. Cardiac compressions should be given at a rate of 100–120 compressions a minute. Compress the lower half of the sternum one finger breadth above the xiphisternum using 1–2 hands depending on the size of the child and the size of your hands. Aim to depress the chest by one-third.
- If no one responds to your initial shout for help, perform **one minute of CPR** before leaving the patient to get help. However, if the arrest is sudden and witnessed the cause may be cardiac and help should be summoned before any resuscitation.

## Further reading

Resuscitation council (UK). Resuscitation guidelines 2015. Available at https://www.resus.org.uk/resuscitation-guidelines/adult-advanced-life-support/#algorithm (accessed 9 January 2016).

# Advanced life support: adult resuscitation

A 73-year-old man experienced a witnessed cardiac arrest on the day of his admission to hospital with chest pain. An ECG performed prior to collapse did not show ST elevation. Successful return of spontaneous circulation was achieved following two attempts at defibrillation, but the patient remained comatose. No drugs were administered during the cardiac arrest.

**Which one of the following statements best describes a principle of his post-resuscitation care?**

a)  Intensive glycaemic control should aim to achieve a blood glucose concentration of 4.5–6.0 mmol/l
b)  Hyperoxaemia should be avoided as it is associated with worse outcomes than mild hypoxaemia
c)  Evidence supports maintaining an arterial partial pressure of carbon dioxide ($PaCO_2$) at the higher end of the normal range
d)  Because ST elevation was not demonstrated on the ECG pre-collapse, coronary angiography is not indicated
e)  As seizures are common in cardiac arrest patients who remain comatose, seizures should be prevented with prophylactic anticonvulsant drugs

Answer: b)

Post-cardiac-arrest syndrome comprises brain injury, myocardial dysfunction, the systemic ischaemia/reperfusion response and the persistence of precipitating pathology. As a result, post-resuscitation care is understandably complex. Hypoxaemia can lead to subsequent cardiac arrest and contribute to secondary brain injury. Studies have also shown that hyperoxaemia is detrimental and, in fact, associated with a worse outcome than mild hypoxaemia. Therefore, arterial blood gas analysis should be monitored as soon as possible to maintain a normal concentration of arterial oxygen and inspired oxygen titrated to achieve $SpO_2$ of 94–98%.

Hypercarbia is also associated with further cardiac arrest and secondary brain injury. There are no data to suggest targeting a specific $PaCO_2$, but the Resuscitation Council (UK) recommends aiming for normocarbia.

Up to 40% of patients who remain comatose post-cardiac arrest will experience seizures or myoclonus. Despite this, prophylactic anticonvulsants are not recommended. Seizures should be treated expediently to minimize the effect of an increase in cerebral metabolism. Appropriate treatment options include benzodiazepines, phenytoin, sodium valproate, propofol or a barbiturate.

A strong association exists between blood glucose control post-resuscitation and neurological outcome. Current recommendations outline a target blood glucose concentration of ≤10 mmol/l. Intensive glycaemic control (4.5–6.0 mmol/l) is not recommended, as studies have shown a significantly increased risk of hypoglycaemia. Severe hypoglycaemia is associated with increased mortality in the critically ill.

Studies have shown an improvement in neurological outcome with mild therapeutic hypothermia in comatose survivors of out-of-hospital arrest caused by ventricular fibrillation. This is attributed to a reduction in the cerebral metabolic rate in response to cooling. Although there are no randomized trials studying therapeutic hypothermia in other cardiac arrests, it may be considered a reasonable management option for both in- and out-of-hospital arrests due to shockable and non-shockable rhythms.

Coronary angiography should be considered in all post-cardiac-arrest patients whose suspected primary pathology is coronary artery disease. In this patient population the incidence of atherosclerotic disease amenable to treatment is high even without the presence of ST elevation.

## Further reading

Bouch D. C., Thompson J. P., Damian M. S. Editorial I: Post-cardiac arrest management: more than global cooling? *Br J Anaesth* 2008; 100(5): 591–4.

## Advanced life support: paediatric resuscitation

As part of the resuscitation team, you are called to the cardiac arrest of a 7-year-old child with cystic fibrosis.

**Which of the following statements is most correct regarding the likely arrhythmia?**

a) The most likely associated rhythm is either asystole or pulseless electrical activity (PEA)
b) The most likely associated rhythm is ventricular fibrillation
c) The most likely associated rhythm is Torsades de pointes
d) The most likely associated rhythm is ventricular tachycardia (VT)
e) The most likely associated rhythm is a supraventricular tachycardia (SVT)

Answer: a)

The most common rhythm observed at a paediatric cardiac arrest is either asystole or PEA. In this setting, CPR is performed by providing five initial rescue breaths followed by chest compression at a rate of 100–120 per minute and ventilation in a ratio of 15:2. Intravenous or intraosseous access should be established and adrenaline 10 mcg/kg is administered every 3–5 minutes. Reversible causes should be considered. There is no role for giving atropine in this setting. Please refer to the paediatric advanced life support algorithm in Section 3.

Recent studies have failed to show any increase in the risk of complications associated with cuffed tracheal tubes compared to uncuffed. In fact, the use of cuffed tubes increases the chance of selecting the correct size tube at the first attempt. Capnography is strongly encouraged to confirm tube placement and optimize ventilation after return of spontaneous circulation. Once intubated the child should have uninterrupted compressions and be ventilated at a rate of 10–12 breaths/min.

In the post-resuscitation period, the child should be assessed using the ABC approach. Oxygen delivered should be closely monitored to reduce the risk of hyperoxaemia. Temperature control should involve cooling in the presence of hyperthermia, as this is associated with a poorer outcome. A period of mild therapeutic hypothermia may be considered, although trials to assess the mortality benefits of therapeutic hypothermia after cardiac arrest in children are ongoing. As in adults, blood glucose should be controlled carefully to minimize the risks of both hyper and hypoglycaemia.

Many parents may wish to be present during a resuscitation attempt. Studies have shown that bereaved parents who were present in the resuscitation room experience less anxiety and depression several months after the death of their child. However, it is the team leader, not the parents, who decides when it is appropriate to stop resuscitation efforts.

## Further reading

Resuscitation Council (UK). Paediatric advanced life support. Resuscitation Guidelines 2010. Available at www.resus.org.uk/pages/guide.htm (accessed 17 April 2015).

## Advanced life support: tachyarrhythmias

An 82-year-old lady attends for day case fluoroscopy-guided facet joint injections under local anaesthesia. She has had hypertension for 20 years and atrial fibrillation (AF) for the past 8 years. She takes ramipril 5 mg for blood pressure (BP) control. On admission, her heart rate (HR) is recorded as 92 bpm and BP is 132/87 mmHg. In the operating theatre, her HR is found to be irregular with a rate of 140–155 bpm, BP is 140/91 mmHg and $SpO_2$ 95% on air. She describes having increased palpitations with slight shortness of breath on climbing stairs for the last 4 days. An ECG confirms fast AF.

**What is the appropriate management of this patient?**

a) Administer a small dose of midazolam and wait to see if HR decreases, then proceed with the procedure only if HR decreases

b) Consider electrical cardioversion in theatre under sedation

c) Control the rate with intravenous beta blocker and if stable, proceed with the injections and refer her to the cardiologist

d) Cancel the procedure. Transfer the patient to a monitored area and give a loading dose of digoxin

e) Cancel the procedure, commence an infusion of intravenous amiodarone 300 mg over one hour and transfer to CCU/ICU

Answer: d)

In people over 75 years old, the incidence of AF is greater than 15%, with rate control being the primary aim of treatment. From her retrospective history it was evident that the patient had been in fast AF for a few days. She did not have any symptoms suggestive of shock, syncope or myocardial ischaemia but slight dyspnoea suggests a degree of heart failure without haemodynamic instability. Sedation is unlikely to help, as the onset of AF almost certainly occurred more than 24 hours ago. Facet joint injections are elective procedures with the intention of providing analgesia, and therefore can be postponed if the patient's condition is suboptimal. Although this lady was assessed on admission, her tachycardia was undetected. A pulse rate check and/or ECG would be needed to diagnose her AF.

Regarding the management of fast AF, electrical cardioversion is indicated in patients with life-threatening haemodynamic instability. This lady is most likely to have long-standing AF without haemodynamic instability or anticoagulation, hence electrical cardioversion is not indicated.

Rate control should be offered as the first-line strategy to people with AF, *except* in those whose AF has a reversible cause, who have heart failure primarily due to AF, those with new onset AF and for whom a rhythm control strategy would be more suitable based on clinical judgement. Standard beta blockers (i.e. not sotalol) or a rate-limiting calcium-channel blocker should be offered as initial monotherapy. Digoxin is considered for patients with non-paroxysmal AF leading a sedentary lifestyle, and may be preferable if there is evidence of heart failure. If there is failure of symptom control on monotherapy, a combination of any two of the above is advised. Amiodarone is unsuitable for long-term rate control.

Rhythm control is most suitable for people with AF whose symptoms continue despite rate control or when a rate-control strategy has failed. Seek advice from a cardiologist; the patient should be managed on CCU/HDU.

## Further reading

www.nice.org.uk/guidance/cg180 (accessed 9 January 2016).
https://www.resus.org.uk/pages/tachalgo.pdf (accessed 26 May 15).

## Peri-operative emergencies: bronchospasm

A 29-year-old woman presents for open reduction and internal fixation of a fractured radius. Soon after induction of anaesthesia and tracheal intubation she becomes difficult to ventilate. She is a known smoker and has recently had an upper respiratory tract infection.

a) **What is your differential diagnosis?**
After checking the equipment, no problem is detected. On examination, there is widespread, bilateral wheeze throughout the chest.

b) **How would you manage this patient?**
The history and examination suggest bronchospasm to be the most likely cause.
- ABC approach
- Call for help

- Oxygen 100%
- Remove any causative agents (drugs, check endotracheal tube position, secretions)
- Avoid histamine releasing agents (e.g. atracurium)
- Maintain adequate anaesthesia preferably with a bronchodilating agent (sevoflurane or isoflurane)
- Hand ventilate to assess compliance
- Allow sufficient time for expiration.

The management of anaphylaxis has been discussed above and is also covered in Chapter 25. If it is more likely that increased airway reactivity is the cause, current British Thoracic Society guidelines for the management of acute asthma suggest:

- Inhaled beta-2 agonist if possible (salbutamol or terbutaline)
- Consider steroid
- Add inhaled ipratropium
- IV 1.2–2 g magnesium sulphate
- Consider IV aminophylline.

Other treatments that may help if conventional treatment fails include ketamine, IV adrenaline and heliox (no evidence for use in acute asthma).

**Table 8.1** Differential diagnosis of difficulty ventilating under anaesthesia

| Equipment problems | Patient problems |
|---|---|
| • Circuit blockage<br>• Endotracheal tube too narrow<br>• Misplaced endotracheal tube:<br>  • oesophageal intubation<br>  • endobronchial intubation<br>• Inappropriate ventilator settings | • Foreign body, including aspiration of gastric contents and mucous plug<br>• Bronchospasm:<br>  • anaphylaxis<br>  • hyperreactive airways<br>  • endotracheal tube irritating the carina<br>• Pulmonary oedema<br>• Tension pneumothorax<br>• Gastric insufflation<br>• Insufficient depth of anaesthesia or muscle relaxation |

# Further reading

Association of Anaesthetists of Great Britain and Ireland. Management of a Patient with Suspected Anaphylaxis during Anaesthesia Safety Drill. 2009. Available at http://www.aagbi.org/sites/default/files/ana_laminate_2009.pdf (accessed 2 January 2016).

British Thoracic Society/Scottish Intercollegiate Guidelines Network. British guideline on the management of asthma. A national clinical guideline. 2014. Available at https://www.brit-thoracic.org.uk/document-library/clinical-information/asthma/btssign-guideline-on-the-management-of-asthma/ (accessed 2 January 2016).

Hemmingsen C., Nielsen P. K., Odorico J. Ketamine in the treatment of bronchospasm during mechanical ventilation. *Am J Emerg Med* 1994; 12(4): 417–20.

Linck S. L. The use of heliox for perioperative bronchospasm: a case report. *AANA J* 2007; 75(3): 189–92.

Rooke G. A., Choi J. H., Bishop M. J. The effect of isoflurane, halothane, sevoflurane and thiopental/nitrous oxide on respiratory system resistance after tracheal intubation. *Anesthesiology* 1997; 86(6): 1294–9.

Woods B. D., Sladen R. N. Perioperative considerations for the patient with asthma and bronchospasm. *Br J Anaesth* 2009; 103: i57–65.

# Perioperative emergencies: equipment failure

You are anaesthetizing a patient for foot correction surgery and maintaining anaesthesia with an oxygen, air and desflurane mix, with the patient breathing spontaneously through a laryngeal mask airway (LMA). Midway through the operation there is a sudden loss of power supply. The back-up batteries to the ventilator and monitoring are working.

**What is the best course of action?**

a) Allow the patient to continue to breathe spontaneously with an oxygen, air and desflurane mix

b) Hand-ventilate the patient and maintain anaesthesia with an oxygen, air and desflurane mix

c) Allow the patient to continue to breathe spontaneously with an oxygen, air and isoflurane mix

d) Hand-ventilate the patient with 100% oxygen via a Mapleson C circuit and wake the patient up

e) Allow the patient to continue to breathe spontaneously with an oxygen and air mix, but maintain anaesthesia with a total intravenous anaesthetic (TIVA) technique

Answer: c)

Prolonged and continued power failure is a rare event mid-operation owing to back-up generators within most hospitals. However, it is important to have a grasp of how to deal with such an event should it occur.

It is important to understand which pieces of equipment have back-up batteries to provide emergency power. Although this may vary worldwide, it is common that the ventilator, monitoring equipment and pumps delivering TIVA all have back-up battery supplies. One piece of equipment which does have an internal battery, but which does not supply emergency power in a power failure, is the desflurane vaporizer. This internal battery is solely for its alarm. Therefore, if anaesthesia is being maintained with desflurane during a power failure, an alternative method of maintenance should be sought. This could be an alternative vapour or switching to a TIVA technique.

Concerning switching to a TIVA technique in this case, there are two main problems that are likely to arise, meaning it may not be the best option. Firstly, setting up the TIVA would take some time (locating pumps and drawing up the drugs) meaning that an alternative method of anaesthesia would be needed while this was being done. Secondly, breathing spontaneously using a TIVA technique can be challenging because of the potent opioids used, resulting in apnoea/hypopnoea and therefore manual ventilation would be required.

With regard to maintaining anaesthesia with an alternative vapour, in this case this is the best option, as the patient can continue to breathe spontaneously while anaesthesia is maintained. The choice of which alternative vapour is chosen is likely to be dictated by which vaporizer is present on the back bar at the time of the failure – isoflurane in this case.

## Further reading

Carpenter T., Robinson S. T. Case reports: response to a partial power failure in the operating room. *Anesth Analg* 2010; 110: 1644–6.

Miles L. F., Scheinkestel C. D., Downey G. O. Environmental emergencies in theatre and critical care areas: power failure, fire, and explosion. *Contin Educ Anaesth Crit Care Pain* 2015; 15(2): 78–83.

# Perioperative emergencies: laryngospasm

An 8-year-old asthmatic boy is undergoing surgery for the initial management of 8% lower limb flame burns that occurred 3 hours ago. He is breathing spontaneously (isoflurane/oxygen/air) via a size 2.5 laryngeal mask airway (LMA) when he suddenly becomes apnoeic and desaturates as the surgeon begins debridement of the burn. Ventilation is possible but extremely difficult because of high airway pressures. You instruct the surgeon to stop operating and switch to 100% high-flow oxygen.

**What is the most appropriate next step in the ongoing anaesthetic management?**

a) Deepen anaesthesia with isoflurane
b) Switch to sevoflurane to deepen anaesthesia
c) Deepen anaesthesia with isoflurane and a bolus of fentanyl (1 mcg/kg)
d) Deepen anaesthesia with a propofol bolus (0.5–1 mg/kg)
e) Administer a dose of suxamethonium (2 mg/kg)

Answer: d)

Laryngospasm is glottic closure due to reflex constriction of laryngeal muscles and a common cause of airway obstruction during anaesthesia. It is more common in paediatric practice, with incidences two times greater in older children and three times greater in younger children compared to adults. Other risk factors include upper respiratory tract infections, obstructive lung disease, passive smoke exposure and management by less experienced anaesthetists. It results either from failure to obtund laryngeal reflexes because of inadequate depth of anaesthesia, or from increased direct or external stimuli.

Laryngospasm is often categorized as either partial or complete. In partial laryngospasm the vocal cords are adducted but there is some movement of gas through the posterior commissure: stridor is present but some movement of gas is possible. In complete laryngospasm both true and false vocal cords are opposed and other laryngeal structures oppose to effectively close the laryngeal inlet: ventilation is impossible, and no movement of gas occurs. The distinction between partial and complete laryngeal spasm is an important one, as it guides immediate management. Initial management requires application of 100% oxygen and continuous positive airway pressure (CPAP) with assessment of ventilation. If partial laryngospasm is present then there is likely to be some oxygen transfer and an improvement in saturations. Here, it may be possible to deepen anaesthesia by using an inhalational agent, as there is some gas transfer. As sevoflurane is the least irritant to the airways, this would be the agent of choice. If laryngospasm is near-complete or complete then there will be little or no gas flow.

In this scenario, the patient is bordering on complete obstruction, as very high pressures are required to get any air flow. Subsequent stepwise management is to deepen anaesthesia with propofol (0.5–1 mg/kg) and then give intravenous suxamethonium (1–2 mg/kg) or intramuscular (4 mg/kg) if there is no IV access. Suxamethonium should not be used once 24 hours has passed from the time of the initial burn. Special manoeuvres include pressure in the laryngospasm notch (between mastoid process and mandible).

Effectively deepening anaesthesia with inhalational agents requires unobstructed gas flow, and short-onset opioids such as alfentanil can be used. Fentanyl may be too long in onset and result in a worsening of apnoea.

## Further reading

Gavel G., Walker R. W. M. Laryngospasm in anaesthesia. *Contin Educ Anaesth Crit Care Pain* 2014; 14(2): 47–51.

## Perioperative emergencies: malignant hyperthermia management

You have anaesthetized a slim 30-year-old for a knee arthroscopy. Anaesthesia is maintained with an oxygen, air and sevoflurane mix. Volume-controlled ventilation is delivering a minute volume of 10 l/min. Just before transfer into theatre, you notice the end-tidal $CO_2$ ($EtCO_2$) is 12 kPa and heart rate is 130 bpm.

**What is the best course of action?**

a) Proceed to theatre as planned, increase the minute ventilation and maintain anaesthesia with sevoflurane

b) Proceed to theatre as planned, increase the minute ventilation and maintain anaesthesia with a propofol infusion

c) Remain in the anaesthetic room, increase the minute ventilation and maintain anaesthesia with sevoflurane

d) Remain in the anaesthetic room, use a Mapleson C circuit and ancillary oxygen to increase the minute ventilation and wake the patient up

e) Remain in the anaesthetic room, use a Mapleson C circuit and ancillary oxygen to increase the minute ventilation and maintain anaesthesia with a propofol infusion

Answer: e)

Until proven otherwise, this patient is developing a malignant hyperthermia (MH) crisis. He has an unexplained high $EtCO_2$ and tachycardia. His high $EtCO_2$ cannot be explained by under-ventilation as his minute volume should be sufficient and his tachycardia cannot be explained by surgery or pain as you are still in the anaesthetic room. Initial treatment of MH is to stop all triggering agents (sevoflurane here), call for help, maintain anaesthesia with an intravenous agent and hyperventilate the patient using a clean breathing system and 100% oxygen. If the patient were already in theatre, surgery should be abandoned or finished as soon as possible with any further muscle relaxation that may be necessary provided using a non-depolarizing neuromuscular blocking drug.

MH is a rare autosomal dominant condition (1 in 5000–200 000) that results from a defect in the ryanodine–dihydropyridine receptor complex found in striated muscle. The receptor is responsible for control of calcium movement in and out of the sarcoplasmic reticulum, which is lost in MH.

MH develops following exposure to triggering agents, these being volatile anaesthetic agents and suxamethonium. Importantly, MH may occur in patients who have previously had an uneventful general anaesthetic and may not present immediately. Reactions have been reported up to 11 hours post-operatively. MH should be suspected in cases where there are unexplained rises in $EtCO_2$, heart rate or oxygen requirement. Of note, a rise in temperature is often a late sign and a diagnosis of MH should not be ruled out if this is not present. Early recognition and prompt treatment is key (see Section 3, Chapter 25).

The third phase of managing a MH crisis is treating the consequences of the condition, which entails giving dantrolene 2.5 mg/kg bolus (repeating 1 mg/kg boluses up to 10 mg/kg), initiating cooling but avoiding vasoconstriction and checking creatinine kinase levels. Hyperkalaemia, arrhythmias, metabolic acidosis, myoglobinaemia and disseminated intravascular coagulation should be monitored for and treated if present. Finally, the patient should be transferred to the ICU once stabilized, where monitoring and treatment can be continued and subsequent referral to the MH unit made.

## Further reading

Association of Anaesthetists of Great Britain and Ireland. Safety Guideline: Malignant Hyperthermia Crisis. 2011. Available at http://www.aagbi.org/sites/default/files/MH%20guideline%20for%20web%20v2.pdf (accessed 2 January 2016).

**Chapter**

**9**

# Airway management

*Airway skills are fundamental to our clinical practice as anaesthetists. This chapter aims to guide you through airway assessment, predicting the difficult airway and how to perform an awake fibre-optic intubation. Management of the obstructed airway is covered in depth, with a helpful table to target your management appropriately.*

## Scoring systems: predicting a difficult airway

You are seeing a patient preoperatively who is scheduled for an elective reversal of an ileostomy. He is starved and has no reflux. His BMI is 23 kg/m$^2$. Whilst assessing his airway you make the following observations: mouth opening 6 cm, Mallampati class 2 view of the pharynx, class A jaw subluxation with a normal jaw, normal head and neck movements, thyromental distance 6.5 cm, sternomental distance 13 cm, presence of two crowns in the upper right 7 and 8 positions but no other dental abnormalities.

**Which one of the following statements would represent your airway assessment findings?**

a) I am concerned that he may be difficult to intubate, so I will plan an awake fibre-optic intubation

b) His airway assessment is not concerning

c) I am concerned that he may be difficult to ventilate, so I will have the difficult airway trolley nearby and another trained assistant

d) I am concerned that he may be difficult to intubate, so I will plan an asleep fibre-optic intubation

e) There is a high chance of a grade 3 or 4 view at laryngoscopy

Answer: b)

The airway assessment details given in the scenario are not associated with either a difficult intubation or ventilation. The crowns, being posterior and to the side, do not represent a great hazard to intubation. His airway assessment is therefore not concerning.

Airway assessment is mandatory before any anaesthetic. The 4th National Audit Project (NAP4) looked at major complications of airway management in the UK, and identified poor airway assessment as a contributing factor in poor airway outcomes. This was due to omission of the assessment, incomplete assessment or failure to alter airway management techniques in response to the assessment.

*Returning to Work in Anaesthesia*, ed. Emma Plunkett, Emily Johnson and Anna Pierson.
Published by Cambridge University Press. © Cambridge University Press 2016.

There is no one best test to perform that will accurately predict the patients in whom either ventilation or intubation will be difficult, and so a variety will need to be done. It should be possible to assess a patient's airway in less than 2 minutes in the majority of cases. Common tests chosen are the ones in the scenario above.

Mouth opening is best performed with the patient sat opposite you; the gap between the teeth should permit the insertion of the patient's middle three fingers (i.e. 4–6 cm). The Mallampati view of the pharynx should be assessed with the tongue protruded without phonation. A class 1 view is one in which the entire uvula may be visualized, and in a class 2 view a portion of the uvula may still be seen, with the fauces. A class 3 view means that the base of the uvula is just visualized and the hard and soft palate are seen, and in a class 4 view (a modification by Samsoon and Young) only the hard palate is seen. Class 3 and 4 views are associated with difficult intubations, but not class 1 and 2.

Jaw subluxation is classed A when the patient's lower jaw can protrude in front of the upper, class B is when they can meet in the middle and class C, when the lower jaw cannot be moved much at all, is the worst. Thyromental distance (Patil distance) is normal when >6 cm, and sternomental distance (Savva distance) is normal when >12.5 cm.

A Wilson's score of zero can be calculated from the information given in the scenario, i.e. low risk of a difficult intubation. (Wilson's score uses a combination of weight, buck teeth, jaw movement, head and neck movement and receding jaw.)

## Further reading
Crawley S. M., Dalton A. J. Predicting the difficult airway. *Contin Educ Anaesth Crit Care Pain* 2014. Available at http://dx.doi.org/10.1093/bjaceaccp/mku047 (accessed 2 January 2016).
4th National Audit Project of the Royal College of Anaesthetists and the Difficult Airway Society. Major complications of airway management in the UK. 2011. Available at http://www.rcoa.ac.uk/NAP4 (accessed 2 January 2016).

# Basic airway management: timing of neuromuscular blockade administration

You are anaesthetizing a 44-year-old lady on a general surgical list for a laparoscopic cholecystectomy. She is obese with a BMI of 38 kg/m$^2$, with no other co-morbidities. She suffers from no reflux symptoms, does not snore and is starved appropriately. Airway assessment: good neck extension, Mallampati score 3, mouth opening and thyromental distance greater than 3 finger widths. You choose to perform tracheal intubation following induction of anaesthesia with propofol. You are not unduly concerned, but have made sure that the difficult airway trolley is available should additional equipment be required. You are deciding on the timing and choice of muscle relaxant.

**The most appropriate choice is:**

1. Induce then check that ventilation is adequate before administering a medium- to long-acting muscle relaxant such as atracurium.
2. Induce then check that ventilation is adequate before administering a medium- to long-acting muscle relaxant such as rocuronium.
3. Induce then check that ventilation is adequate before administering a short-acting muscle relaxant such as suxamethonium. Administer longer-acting muscle relaxant following tracheal intubation.

4. Induce and administer a short and rapidly acting muscle relaxant such as suxamethonium. The relaxant will wear off if ventilation is not adequate.
5. Induce and administer a medium- to long-acting muscle relaxant such as atracurium to facilitate ease of ventilation.
6. Induce and administer a medium- to long-acting muscle relaxant such as rocuronium to facilitate ease of ventilation.

Answers: 2 and 6

If a decision has been made preoperatively that ventilation and/or intubation is likely to be challenging, then elective awake fibre-optic intubation may be the optimum choice. For all other patients, the debate about whether adequacy of ventilation should be assessed prior to administration of muscle relaxant has been argued on both sides, without clear consensus – making either choice reasonable, as long as the decision is well reasoned. It is important to bear in mind however that checking ventilation does not guarantee adequacy of ventilation following muscle relaxation, which tends to be easier, but may be more difficult as pharyngeal structures relax. A suggested plan for 'checkers' and 'non-checkers' is detailed below:

*Checkers:*

It is essential to have a pre-constructed strategy if ventilation is difficult following induction of anaesthesia. One option is to wake the patient up and perform an awake fibre-optic intubation. Research suggests however that most patients will become easier to ventilate following administration of a muscle relaxant, and appears to be the practice of most 'checkers'. In this case, it would be sensible to use a short-acting muscle relaxant, or one which can be readily reversed with sugammadex.

*Non-checkers:*

If any concern exists about possible adequacy of ventilation, conditions should be optimized with careful positioning and the early use of airway adjuncts. The view of 'non-checkers' is that the use of a muscle relaxant is a core part of optimization. As for the 'checkers' technique, choosing a muscle relaxant readily reversible with sugammadex would seem sensible. Suxamethonium would be an alternative, although its adverse event and side effect profile make it a less suitable drug for routine and day case use.

# Advanced airway management: awake fibre-optic intubation

You have been asked to anaesthetize a 70-year-old gentleman who has sustained a fracture to his proximal humerus. He has previously undergone localized radiotherapy for a laryngeal tumour, which has led to remission. He has undergone a previous anaesthetic within the last 6 months, during which he was noted to be difficult to ventilate using a bag and mask, and was Cormack and Lehane grade 3 at intubation. He has agreed to undergo an awake fibre-optic intubation.

**Is it acceptable to use a sedating agent during 'awake' fibre-optic intubation?**

No two cases are exactly the same when preparing for the management of a potentially difficult airway. When deciding whether to use sedation or not, one should consider the level of patient anxiety and the risk of airway compromise with sedation. Most patients respond well without sedation if the procedure is competently and confidently performed with adequate communication at all stages. If the airway is not deemed critically compromised, then short-acting sedating agents such as propofol or remifentanil target-controlled infusions at low predicted concentrations have been used effectively.

**How would you anaesthetize the airway, and how much local anaesthetic is it safe to use?**

There are a number of ways to anaesthetize the airway in preparation for tracheal intubation. One 'spray as you go' technique is described here. Other techniques may include direct blockade of nerves supplying the airway, and trans-tracheal injection of local anaesthetic.

Patient preparation:

1. Explain the procedure thoroughly, and gain consent prior to arriving in theatres.
2. Position patient in sitting position on a trolley, gain intravenous access and administer 200 mcg glycopyrrolate to reduce secretions.
3. Consider using low dose sedation if deemed safe to do so.
4. Administer oxygen via nasal sponge into least patent nostril.

Local anaesthesia:

The use of 4% lidocaine is recommended to effectively anaesthetize the upper airway. Careful calculation of dosage and syringe preparation is required to prevent excessive dosage.

Local anaesthetic solution preparation below is a safe dose for an adult above 55 kg – reduce volume for smaller patients using maximum of 9 mg/kg lidocaine.

**Nasal solution:** 5 ml syringe: 4.5 ml 4% lidocaine, 0.5 ml 1:1000 adrenaline, 0.5 ml 8.4% sodium bicarbonate

**Oral solution:** 5 ml syringe: 5 ml 4% lidocaine

**Spray as you go solution:** $3 \times 10$ ml syringe: 1 ml 4% lidocaine solution, 9 ml air (to flush).

Set up a local anaesthetic atomizer using an 18G cannula with trocar removed, attached to oxygen tubing running at 2 l/min. Local anaesthetic is delivered slowly down injection port of cannula.

1. Nasal preparation: care and patience is employed to anaesthetize the nostril, by slowly advancing the cannula, moving the tip to coat the nasopharynx. Encourage the patient to breathe through the nostril to facilitate coating of deeper structures.
2. Oropharyngeal preparation: spray solution onto oropharynx with patient breathing through mouth. Ask patient to say 'aah' to visualize and anaesthetize the posterior oropharynx.
3. Consolidation: repeat nasal spray to reassure patient that nose is numb.

**What type of endotracheal tube would you use, and how would you anaesthetize the vocal cords?**

Lubricate and mount a size 6 or 6.5 mm reinforced endotracheal tube onto fibrescope. Advance scope under direct vision through nostril to level of vocal cords. Feed 16G epidural catheter through suction channel of scope, and position above cords. Inject first 'spray as you go' syringe, including air flush. Repeat after advancing epidural catheter through vocal cords. Repeat again at this level if significant cough response previously. Remove epidural catheter and advance fibrescope through vocal cords. Advance endotracheal tube using 'corkscrew' action to prevent hold-up on entering the larynx. Visualize the carina to confirm correct positioning. Perform usual checks to confirm correct tube placement, then induce anaesthesia.

## Further reading

'Spray as you go' awake fibre-optic intubation method adapted from the BASDART difficult airway guidelines, devised by Dr Julian Berlet, Worcestershire Acute Hospitals NHS Trust, UK. Contact details available at www.basdart.co.uk (accessed 9 January 2016).

## Management of the obstructed airway: options for induction of anaesthesia

A 24-year-old man presents to the emergency department with a history of fever, sore throat and increasing inability to swallow saliva. He has stridor at rest. Nasendoscopy reveals supraglottitis.

1. **What are the different options for inducing anaesthesia in the patient with an obstructed airway?**
2. **What are the advantages and disadvantages of each option?**

## Management of the obstructed airway

Is the presentation acute (inability to lie flat, stridor, tachypnoea, accessory muscle use, tracheal tug and hypoxia) or chronic (no obvious signs or symptoms at rest)?

Primary medical management of acute airway obstruction is to maintain oxygenation. This may involve humidified oxygen, nebulized adrenaline and intravenous corticosteroids to reduce airway oedema, and in some cases a helium/oxygen mix to improve gas flow. If time permits imaging (CT or MRI) and/or nasendoscopy will determine the site, size, level, extension and nature of airway obstruction.

## Anaesthetic options

It is important to consider the expertise of the anaesthetist and the surgeon, the team available, the urgency, the patient's co-morbidity and the site and extent of airway obstruction. Whatever option is chosen (Table 9.1) to manage the airway a plan B must always be considered.

*Will I be able to mask ventilate the patient?*
No – an awake technique should be used.
*Will I be able to pass an endotracheal tube through the obstruction?*
No:

- Glottic/supraglottic lesion – tracheostomy required.
- Infraglottic, extrathoracic lesion – facilities to perform rigid bronchoscopy and jet ventilation available.
- Infraglottic, intrathoracic lesion – ideally should be managed in a cardiothoracic centre.

**Table 9.1** Options for inducing anaesthesia when the airway is obstructed

| Anaesthetic technique | Advantages | Disadvantages |
|---|---|---|
| Inhalational induction without neuromuscular blockade | Theoretically: | – inhalational induction slow in the presence of an obstructed airway<br>– apnoea may occur and patient may not waken |
| | – maintenance of spontaneous ventilation | – mask ventilation then required and theoretical advantages of technique lost |
| | – patient will waken from anaesthesia rapidly if agent delivery stopped | – neuromuscular blocking agents may be required to aid ventilation<br>– laryngoscopy may cause trauma or fail<br>– may lead to can't intubate, can't ventilate (CICV) situation |
| Intravenous induction with neuromuscular blockade | – likely to facilitate mask ventilation | – laryngoscopy may cause trauma or fail |
| | – abolishes laryngeal reflexes making tracheal intubation less traumatic | – may lead to CICV situation |
| Awake fibre-optic intubation | – avoids general anaesthesia | – complete airway obstruction may occur when used for glottic/subglottic lesions ('cork in bottle') |
| | – may be able to pass fibre-optic scope around a supraglottic lesion which may otherwise make mask ventilation difficult | – local anaesthesia of the airway may be challenging, cause coughing and airway obstruction |
| Tracheostomy under local anaesthesia | – avoids general anaesthesia | – may be challenging in a patient with obstructed airway who may have difficulty lying flat and extending neck |
| Trans-tracheal catheter/cricothyroidotomy under local anaesthesia | – will allow jet ventilation in situation of CICV<br>– may be able to bypass infraglottic lesion with catheter | – may be challenging to identify cricothyroid membrane<br>– jet ventilation may cause barotrauma |

# Further reading

Patel A., Pearce A. Progress in management of the obstructed airway. *Anaesthesia* 2011; 66 (Suppl 2): 93–100.

Prout J., Jones T., Martin D. *Advanced Training in Anaesthesia: The Essential Curriculum.* Oxford: Oxford University Press, 2014, pp. 208–9.

# General principles

## 10

*In this next chapter, a variety of question styles cover a broad range of topics. These include important issues and guidance relevant to preoperative assessment, advanced patient monitoring, sedation and patient transfers. In particular, we aim to provide a useful reference point for those situations encountered less frequently, such as anaesthesia in the MRI scanner. Well-informed decision making is paramount when considering when and if to continue with anaesthesia. These questions are here to make you think, and to provide some pointers on how to proceed in such situations.*

## Preoperative assessment and preparation for surgery: CPET

A 68-year-old female patient is scheduled for a Whipple's procedure, as curative treatment for pancreatic cancer. As part of her preoperative assessment, she undergoes cardiopulmonary exercise testing (CPET), which elicits an anaerobic threshold of 14.6 ml/kg/min and a peak $VO_2$ (oxygen consumption) of 25.6 ml/kg/min.

**What would be the most appropriate management plan for this patient?**

a) Advise the surgical team that the patient is unsuitable for any surgical procedure
b) Advise the surgical team that the patient is unsuitable for major surgery, but could undergo a less invasive palliative procedure
c) Advise the surgical team that the patient would only tolerate the procedure if it is performed laparoscopically
d) Continue with the operation, with an HDU bed arranged post-operatively
e) Continue with the operation, but arrange for the patient to go to ICU ventilated after the procedure

Answer: d)

In this scenario the anaerobic threshold (AT) exceeds 11 ml/kg/min and the peak $VO_2$ exceeds 20 ml/kg/min, so the operation should continue and the aim would be for the patient to be extubated and transferred to an HDU bed post-operatively. Cardiopulmonary exercise testing (CPET) is an established form of preoperative assessment, and allows risk stratification and appropriate perioperative planning. CPET is non-invasive, reproducible and includes measurement of variables, which are both dependent on and independent of patient effort.

*Returning to Work in Anaesthesia*, ed. Emma Plunkett, Emily Johnson and Anna Pierson.
Published by Cambridge University Press. © Cambridge University Press 2016.

The AT marks the onset of anaerobic metabolism, and is the point below which oxygen delivery is insufficient to meet the oxygen demand. The AT is independent of effort, and therefore provides an objective measure of a patient's exercise tolerance. The peak $VO_2$ (oxygen consumption) is usually the measured oxygen consumption at the termination of exercise, and is greatly affected by patient motivation.

An AT $< 11$ ml/kg/min and peak $VO_2$ $< 20$ ml/kg/min is associated with increased post-operative complications following major surgery, and suggests a planned post-operative ICU admission to try to minimize these complications. An AT $> 11$ ml/kg/min and peak $VO_2$ $> 20$ ml/kg/min suggests that a patient is much more likely to cope with the demands of major surgery, and is at low risk of developing post-operative cardiorespiratory complications.

CPET allows rationalization of critical care beds. In the scenario described, the patient easily exceeds these values, therefore the operation should continue. The patient could return to the ward post-operatively.

## Further reading

Agnew N. Preoperative cardiopulmonary exercise testing. *Contin Educ Anaesth Crit Care Pain* 2010; 10: 33–7.

# Perioperative management of the patient with diabetes

Please answer true or false to the following statements regarding the perioperative management of patients with diabetes.

1. Glycaemic control has been implicated in the rate of surgical site infections in a number of surgical specialties
2. Patients on insulin should be started on a variable-rate insulin infusion as soon as they are 'nil by mouth'
3. Capillary blood glucose levels should be checked every 2 hours
4. The target blood glucose range should be 6–10 mmol/l, with an acceptable range up to 12 mmol/l
5. Patients with an HbA1c of $\geq 69$ mmol/mol should not proceed with elective surgery
6. Hartmann's should be avoided in diabetic patients
7. Metformin can usually be safely continued in the perioperative period

Answers: TFFTTFT

In April 2011, the Joint British Diabetes Societies Inpatient Care Group published guidance regarding the management of patients with diabetes having surgery or elective procedures. This guidance has since been adapted by an Association of Anaesthetists of Great Britain and Ireland (AAGBI) Working Party to produce the AAGBI Guideline Peri-operative management of the surgical patient with diabetes 2015. Diabetic patients are known to have an increased morbidity and mortality associated with surgery so it is imperative that anaesthetists do all they can to mitigate these risks.

The overriding principles governing the management of the diabetic patient are that the fasting period should be minimized, hypo and hyperglycaemia should be avoided and the anaesthetic technique should be adapted to reduce nausea and vomiting. If optimally managed these will lead to minimal interruption to the patients' diabetic regimens and also can avoid the need for variable-rate intravenous insulin infusions (VRIIIs).

Here are some key points from the guidance:

- Diabetic control should be assessed by HbA1c levels at the time of listing for surgery.
- Urea and electrolytes and an ECG should be done preoperatively for all diabetic patients.
- Diabetic patients should be booked first on the list and if only one meal is missed then modification of their usual regimen is usually all that is required. There are two tables in the guideline regarding management of insulin and oral hypoglycaemics in the perioperative period. (Please see Tables 10.1 and 10.2 at the end of the question).
- Agents which can cause hypoglycaemia should be given at a lower dose or stopped perioperatively. These include sulphonylureas, meglitinides, thiazolidinediones and insulin.
- Agents which prevent glucose from rising may be continued (metformin, glucagon-like peptide-1 analogues and dipeptidyl peptidase-4 inhibitors).
- Indications for use of a VRIII are: emergency surgery; elective patients who have poor control (if surgery cannot be deferred); patients who will miss more than one meal; type 1 diabetic patients with no background insulin.
- Target capillary blood glucose (CBG) should be 6–10 mmol/l (up to 12 mmol/l being acceptable), and levels should be monitored hourly.
- Hartmann's is safe to administer to diabetic patients. If available, the recommended solution to accompany a VRIII is 0.45% saline with 5% glucose and potassium chloride (0.15% or 0.3%).
- The plan for returning to normal medication must be clear. In general if switching from a VRIII, there should be an overlap of 30–60 minutes.
- Doses of hypoglycaemic agents may need to be adjusted if normal diet is not resumed or to account for post-operative stress or infection.

### Management of hyperglycaemia

- Check for ketones (capillary ketones > 3 mmol/l or > 2+ ketones on urine dipstick).
  - If present, treat as diabetic ketoacidosis.
  - If absent, correct with up to 6 IU of subcutaneous insulin (1 IU will decrease CBG by 3 mmol/l).

### Management of hypoglycaemia

- CBG 4–6 mmol/l: Give 50 ml of 20% glucose IV
- CBG < 4 mmol/l: Give 100 ml of 20% glucose IV

# Further reading

Association of Anaesthetists of Great Britain and Ireland. Peri-operative management of the surgical patient with diabetes 2015. *Anaesthesia* 2015; 70(12): 1427–40. Available at http://onlinelibrary .wiley.com/doi/10.1111/anae.13233/full (accessed 2 January 2016).
Joint British Diabetes Societies Inpatient Care Group on behalf of NHS Diabetes. Management of adults with diabetes undergoing surgery or elective procedures. 2011.

**Table 10.1** Guideline for peri-operative adjustment of insulin (short starvation period – no more than one missed meal). Reproduced with permission from John Wiley and Sons

| Insulin | Day before admission | Day of surgery | | Whilst a VRIII is being used* |
| --- | --- | --- | --- | --- |
| | | Surgery in the morning | Surgery in the afternoon | |
| Once daily (e.g. Lantus®, Levemir®, Tresiba®, Insulatard®, Humulin I®, Insuman®) | | | | |
| Evening | Reduce dose by 20% | Check blood glucose on admission | Check blood glucose on admission | Continue at 80% of usual dose |
| Morning | Reduce dose by 20% | Reduce dose by 20%; check blood glucose on admission | Reduce dose by 20%; check blood glucose on admission | Continue at 80% of usual dose |
| Twice daily | | | | |
| Biphasic or ultra-long-acting (e.g. Novomix 30®, Humulin M3®, Humalog Mix 25®, Humalog Mix 50®, Insuman® Comb 25, Insuman® Comb 50, Levemir®, Lantus®) by single injection, given twice daily | No dose change | Halve the usual morning dose; check blood glucose on admission; leave evening meal dose unchanged | Halve the usual morning dose; check blood glucose on admission; leave the evening meal dose unchanged | Stop until eating and drinking normally |
| Short-acting (e.g. animal neutral, Novorapid®, Humulin S®, Apidra®) and intermediate-acting (e.g. animal isophane, Insulatard®, Humulin I®, Insuman®) by separate injections, both given twice daily | No dose change | Calculate total dose of morning insulin(s); give half as intermediate-acting only in the morning; check blood glucose on admission; leave evening meal dose unchanged | Calculate total dose of morning insulin(s); give half as intermediate-acting only in the morning; check blood glucose on admission; leave evening meal dose unchanged | Stop until eating and drinking normally |
| Three to five injections daily | No dose change | Basal bolus regimens: Omit morning and lunchtime short-acting insulins; keep basal unchanged* Premixed morning insulin: Halve morning dose and omit lunchtime dose; check blood glucose on admission | Give usual morning insulin dose(s); omit lunchtime dose; check blood glucose on admission | Stop until eating and drinking normally |

* If the patient requires a VRIII then the long-acting background insulin should be continued but at 80% of the dose the patient usually takes when he/she is well. VRIII, variable-rate intravenous insulin infusion.

**Table 10.2** Guideline for peri-operative adjustment of oral hypoglycaemic agents (short starvation period – no more than one missed meal). Reproduced with permission from John Wiley and Sons

| Agent | Day before admission | Day of surgery — Surgery in the morning | Day of surgery — Surgery in the afternoon | Whilst a VRIII is being used |
|---|---|---|---|---|
| **Drugs that require omission when fasting owing to risk of hypoglycaemia** | | | | |
| Meglitinides (e.g. repaglinide, nateglinide) | Take as normal | Omit morning dose if nil by mouth | Give morning dose if eating | Stop until eating and drinking normally |
| Sulphonylurea (e.g. glibenclamide, gliclazide, glipizide) | Take as normal | Omit morning dose (whether taking once or twice daily) | Omit (whether taking once or twice daily) | Stop until eating and drinking normally |
| **Drugs that require omission when fasting owing to risk of ketoacidosis** | | | | |
| SGLT-2 inhibitors* (e.g. dapagliflozin, canagliflozin) | No dose change | Halve the usual morning dose; check blood glucose on admission; leave evening meal dose unchanged | Halve the usual morning dose; check blood glucose on admission; leave the evening meal dose unchanged | Stop until eating and drinking normally |
| **Drugs that may be continued when fasting** | | | | |
| Acarbose | Take as normal | Omit morning dose if nil by mouth | Give morning dose if eating | Stop until eating and drinking normally |
| DPP-IV inhibitors (e.g. sitagliptin, vildagliptin, saxagliptin, alogliptin, linagliptin) | Take as normal | Take as normal | Take as normal | Stop until eating and drinking normally |
| GLP-1 analogues (e.g. exenatide, liraglutide, lixisenatide) | Take as normal | Take as normal | Take as normal | Take as normal |
| Metformin (procedure not requiring use of contrast media†) | Take as normal | Take as normal | Take as normal | Stop until eating and drinking normally |
| Pioglitazone | Take as normal | Take as normal | Take as normal | Stop until eating and drinking normally |

\* Also omit the day after surgery.

† If contrast medium is to be used or the estimated glomerular filtration rate is under 60 ml.min$^{-1}$.1.73 m$^{-2}$, metformin should be omitted on the day of the procedure and for the following 48 h.

VRIII, variable-rate intravenous insulin infusion; SGLT-2, sodium-glucose co-transporter-2; DPP-IV, dipeptidyl peptidase-IV; GLP-1, glucagon-like peptide-1.

# Preoperative assessment and preparation for surgery: hypertension guidelines

A 72-year-old man presents on the morning of surgery for transurethral resection of the prostate (TURP) for suspected benign prostatic hypertrophy. He has no additional medical history and is generally fit and well. His blood pressure taken on the morning of surgery is 187/112 mmHg. He was seen in the preoperative assessment clinic where three BP readings were taken, the lowest of which was 170/100 mmHg. There is no documented recording of BP from his GP within the last year.

**What is the best course of action?**

a) Proceed with the surgery as planned with anaesthesia of your choice, and ensure the patient has his hypertension followed up by his GP
b) Recheck the blood pressure in 30 minutes, and proceed with the surgery only if there is a further drop in blood pressure
c) Postpone the surgery until better blood pressure control can be established
d) Give a dose of metoprolol 200mg orally, and proceed with the surgery when blood pressure has reduced

Answer: a)

This patient has stage 3 hypertension, defined as having a systolic BP 180–209 mmHg or diastolic BP 110–119 mmHg. The guidelines for management of primary hypertension before elective surgery have recently been published. This patient, according to the new guidelines, would be able to undergo elective surgery without further intervention. There is little evidence to suggest that having raised BP prior to planned surgery significantly affects postoperative outcomes, but hypertension still seems to be a common reason for cancellation. Management of hypertension is complex and must balance the risk of delaying the operation for that individual and the risks of anaesthesia without appropriate treatment. Implications for cancelling surgery extend beyond the obvious disappointment; psychological, social and financial factors all play a part.

There is currently no clear evidence that lowering BP preoperatively affects the rate of cardiac events beyond those expected in a month in primary care. Indeed, BP readings may be more accurate with the GP. There is little guidance on a 'safe' BP for planned anaesthesia and surgery. However, it does seem that those with stage 1 or 2 hypertension (without evidence of end organ damage) are not at an increased perioperative cardiovascular risk.

When referring a patient for elective surgery, they should ideally have documented BP readings from their GP within the past 12 months. These should be requested as soon as possible. Surgery can proceed if the BP in primary care is <160/100 mmHg. If this is not the case, BP may be measured in the preoperative assessment clinic up to three times. If the lowest reading is SBP <180 mmHg and DBP <110 mmHg, surgery may proceed. Otherwise, the patient warrants referral back to the GP for treatment. Here, the elevated reading on the morning of surgery would not be a reason for cancellation and there is no evidence that acutely lowering BP with β-blockers is in the patient's interest.

Perioperative β-blockers were used in the POISE trial, and although this was associated with a reduction in cardiac morbidity, there was an overall increase in mortality. The study does not support the routine use of perioperative β-blockers, but they may have a role to play in patients with risk factors for ischaemic heart disease.

# Further reading

Hartle A., McCormack T., Carlisle J., Anderson S., et al. The measurement of adult blood pressure and management of hypertension before elective surgery. Joint guidelines from the Association of Anaesthetists of Great Britain and Ireland and the British Hypertension Society. *Anaesthesia* 2016; 71: 326–37

Fleisher L. A., Beckman J. A., Brown K. A., et al. ACC/AHA 2007 guidelines on perioperative cardiovascular evaluation and care for non-cardiac surgery. *Circulation* 2007; 116: e418–99.

Sear J. W., Giles J. W., Howard-Alpe G., Foëx P. Perioperative beta-blockade, 2008: what does POISE tell us, and was our earlier caution justified? *Br J Anaesth* 2008; 101: 135–8.

Hypertension: management of hypertension in adults in primary care; NICE Clinical Guideline (August 2011). Available online at http://www.nice.org.uk/guidance/CG127 (accessed 28/4/15).

# Preoperative assessment and preparation for surgery: recent myocardial infarction and stents

A 65-year-old man is seen in a preoperative assessment clinic. He is listed for a craniotomy for an astrocytoma in 2 weeks. His past medical history includes an ST-elevation myocardial infarction 6 months ago which was treated with a drug-eluting stent to his left main stem coronary artery. He is currently taking aspirin 75 mg OD and clopidogrel 75 mg OD.

**Regarding the management of his antiplatelet medication, which ONE option would be most suitable?**

a)  Continue both aspirin and clopidogrel throughout
b)  Stop both aspirin and clopidogrel 10 days preoperatively
c)  Stop clopidogrel 5 days preoperatively and continue the aspirin throughout
d)  Stop aspirin and clopidogrel the day before surgery and start bridging therapy
e)  Continue aspirin throughout, stop clopidogrel 5 days pre-op and start bridging therapy

Answer: e)

Percutaneous coronary intervention (PCI) is a common and effective method of coronary revascularization. The vast majority of PCIs involve placement of one or more stents. There are two types of coronary stents used; bare-metal stents (BMS) and drug-eluting stents (DES). DES are coated with a material which slowly releases an anti-proliferative drug; this inhibits smooth muscle proliferation, thus preventing the formation of a neo-intima which can cause stent re-stenosis. Re-endothelialization is consequently slowed down compared with BMS.

Stent thrombosis is a rare but catastrophic complication resulting in myocardial ischaemia or death. The majority occur before re-endothelialization is complete; dual antiplatelet therapy (DAPT) is therefore recommended during this time (6–12 weeks for BMS and at least 12 months for DES). DAPT commonly consists of aspirin and clopidogrel. These both irreversibly inhibit platelet function. Stopping clopidogrel during this time results in a 30-fold increased risk of stent thrombosis.

Wherever possible, elective surgery should be postponed until DAPT is no longer required. Essential surgery will require careful management and a multidisciplinary team approach. For the majority of operations, aspirin is not associated with an increased risk of surgical bleeding, unlike clopidogrel. Careful discussion of the risks of surgical bleeding versus stent thrombosis should be made in collaboration with anaesthetists, surgeons, and cardiologists. Continuing DAPT is often the safest option and is recommended in cases of low/intermediate surgical bleeding risk. This category includes visceral surgery, major orthopaedic surgery, ENT, cardiac surgery, etc. However, continuing DAPT is not appropriate where there is a high risk of surgical bleeding (or serious consequences of this bleeding, e.g. neurosurgery, spinal surgery and posterior eye surgery). In these situations, clopidogrel should be stopped 5 days preoperatively, and bridging therapy started the following day.

Various regimes for bridging therapy have been suggested, including unfractionated heparin, low molecular weight heparin (LMWH), and more commonly glycoprotein (GP)IIb/IIIa inhibitors such as tirofiban. The bridging therapy is then stopped pre-op (4 hours pre-op for tirofiban), and restarted post-op until clopidogrel is reloaded. Aspirin should be continued throughout. Thromboelastography (TEG) can be used to titrate the dosing of GPIIb/IIIa inhibitors.

Emergency surgery in the presence of DAPT can be challenging and requires expert management; major uncontrolled haemorrhage may warrant platelet transfusion to reverse the antiplatelet agents.

## Further reading

Fleischer L. A., Fleischmann K. E., Auerbach A. D., American College of Cardiology; American Heart Association. 2014 ACC/AHA guideline on perioperative cardiovascular evaluation and management of patients undergoing non-cardiac surgery. *J Am Coll Cardiol* 2014; 64(22): e77–137.

# Preoperative assessment and preparation for surgery: anaesthetic machine check

You are anaesthetizing for an ENT list.

**Which one of the following statements regarding the anaesthetic machine check is true?**

a) A full machine check should be completed before each patient
b) The anaesthetist is primarily responsible for checking the anaesthetic machine and equipment
c) The ODP is responsible for documentation of each check
d) There is no need to perform a check straight after it has been serviced
e) Training on any new equipment can take place during the first case

Answer: b)

The pre-use check of anaesthetic equipment is essential to maintain patient safety. It is the primary responsibility of the anaesthetist and forms part of the World Health Organization (WHO) Surgical Safety Checklist. The AAGBI has produced guidelines and an abbreviated checklist that are suitable for all modern anaesthetic workstations. These should be available in laminated form.

The anaesthetist has a responsibility to ensure that they are familiar with all the equipment; formal training and induction should be given for any new or unfamiliar equipment. At the start of every operating session a full check should be carried out. Further specific checks should be performed before every new patient or after a change in equipment. Checks should be documented in a record kept with the anaesthetic machine and in the patient's notes. The first user check after servicing is particularly important and must be documented.

The pre-use check starts with ensuring the availability of a self-inflating bag – a potentially life-saving alternative means of ventilation. The manufacturer's machine check should then be performed; this usually occurs automatically on start-up. The power supply should be checked. An adequate gas supply should be confirmed; a pipeline tug test is now recommended to avoid potential Schrader socket and probe failure. A reserve cylinder of oxygen must be present and adequately filled. The flowmeters, hypoxic guard, emergency oxygen bypass control (oxygen flush) and suction should be working.

The breathing system should then be checked. After visual inspection and checking of connections, a pressure leak test checks the adjustable-pressure limiting (APL) valve. The vaporizers must be adequately filled, siting correctly, plugged in and leak free. The contents, connections and colour of the soda lime should be checked. Any alternative breathing systems should be checked. The correct gas outlet should be selected; this is especially relevant during lists where the breathing systems are regularly changed. The ventilator, scavenging, and monitors must be checked and the settings selected, including audible alarms.

The two-bag test is performed after the breathing system, vaporizer and ventilator have been checked, checking for patency of the breathing system, the function of the unidirectional and APL valves and any leaks. Finally the airway equipment should be checked, including the availability of difficult airway equipment.

The checks to be performed prior to every new patient include those of the breathing system, ventilator, airway equipment and suction.

Despite satisfactory pre-use checks, equipment faults can develop or manifest during anaesthesia. A logical, stepwise approach to checking the equipment during anaesthesia should be adopted in the event of a critical incident.

## Further reading

Association of Anaesthetists of Great Britain and Ireland. Checking Anaesthetic Equipment 2012. *Anaesthesia* 2012; 67: 660–8.

# Advanced patient monitoring techniques: cardiac output monitoring

An 82-year-old lady is undergoing emergency laparotomy for bowel obstruction.

1. What devices are available to monitor her cardiac output perioperatively?
2. What are the advantages and disadvantages of each device?
3. What is goal-directed fluid therapy?

**Table 10.3** Normal values

| | | |
|---|---|---|
| Cardiac output (CO) | HR × SV/1000 | 4–8 l/min |
| Cardiac index (CI) | CO/BSA | 2.5–4 l/min/m$^2$ |
| Stroke volume (SV) | CO/HR × 1000 | 60–100 ml/beat |
| Stroke volume index (SVI) | SV/BSA | 33–47 ml/beat/m$^2$ |
| Systemic vascular resistance (SVR) | 80 × (MAP – CVP)/CO | 800–1200 dynes/s/cm$^{-5}$ |
| Systemic vascular resistance index | SVR/BSA | 1970–2390 dynes/s/cm$^{-5}$/m$^2$ |

BSA = body surface area; CVP = central venous pressure; MAP = mean arterial pressure.

**Table 10.4** Cardiac output monitors

| Cardiac output monitor | Principle | Advantages | Disadvantages |
|---|---|---|---|
| **Pulmonary artery flotation catheter** | *Thermodilution*: a change in blood temperature is measured by a thermistor in the pulmonary artery following injection of a known volume of cold saline into the right atrium. This allows calculation of right heart CO | Gold standard<br>Automated system now available to give continuous readings of CO | Invasive<br>Risk of damage to cardiac valves with prolonged use, catheter knotting, pulmonary artery rupture and pulmonary infarction |
| **Pulse contour analysis**<br>PiCCO [™Pulsion Medical Systems, Munich, Germany]<br>FloTrac/Vigileo [™Edwards Lifesciences, Irvine, CA, USA] | *Pulse contour analysis of the aortic waveform*: CO is proportional to arterial pulse pressure, therefore the contour of the systolic portion of the arterial pressure waveform can be related to SV and SVR | Continuous<br>Less invasive and useful in both conscious and unconscious patients. The FloTrac/Vigileo system only requires an existing arterial line and does not require external calibration<br>Provides SVV measurements: SVV is the change in SV over the respiratory cycle caused by alterations in preload as intrathoracic pressure changes. SVV can be used as an indicator of fluid responsiveness. Patients with an SVV > 15% are likely to benefit from fluids | PiCCO requires a specific thermistor-tipped arterial line in a proximal artery and a CVC to calibrate the system using a transpulmonary thermodilution technique which measures left heart CO<br>Less accurate for absolute measurement if uncalibrated FloTrac/Vigileo system but useful for trends |
| **Pulse power analysis**<br>LiDCO [™LiDCO, Cambridge, UK] | *Lithium dilution and pulse power analysis*: uses lithium dilution for initial calibration followed by a pulse power algorithm to determine beat to beat SV from a mathematical analysis of the peripheral arterial waveform | Only requires standard arterial catheterization<br>Continuous<br>Useful in conscious and unconscious patients<br>Can be calibrated using lithium dilution or used uncalibrated to monitor trends<br>Measures SVV | Non-depolarizing muscle relaxants may interfere with the lithium ion sensing electrode<br>Contraindicated with concurrent lithium use or in first trimester of pregnancy. If using lithium dilution |
| **Oesophageal Doppler monitor** | *Doppler shift*: the frequency of reflected ultrasound waves changes with the velocity of flow. This change in frequency is proportional to flow and when the cross-sectional area of flow is known CO can be calculated. The oesophageal Doppler measures flow in the descending aorta | Minimally invasive<br>Continuous measurement | Probes uncomfortable in awake patients<br>Contraindicated in patients with severe oesophageal pathology<br>A correction factor is required to take account of the fact that it measures CO to the lower body. Alternatively CO is calculated from a nomogram using aortic blood velocity, height, weight and age |
| **Supra-sternal Doppler** | *Doppler shift*: a probe in the jugular notch is used to measure blood velocity in the ascending aorta. Measurement of the cross-sectional area of the aortic outflow tract is used to calculate SV and CO | Non-invasive alternative to oesophageal Doppler<br>Measurements are taken from the aortic root and therefore unaffected by distribution of CO to upper and lower body | May be difficult to identify aortic root in some subjects<br>May have greater interobserver variability than other methods |

Transoesophageal echocardiography (TOE) also uses the principles of Doppler shift to measure CO. Other methods of measuring CO using pulmonary gas clearance and electrical impedance are available but are less often used in clinical practice.

Cardiac output (CO) is defined as the volume of blood ejected by the left ventricle per minute and is determined by heart rate (HR), preload, afterload and myocardial contractility. Inadequate CO will lead to cellular hypoxia and predicts a poor outcome following major surgery. Knowledge of a patient's CO therefore has potential significant influence on perioperative management and can be used to direct fluid, vasoactive and inotropic therapy. Its estimation using clinical parameters may be unreliable and blood pressure (BP) measurements correlate poorly with CO since CO is a measure of flow rather than pressure. Several different methods of measuring CO have been developed and are discussed below.

## Goal-directed fluid therapy (GDFT)

The perioperative 'goal' is to maintain tissue perfusion and cellular oxygenation by optimizing CO. GDFT has assumed that the optimum circulating volume for an individual is that defined by the preload required to produce maximal SV. Repeated fluid challenges are given to increase the preload until the patient is at the top of the Starling curve and further fluid challenges no longer produce an increase in SV.

On the basis of a series of small studies which used the Doppler monitor to guide fluid management during surgery NICE (National Institute for Health and Clinical Excellence) recommended that: 'The CardioQ-ODM [$^{TM}$ Deltex Medical, West Sussex, UK] should be considered for use in patients undergoing major or high-risk surgery or other surgical patients in whom a clinician would consider using invasive cardiovascular monitoring' as there was 'a reduction in post-operative complications, use of central venous catheters and in-hospital stay'. The NHS Commissioning Board has subsequently used financial incentives to encourage trusts to invest in and use fluid management technology by linking their use to CQUIN (Commissioning for Quality and Innovation) payments.

The more recent OPTIMISE trial found no difference in outcome when GDFT was used, and a Cochrane review found that GDFT does not reduce mortality perioperatively but may reduce complications and length of stay. A further study found that in an aerobically fit population those in the GDFT group had an increased hospital stay.

It is still unclear therefore, when and in whom GDFT is beneficial. Other questions also remain unanswered regarding the best haemodynamic goal to aim for as well as which CO monitor and fluids should be used, and the addition of inotropes. Surgical technique and perioperative care is constantly evolving and the use of GDFT in laparoscopic abdominal surgery and enhanced recovery programmes also remains to be defined.

## Further reading

Allsager C., Swanevelder J. Measuring cardiac output. *BJA CEPD Rev* 2003; 3(1): 15–19.

Challand C., Struthers R., Sneyd J. et al. Randomized controlled trial of intraoperative goal-directed fluid therapy in aerobically fit and unfit patients having major colorectal surgery. *Br J Anaesth* 2012; 108(1): 53–62.

Drummond K., Murphy E. Minimally invasive cardiac output monitors. *Contin Educ Anaesth Crit Care Pain* 2012; 12(1): 5–10.

Ghosh S., Arthur B., Klein A. A. NICE guidance on CardioQTM oesophageal Doppler monitoring. *Anaesthesia* 2012; 67(2): 1081–3.

Grocott M. P., Dushianthan A., Hamilton M. A. et al. Perioperative increase in global flow to explicit defined goals and outcomes after surgery: a Cochrane systematic review. *Br J Anaesth* 2013; 11(4): 535–48.

Jhanji S., Dawson S., Pearse R. Cardiac output monitoring: basic science and clinical application. *Anaesthesia* 2008; 63: 172–81.

National Institute for Health and Clinical Excellence (NICE). Medical technologies guidance MTG3: CardioQ-ODM oesophageal doppler monitor. London: NICE, 2011. https://www.nice.org.uk/Guidance/MTG3 (accessed 2 January 2016).

O'Neal J., Shaw A. Goal directed therapy what we know and what we need to know. *Perioper Med* 2015; 4: 1.

Pearse R. M., Harrison D. A., MacDonald N. et al. Effect of a perioperative, cardiac output-guided haemodynamic therapy algorithm on outcomes following major gastrointestinal surgery: a randomised clinical trial and systematic review. *JAMA* 2014; 311(21): 2181–90.

# Advanced patient monitoring techniques: depth of anaesthesia monitoring

Following a complaint about intraoperative awareness, the anaesthetic department has decided to invest in some depth-of-anaesthesia monitoring equipment. Various devices are being considered, among which is the Bispectral Index (BIS) monitor.

**During maintenance of anaesthesia which of the following BIS values is most appropriate to be aimed for?**

a) 100
b) 10
c) 50
d) 30
e) 80

Answer: c)

The Bispectral Index (BIS) monitor is probably the most widely available depth-of-anaesthesia monitor in UK anaesthetic practice. BIS converts raw EEG data captured from a forehead electrode into a dimensionless number between 0 and 100. A BIS value of 100 represents normal cortical activity, and 0 represents cortical silence. The BIS monitor also displays a measure of signal quality and the degree of electromyographic interference. The BIS algorithm was developed by studying the EEG of healthy volunteers who repeatedly underwent transition from consciousness to unconsciousness. The raw EEG data were time-stamped with various clinical endpoints and the features that best correlated to various depths of anaesthesia were fitted to a model by multivariate regression analysis. No particular BIS value predicts loss or recovery of consciousness, and there is wide inter-patient variability and overlap, but suggested interpretation of BIS values is as follows:

- 100–85: awake, aware, capable of memory processing and explicit recall
- 85–60: increasing sedation and impairment of memory processing; responds to stimulation
- 60–40: surgical anaesthesia; decreasing probability of post-operative recall; auditory processing and reflex movement still occur
- 40–0: increasing frequency of burst suppression.

BIS values correlate with measurement of the hypnotic element of anaesthesia; they display an inverse dose–response relationship with all intravenous and inhaled anaesthetic agents with the exception of ketamine, which causes an increase in measured BIS values.

Nitrous oxide has no effect on baseline BIS values at concentrations up to 50%, and in the absence of surgical stimulus, has no effect on BIS values if used in balanced anaesthesia. In the absence of surgical stimulus BIS values are also unaffected by opioids, despite the observed clinical effect on depth of anaesthesia or sedation they may have. However, when opioids are given during surgical stimulus, BIS values do decrease, reflecting the ablation of noxious stimuli.

Paediatric EEG approaches an adult pattern by the age of 5 years, but BIS was developed in studies of adult patients, and therefore its efficacy in children is unclear. BIS monitoring is likely to be valid in older children, but its use in infants cannot be supported.

## Further reading

Davidson A. J. Monitoring the anaesthetic depth in children: an update. *Curr Opin Anaesthesiol* 2007; 20: 236–43.

Goddard N., Smith D. Unintended awareness and monitoring of depth of anaesthesia. *Contin Educ Anaesth Crit Care Pain* 2013; 13(6): 213–17.

## Blood product usage: point-of-care coagulation testing

On the cardiac intensive care unit, you have been asked to review a 75-year-old patient who has returned following difficult aortic valve surgery. You are shown a significant amount of blood in the drain, and the patient is haemodynamically unstable. A viscoelastic point-of-care test (thromboelastography (TEG)) is as shown (Figure 10.1).

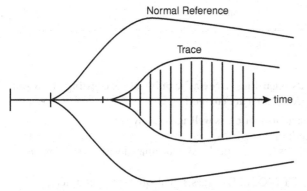

Normal Reference

Trace

time

**Figure 10.1** Example thromboelastography trace.

**Which of the following statements is most accurate?**

a) The primary concern is platelet failure – either qualitative or quantitative. Treatment should be with platelet infusion

b) The primary concern is excessive thrombolysis, and the patient may have developed disseminated intravascular coagulopathy

c) The primary concern is a prolonged R-time, and the treatment should include fresh frozen plasma (FFP)

d) Before any blood product is administered, the patient's temperature, haemoglobin, international normalized ratio (INR), APTT (or ACT), fibrinogen and platelet count should be measured formally in the laboratory

e) The treatment of choice is cryoprecipitate due to a relative inefficiency of fibrin formation

Answer: c)

TEG* parameters: R – reaction time; K – kinetics; α – alpha angle; MA – maximum amplitude; CL – clot lysis. ROTEM* parameters: CT – clotting time; CFT – clot formation time; α – alpha angle; MCF – maximum clot firmness; LY – clot lysis.

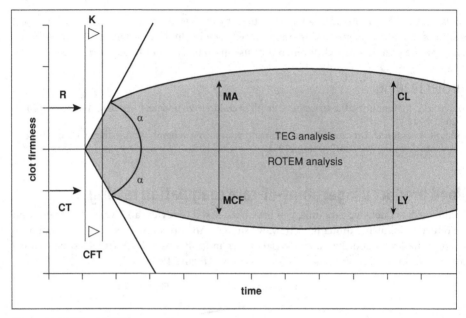

**Figure 10.2** TEG and ROTEM traces with parameters.

**Which of the following statements regarding viscoelastic point-of-care testing (TEG and rotational thromboelastometry (ROTEM)) are correct?**

a) TEG and ROTEM test both fibrin formation as well as fibrinolysis
b) The tests compensate for hypothermic patients
c) Both tests compensate for patients therapeutically anticoagulated with unfractionated heparin
d) A prolonged R-time (TEG) or CT (ROTEM) suggests inadequate platelet function (quality or quantity)
e) The treatment for a reduced maximum amplitude (MA; TEG) or maximal clot firmness (MCF; ROTEM) could be fibrinogen

Answers: TFTFT

Point-of-care testing (POCT) for coagulation has become a standard operating procedure in a number of areas of medicine. Owing to the relatively long turnaround time for laboratory testing, POCTs have guided clinicians in the use of blood products – producing better patient outcomes and reducing blood product usage.

The abnormal trace shows a delay in onset of clot formation (R-time/CT). This is often as a result of anticoagulation with heparin, for example (effect of heparin can be compensated for by use of heparinase and determines need for further protamine). However, it may also be due to a relative clotting factor deficiency. In this case the patient requires initial treatment with FFP. Although a formal sample should be set to ascertain coagulation status, this should not delay treatment in a bleeding, unstable patient. The cardiothoracic surgeon should be informed as the patient may need to return to theatre.

A reduction in maximal amplitude (MA or MCF) compared with the reference trace suggests a deficiency in clot formation, dependent on fibrin polymerization, platelet function and factor XIII (FXIII). A reduced MA/MCF is mostly due to reduced platelet function (quality or quantity), but lack of fibrin may be a contributory factor. Therefore, although bleeding may reduce with FFP only, it is advisable to administer a combination of packed red cells, FFP, platelets and cryoprecipitate in the haemodynamically unstable, bleeding patient. Hypothermia and hypocalcaemia should be corrected to aid clotting.

The tested blood sample is warmed to 37 °C, but does not take into account that the patient's own hypothermia may be a contributory factor to their coagulopathy. Figure 10.3 shows a variety of different traces, and their explanation.

## Further reading

Sankarankutty A., Nascimento B., Teodora da Luz L., Rizoli S. TEG® and ROTEM® in trauma: similar test but different results? *World J Emerg Surg* 2012; 7(Suppl 1): S3.

## Anaesthesia for non-operative procedures: MRI

You are anaesthetizing a patient for an MRI scan. She is breathing spontaneously through a laryngeal mask airway (LMA), with sevoflurane in 50% oxygen delivered via a circle system attached to an MR-unsafe anaesthetic machine situated outside the scanner. During the scan, the oxygen failure alarm sounds on the anaesthetic machine. You decide to stop the scan and wake the patient up.

**What is the most appropriate method to do this?**

a) Ventilate the patient with a bag-valve-mask circuit using 15 l/min oxygen from a portable cylinder and remove her from the MRI room
b) Attach a T-bag with 5 l/min of oxygen from a portable cylinder delivered via the side port to the LMA and remove the patient from the MRI room
c) Allow the patient to breath air spontaneously, remove her from the MRI room and attach her to a breathing circuit outside the MRI room
d) Ventilate the patient with a Mapleson C type circuit in the MRI room with 15 l/min of oxygen from a portable cylinder
e) Allow the patient to breathe spontaneously using 100% oxygen delivered through the circle attached to the anaesthetic machine

Answer: c)

The scenario in this question may be unfamiliar to many trainees, either because they have not given an anaesthetic to patients requiring an MRI scan, or because they are used to having an MR-safe anaesthetic machine within the MRI room. But there are many hospitals where the anaesthetic machine is placed in the scanner's control room because it is not MR-safe. Where this is the case, the patient is often anaesthetized in a room adjacent to the scanner room (outside the 50 gauss line) using a standard anaesthetic machine (MR-unsafe), but on an MR-safe trolley.

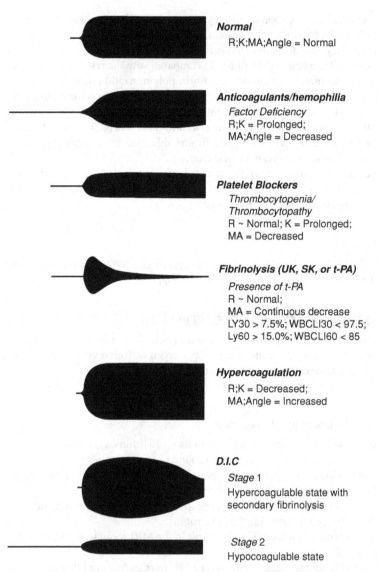

**Figure 10.3** Abnormal thromboelastography traces. Reproduced with permission from TEG and ROTEM: Technology and clinical applications. D. Whiting and J. A. DiNardo. *American Journal of Haematology* 89(2). 2014. John Wiley and Sons.

Once anaesthetized, the patient is transferred to the MRI scanning room and connected to an anaesthetic machine situated in the MRI control room. This therefore means that there is a large distance between the anaesthetic machine and the patient, requiring a long breathing circuit, bringing with it the problems of breathing through long tubing. Additionally, as the patient and anaesthetic machine are in separate rooms, two anaesthetists need to be present – one with the patient, the other controlling the anaesthetic machine. Faced with this arrangement, it is important to realize that in an emergency, most of the equipment you may need to resuscitate or treat a patient will be metallic and not safe to take into the scanning room (within the 50 Gauss line) – e.g. oxygen cylinders, defibrillator, laryngoscope. When an emergency occurs during a scan, it is therefore best to stop the scan and remove the patient from the MRI room. In the case presented here it would not be safe to keep the patient attached to the anaesthetic machine, given that the oxygen failure alarm has sounded. Any strategy that involves taking an oxygen cylinder into the MRI room can be ruled out, as the cylinder will be pulled into the scanner, endangering the patient. Therefore, of the options presented, the best course of action would be to take the patient outside the 50 gauss line before attaching her to an appropriate breathing circuit.

## Further reading

Association of Anaesthetists of Great Britain and Ireland. Safety in magnetic resonance units: an update. *Anaesthesia* 2010; 65: 766–70.

Association of Anaesthetists of Great Britain and Ireland. Provision of anaesthetic services in magnetic resonance units. 2002. Available at http://www.aagbi.org/sites/default/files/mri02.pdf (accessed January 2016).

Stuart G. Understanding magnetic resonance imaging. Anaesthesia Tutorial of the Week 177. Available at http://www.aagbi.org/sites/default/files/177-Understanding-Magnetic-resonance-imaging.pdf (Accessed 29 April 15).

## Anaesthesia for non-operative procedures: cardioversion

You have been called to the emergency department (ED) to assist with a DC cardioversion of a 75-year-old man who is found to be in fast atrial fibrillation (AF) at a rate of 145 bpm after complaining of palpitations and chest pain for 2–3 days. Currently his blood pressure is 115/60 mmHg, Glasgow Coma Score (GCS) is 15/15 and he is comfortable. The ED consultant asks you to 'give some sedation or a quick general anaesthetic' to facilitate the procedure.

**What are your immediate concerns?**

This situation occurs reasonably frequently in anaesthesia; as part of our service, we are often called to provide "sedation" for procedures outside the theatre/ICU setting. Such scenarios may be a particular cause for concern upon returning to work, simply because of a lack of recent practical experience or unfamiliarity of local protocols.

Upon reviewing this patient, a number of factors should be considered immediately before undertaking any anaesthetic management, and at the very least before any drugs are given:

- Stability of patient – are any adverse signs associated with tachyarrhythmia present, e.g. chest pain, syncope? (Refer to Chapter 30, Advanced life support.) Determine urgency.
- Onset of AF – consider need for anticoagulation if onset >48 hours (see Chapter 8, Advanced life support: tachyarrhythmias)
- Remote site – ED may be a significant distance from theatres
- Pressure to provide anaesthesia in an unprepared patient – starvation time may be unclear, lack of history, availability of cardiologist
- Availability of appropriate back-up and support
- Availability of monitoring/equipment as per AAGBI recommendations
- Potentially high-risk anaesthesia – the reasons above pose a number of clinical and logistical difficulties
- Level of seniority of the attending anaesthetist – often a junior registrar may attend calls to ED. It is vital that in unfamiliar surroundings, or when posed with a clinical decision

with which you may be uncertain, senior help is summoned. Lack of appreciation of the potential pitfalls could result in substandard patient care.

The NAP4 report served to highlight the risks associated with airway management and anaesthesia in locations outside of the theatre environment. These are discussed in Chapter 34 in more detail.

**What would your management be in this situation?**

As with all anaesthetic emergencies, management should follow the basic 'ABC' principle. The points above should give you some idea as to how you should proceed.

- Determine urgency – if adverse signs present, the patient should undergo electrical cardioversion as soon as possible without waiting for adequate starvation time; a rapid sequence induction (RSI) is indicated here.
- Determine location – unless peri-arrest, cardioversion should ideally be booked onto an emergency CEPOD list, rather than performed in ED.
- Choice of drug for hypnosis – different between the anaesthetist and non-anaesthetist, with the latter favouring benzodiazepines, which are poor at providing deep sedation. A survey of anaesthetists in 2003 showed 90% used propofol, 9% used etomidate, 43% using an additional short-acting opiate +/− sevoflurane. Agents with a rapid recovery profile should be used, alongside analgesia.
- This is a short, painful procedure with stimulus intensity similar to that of a surgical incision. Adequate depth of anaesthesia is required to prevent recall of unpleasant experience and to attenuate the catecholamine surge of the stress response (especially important in a population with a high rate of myocardial ischaemia and when the ultimate goal is rhythm stabilization).
- Owing to the narrow therapeutic window between deep sedation and general anaesthesia, the provider must be appropriately trained, with a skilled assistant, i.e. ODP present.
- Airway – variable, case dependent. Face mask/supraglottic devices acceptable if patient starved, otherwise tracheal intubation will be required.
- Monitoring essential.
- Ensure DC shock is delivered safely and at a suitable level.

The Royal College of Anaesthetists (RCoA) have devised audit recipes to monitor adherence to recommended standards for provision of anaesthesia and sedation outside theatres. Common reasons for failure to meet standards include: failure to appreciate importance of appropriate facilities; inadequate staffing/training; inadequate provision of monitoring; failure to be anticoagulated effectively; failure to use paddles and pads correctly and failure to use cardioversion device with biphasic waveform. In this case, the patient is stable enough to wait for the cardioversion to be performed in theatre when fully starved. The onset of atrial fibrillation is unclear, therefore need for prior anticoagulation should be discussed with a cardiologist.

# Further reading

Royal College of Anaesthetists. Raising the Standard: a compendium of audit recipes (3rd edition) 2012, Section 6: Anaesthesia and sedation outside theatres. Available at http://www.rcoa.ac.uk/ARB2012 (accessed 9 January 2016).

# Anaesthesia for non-obstetric procedures in the pregnant patient

A 21-year-old woman is listed on the emergency list for appendicectomy. She is 22 weeks pregnant.

1. **What modifications are you going to make to your standard technique because of the pregnancy?**
2. **At your preoperative visit the patient is extremely anxious about the anaesthetic and wants to know what the risks are to her baby. What do you tell her?**
3. **Are there any drugs that you wish to avoid?**

1. Throughout the anaesthetic you have two patients to consider; optimize maternal physiological function to ensure utero-placental blood flow and oxygen delivery to the baby is maintained. The most important physiological changes of pregnancy to consider perioperatively are:
   - Effects of aortocaval compression from around 20 weeks – left lateral tilt required if supine.
   - Decreased lower oesophageal sphincter tone – risk of aspiration even if adequately starved so requires rapid sequence induction with cricoid pressure. Consider ranitidine and sodium citrate preoperatively.
   - 20% increase in oxygen consumption and 20% decrease in functional residual capacity – risk of rapid desaturation at induction.
   - Increased blood volume (50%) and increased cardiac output (40%). Important to avoid hypotension to ensure adequate utero-placental flow. Use vasopressors (e.g. phenylephrine) if necessary.
   - Ensure thorough assessment of airway preoperatively and have more senior help available if potentially difficult airway.
   - Hypercoagulable state – thromboprophylaxis is essential.

   You also need to avoid any unwanted drug effects on the fetus, avoid stimulating the myometrium and avoid awareness.

   Fetal monitoring should be considered. At 22 weeks the fetus is not viable. The patient should be discussed with the local obstetrician and neonatologist, who will probably recommend a fetal heart rate check prior to surgery and then post-operatively. Delivery will not be appropriate in the event of fetal distress. The patient and her partner may wish to speak to an obstetrician and/or neonatologist prior to giving consent.

   If the fetus is viable then the case should have a multidisciplinary discussion. The patient may require continuous monitoring during the surgery with obstetricians and neonatologists on standby should there be a need for immediate delivery.

   Although not appropriate in this scenario, when faced with a pregnant patient requiring non-obstetric surgery always consider whether a regional anaesthetic technique is possible.

2. There have been many animal studies and observational studies in humans looking at the effects of anaesthetic drugs on the fetus but none have shown any definite link between an anaesthetic drug and long-term effects on the fetus. However, there is a small increased risk of preterm labour or miscarriage. This may be due to the anaesthetic, surgery or the condition warranting the surgery. There is a proven risk of fetal loss with acute appendicitis with peritonitis; therefore, in this case, not having the surgery probably poses a greater risk to the pregnancy than having it.

3. Analgesics: avoid NSAIDs. They may be used in the first or second trimester if benefit outweighs the risk to the fetus but must not be used in the third trimester (risk of premature closure of ductus arteriosus). Consider paracetamol, codeine, morphine, local anaesthetic blocks.
Antibiotics: co-amoxiclav may be associated with necrotizing enterocolitis in neonates; avoid if possible.
Many other drugs are contraindicated in pregnancy but these are the most important ones to consider in this scenario.

## Further reading

Reitman E., Flood P. Anaesthetic considerations for non-obstetric surgery during pregnancy. *Br J Anaesth* 2011; 107(S1): 172–8.
Walton N. K. D., Melachuri V. K. Anaesthesia for non-obstetric surgery during pregnancy. *Contin Educ Anaesth Crit Care Pain.* 2006; 6(2): 83–5.

# Sedation in adults: practicalities of target-controlled infusion (TCI) sedation

You have been asked to provide sedation for an extremely anxious 45-year-old lady to facilitate CT scanning of her abdomen and pelvis. You have chosen to use propofol by infusion to achieve this.

**What would be the most suitable method of drug administration? (Single best answer)**

a) Intermittent boluses
b) Variable-rate continuous infusion
c) Target-controlled infusion (TCI)

Answer: c)

**What are the disadvantages of targeting 'effect site' when using TCI?**

a) Increased risk of cardiovascular and respiratory side effects
b) Slower change in clinical depth of anaesthesia
c) Increased wake up time

Answer: a)

Given that you should not be present in the scanning room during the scan, it would be technically difficult to administer intermittent boluses of propofol in this environment, and this technique suffers from a high risk of under and overdosing, with resultant patient movement or apnoea. As plasma propofol concentrations are estimated using complex multicompartment modelling, although possible to approximate concentrations using a combination of initial drug bolus followed by regularly adjusted rates of continuous infusion, a simpler and more controlled method would be to use an infuser with an inbuilt target-controlled infusion model for propofol delivery.

Two models are currently available commercially for use in adults; the Marsh model and the Schnider model. The Marsh model will estimate propofol concentrations based on the patient's weight, and the Schnider model also uses height, age, and gender in its modelling.

Both models are less accurate in the presence of morbid obesity, and most infusers prevent drug administration for such patients. Propofol sedation in morbid obesity is inherently more risky for this reason, and because of the higher incidence of airway compromise, general anaesthesia may be the preferred option.

Practically speaking, either model may be used, and estimated concentrations are adjusted to clinical effect (usually propofol concentrations between 0.5 and 1.5 mcg/ml are sufficient). Some infusers have the additional capability of allowing 'effect site' estimation. Use of this facility is designed to allow a more rapid achievement of desired effect, by allowing the plasma concentration to over or undershoot, and thus more rapidly achieve target concentrations within the brain. Clinically, however, this may lead to an increased risk of respiratory or cardiovascular side effects.

## Further reading

Sivasubramaniam S. Target controlled infusions (TCI) in Anaesthetic practice. Anaesthesia UK 2007. Available at www.anaesthesiauk.com/article.aspx?articleid=101001 (accessed 9 January 2016).

## Patient transfers

You have been asked to transfer a patient from your emergency department to a nearby tertiary centre with neurosurgical facilities. The patient is a 46-year-old female who was admitted following a seizure. Her Glasgow Coma Score (GCS) on arrival was 7/15. She is intubated and being ventilated. Her CT head confirms a large subarachnoid haemorrhage.

**Which ONE of the following statements regarding her transfer is true?**

a) There is no need to discuss the case with the tertiary hospital prior to departure, as they are obliged to accept the patient
b) In time-critical cases such as this, transfer by air is always preferable
c) Minimum monitoring should include intra-arterial blood pressure (IABP), ECG, $SpO_2$, and capnography
d) To reduce the risk of drug errors, no emergency drugs should be drawn up prior to transfer
e) The patient should be established on the portable ventilator with 100% $O_2$ at least 30 minutes prior to departure

Answer: c)

Interhospital transfer of a critically ill patient can be a difficult and potentially dangerous situation. Optimum planning, preparation, communication and team working are vital to minimize risks and allow a safe transfer.

The decision to transfer a patient should be consultant led. Communication with the accepting hospital should begin as early as possible; a consultant to consultant referral is preferable. Where available, a transfer network may help with identifying an ITU bed and other logistics.

Pre-transfer stabilization should also begin as early as possible. In almost all cases, the patient should have completed their immediate resuscitation and be haemodynamically stable prior to departure. Where there is any risk of airway compromise, the airway should be secured prior to transfer. All necessary lines should be secured and labelled, and any necessary infusions started. Stability on the transfer ventilator should be confirmed prior to patient departure – an arterial blood gas will help guide this setup.

Minimum necessary monitoring for an ICU patient will include IABP, ECG, $SpO_2$ and capnography. The anaesthetist should make themselves familiar with the transfer monitors and increase the alarm volume and display size where possible. Any necessary drugs should be drawn up and well labelled; prefilled syringes are ideal.

All equipment should be lightweight, portable and have a good battery life; additional batteries should always be carried. Other necessary equipment such as additional airway equipment, IV access etc. should be organized and readily available. The AAGBI guideline 'Interhospital Transfer' provides a useful Departure checklist.

The mode of transport will depend on many factors. Transfer by helicopter is not always the fastest, and is often more technically challenging.

Clear and detailed documentation should be completed for any transfer. A formal handover to the accepting team should occur on arrival, including medical history, transfer details, investigations, images and notes. In summary, it may help to consider the following rule of thumb: 'Take the RIGHT patient at the RIGHT time, by the RIGHT people to the RIGHT place, using the RIGHT transport modality and receiving the RIGHT clinical care throughout'.

## Further reading

Association of Anaesthetists of Great Britain and Ireland (AAGBI). AAGBI Safety Guideline: Interhospital Transfer. London: AAGBI, 2009

**Chapter**

# 11

# Obstetrics

*This chapter provides an overview of the common situations and difficulties encountered in the provision of obstetrics anaesthesia. In addition, some questions look at the more commonly encountered complications and their management, from major obstetric haemorrhage to management of dural tap and eclampsia. A question on neonatal resuscitation is also included. The aim is to refresh your knowledge and provide a reference guide for your return to work, leaving you feeling more prepared to provide emergency cover in obstetrics.*

## Analgesia for labour: the poorly functioning epidural

A 38/40-week primiparous lady in spontaneous labour had an epidural sited 2 hours ago when her cervix was 3 cm dilated. The epidural was easy to insert (depth of space 5 cm at L3/4 interspace with 9 cm marking at the skin) and is being maintained on a PCEA of levobupivacaine (0.1%) and fentanyl (2 mcg/ml) with 5 ml boluses and a 10-minute lockout. She is still complaining of pain in the T9–12 dermatomal region, mostly on the left side, despite regular use of the PCEA.

**What would be the most appropriate management option?**

a) 'Top-up' of 10 ml 0.1% levobupivacaine and fentanyl solution in left lateral position
b) 'Top-up' with 5–10 ml bolus of 0.25% levobupivacaine plus 25–50 mcg fentanyl in left lateral position
c) Pull back epidural by 1 cm and give further 'top-up' of 10 ml 0.1% levobupivacaine and fentanyl solution in left lateral position
d) Re-site epidural as a combined spinal–epidural (CSE)
e) Re-site epidural

Answer: b)

The management of inadequate epidural analgesia in labour can be challenging. Key questions to ask are:

1. Is the epidural working at all?
2. Is the block too high or too low?
3. Is the block dense enough?
4. Is the block unilateral?

---

*Returning to Work in Anaesthesia*, ed. Emma Plunkett, Emily Johnson and Anna Pierson.
Published by Cambridge University Press. © Cambridge University Press 2016.

**Table 11.1** Management of poorly functioning epidurals

| Block too high | Sit patient up. Stop epidural. Support blood pressure as necessary |
|---|---|
| Block too low | Top up with low dose mixture |
| Unilateral block, missed segment or breakthrough pain | Top up with stronger local anaesthetic and opioid with 'bad' side down. Consider catheter pull back |
| Low back pain from occipito-posterior presentation | Top up with low dose mix plus additional opioid |
| No block | Re-site epidural or CSE |

In this case, given that there is some evidence of a block, it is worth trying to salvage the epidural in situ. The options are to use a low dose mixture, a higher concentration (with or without opioid), +/− withdrawal of the catheter by 1–2 cm. Which option is best may be debated. A study by Beilin et al. in 1998 compared top-up alone with top-up and catheter pull back (all top-ups using 0.25% bupivacaine) and found both interventions were successful in ¾ of women.

What you need to work out is whether the epidural can be rescued. Giving a low dose top-up on the background of reasonable PCEA use probably won't answer this question as quickly as topping-up using a stronger concentration of local anaesthetic in the appropriate position. Pulling back the catheter also risks pulling it out of the epidural space and introduction of infection, so it is better not to try this initially. However, if your first intervention is ineffective, you might then consider catheter pull-back with a further top-up, or alternatively re-siting the epidural. These decisions will also depend on the stage of labour, likelihood of assisted delivery and ease of initial epidural insertion.

## Further reading

Allman K. G., Wilson I. H. *Oxford Handbook of Anaesthesia*, 2nd edn. Oxford: Oxford University Press, 2007, p. 702.

Beilin Y., Zahn J., Bernstein H. H. et al. Treatment of incomplete analgesia after placement of an epidural catheter and administration of local anesthetic for women in labor. *Anaesthesiology* 1998; 88: 1502–6.

## Alternatives to regional anaesthesia: remifentanil PCA

A patient on prophylactic enoxaparin is requesting an epidural. She is on 40 mg once a day and had her last dose 6 hours ago.

**Are you happy to proceed with the epidural?**

Association of Anaesthetists of Great Britain and Ireland (AAGBI) guidelines (Regional anaesthesia and patients with abnormalities of coagulation, 2013) recommend waiting 12 hours after a prophylactic dose of enoxaparin before attempting regional anaesthesia so it would be inadvisable to site an epidural in this patient. If the patient receives a treatment dose of enoxaparin then recommendations suggest waiting 24 hours before attempting regional anaesthesia.

Since the publication of these guidelines, there is now less focus on adherence to absolute numbers and timings, and rather on an assessment of individual risk. This allows for consideration of regional anaesthesia, should the alternative option be deemed a greater risk.

Consider performing a spinal anaesthetic in a patient with idiopathic thrombocytopenia and a platelet count of $60 \times 10^9$. This is likely to be lower risk than performing a general anaesthetic in a labouring patient with a full stomach and an anticipated difficult airway. A move away from current recommendations allows for an informed discussion of acceptable risk with every woman, and the preferred option for her. Cases such as the example given should always be discussed with a consultant anaesthetist. The seniority of the anaesthetist available to perform the spinal/epidural also influences the degree of risk.

**What other forms of analgesia could you offer her?**

It is important to offer an alternative form of analgesia to reduce the patient's discomfort until the recommended 12 hours has elapsed.

- Pethidine IM – effective in early labour, should not be used near to time of delivery, owing to respiratory depression in neonate
- Entonox – if used appropriately many parturients cope very well. Some women do not like the nausea or light-headedness it causes
- Remifentanil PCA – an ultrashort-acting mu receptor agonist. It has a rapid onset and offset of action when given intravenously. It does cross the placenta but is metabolized rapidly in the neonate so has no clinically adverse effects.

**How would you set up a remifentanil PCA and monitor the patient?**

This is a highly effective form of analgesia but requires a higher level of monitoring than Entonox. Always refer to trust protocols for dosing and monitoring requirements. Most units start with a bolus dose of 40 mcg with a 2- or 3-minute lockout period. Individual trust protocols may vary but generally:

- Requires one-to-one care from midwife
- Only used if fetus >36 weeks (unless non-viable pregnancy) and in established labour
- Do not use within 4 hours of other parenteral opioids
- Administer via dedicated cannula (20G is sufficient)
- Encourage to press PCA button at start of contraction to enable the peak of analgesia to coincide with the peak of the contraction
- Entonox may be used as well
- Monitor oxygen saturations continuously – warn the patient that they may require facial/nasal oxygen if their saturations drop to <94%
- Also monitor sedation score and respiratory rate
- Continuous cardiotocograph (CTG) for first 20 minutes then intermittent
- Recommend that it is discontinued when second stage commences.

# Further reading

Association of Anaesthetists of Great Britain and Ireland, Obstetric Anaesthetists' Association and Regional Anaesthesia UK. Regional anaesthesia and patients with abnormalities of coagulation. *Anaesthesia* 2013; 68: 966–72.

Comparison leaflet on pain relief options in labour. Obstetric Anaesthetic Association, 2014. Available at http://www.labourpains.com/ui/content/content.aspx?id=45 (accessed 2 January 2016).

Examples of remifentanil guidelines. OAA website. http://www.oaa-anaes.ac.uk/ui/content/content .aspx?id=191 (accessed 2 January 2016).

# General anaesthesia for Caesarean section

You are bleeped to anaesthetize a lady for a category 1 lower segment Caesarean section (LSCS) for persistent fetal bradycardia.

**Which one of the following statements is true?**

a) An airway examination is not necessary as it will not alter your management
b) Induction should be with thiopentone 3 mg/kg and suxamethonium 1 mg/kg
c) Pre-oxygenation for 3 minutes or eight vital capacity breaths is necessary
d) An opioid should be given at induction to reduce post-operative pain
e) The risk of awareness is similar to other emergency operations

Answer: c)

Performing a general anaesthetic (GA) for Caesarean section (CS) can be challenging and stressful for even the most experienced anaesthetist. The incidence has fallen to less than 10% of all CS; trainee experience has therefore reduced significantly. The common indications are: urgency; failed attempts at regional anaesthetic (RA); contraindications to RA and obstetric indications.

There are a number of important physiological changes during pregnancy and labour. A significant decrease in functional residual capacity (up to 40%), plus an increase in oxygen consumption, contributes to early desaturation. Airway oedema, fatty deposition and large breasts contribute to an increased risk of difficult intubation (1:300). An increase in intra-abdominal pressure, decrease in lower oesophageal tone and decreased gastric emptying during labour (especially if opioids have been given) all increase the risk of aspiration (1:400–600).

Pre-assessment should be as thorough as possible. This should include any significant medical, drug, family and previous anaesthetic history, allergies, fasting status and a focussed airway examination. Verbal consent should be obtained. Recent bloods should be checked, ensuring that a group and save is available.

Large-bore IV access should be secured and the patient positioned with a left lateral tilt to reduce aortocaval compression. Prophylaxis against acid aspiration includes an $H_2$ receptor antagonist (ranitidine 150 mg PO/50 mg IV), 30 ml sodium citrate 0.3 M, and a head-up tilt.

Pre-oxygenation is essential – 3 minutes or eight vital capacity breaths. Induction is commonly with thiopentone 5 mg/kg LBW and suxamethonium 1–1.5 mg/kg TBW (often more than 100 mg). A short-acting opioid, such as alfentanil or remifentanil, can be given prior to induction in patients with pre-eclampsia to obtund the hypertensive response to laryngoscopy; remember to inform the neonatal team if administered. In general other drugs are withheld until after delivery to avoid placental transfer.

Optimization of your first intubation attempt is important; consider positioning ('ramped' or HELP pillow if obese), correctly placed cricoid pressure, use of bougie and a short handled laryngoscope. Easy access to the difficult airway trolley and protocols is essential. The Difficult Airway Society (DAS) Obstetric Difficult Airway Guideline is available in Chapter 33.

Anaesthesia is usually maintained with volatiles +/− nitrous oxide. The risk of awareness is high; obstetrics was the most over-represented specialty for accidental awareness after general anaesthesia (AAGA) according to NAP5 (see Chapter 34). This is probably because a GA for emergency CS represents a combination of many of the identified risk factors for AAGA: emergency nature, out-of-hours operating, junior anaesthetist, use of neuromuscular blockade, no opioids, rapid commencement of surgery, high patient anxiety and altered physiology and pharmacology.

Paracetamol and NSAIDs can be given intraoperatively. Opioid analgesia is required (often in high doses). Supplemental analgesia can be provided by wound infiltration with local anaesthetic or transversus abdominis plane (TAP) blocks (although there is a paucity of high quality evidence for their efficacy in this situation). Antiemetics should be given.

Extubation should be in the left lateral position or supine and head up, and only after the return of airway reflexes.

## Further reading

McGlennan A., Mustafa A. General anaesthesia for Caesarean section. *Contin Educ Anaesth Crit Care Pain* 2009; 9(5): 148–51.

Richardson A. L., Wittenberg M., Luca D. N. An urgent call to the labour ward. *Contin Educ Anaesth Crit Care Pain* 2015; 15(1): 44–9.

Rucklidge M., Hinton C. Difficult and failed intubation in obstetrics. *Contin Educ Anaesth Crit Care Pain* 2012; 12(2): 86–91.

# Regional anaesthesia for Caesarean: management of high spinal

A 35-year-old requires a category 1 lower segment Caesarean section (LSCS) for fetal distress. She has an epidural in situ, which has been providing adequate analgesia. You top up her epidural with 15 ml 0.5% bupivacaine. Shortly afterwards she complains of tingly fingers and breathlessness. She looks anxious. Her blood pressure (BP) is 90/50 mmHg, heart rate (HR) 105 bpm and $SpO_2$ 97% on air.

**1. Which one of the following options would be the most suitable initial management?**

a) Reassure her and encourage her partner to do the same. Ask the surgeons to proceed – a baby will be the best distraction for her

b) Increase the IV fluid rate, 50–100 mcg bolus phenylephrine, check block and steep head-up positioning

c) Check block to cold, pinprick and touch, then steep head-down positioning

d) Give 30 ml sodium citrate 0.3 M PO, pre-oxygenate with a tight fitting mask and eight tidal volume breaths whilst asking ODP to prepare for a rapid sequence induction (RSI)

Despite your management, she continues to deteriorate. She becomes apnoeic. Her BP is 60/45 mmHg, HR 40 bpm, $SpO_2$ 89% on 15 l oxygen.

**2. Which one of the following actions would not be appropriate?**

a) Call senior help or crash team

b) Considering alternative diagnoses

c) RSI with suxamethonium 100 mg only (no induction agent)

d) Vasopressors, inotropes and vagolytics as required

Answers: b) and c)

A 'high spinal' refers to a spinal block where the level extends higher than anticipated. A 'total spinal' involves the brainstem and cranial nerves. It is an anaesthetic emergency and requires prompt recognition and management.

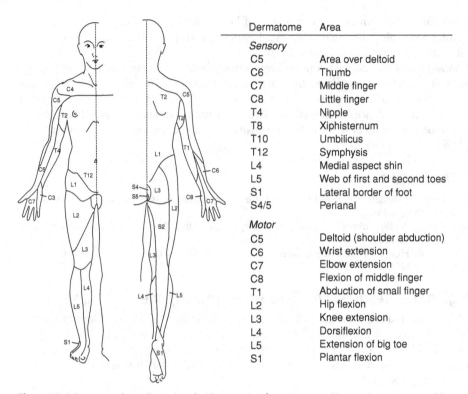

| Dermatome | Area |
|-----------|------|
| *Sensory* | |
| C5 | Area over deltoid |
| C6 | Thumb |
| C7 | Middle finger |
| C8 | Little finger |
| T4 | Nipple |
| T8 | Xiphisternum |
| T10 | Umbilicus |
| T12 | Symphysis |
| L4 | Medial aspect shin |
| L5 | Web of first and second toes |
| S1 | Lateral border of foot |
| S4/5 | Perianal |
| *Motor* | |
| C5 | Deltoid (shoulder abduction) |
| C6 | Wrist extension |
| C7 | Elbow extension |
| C8 | Flexion of middle finger |
| T1 | Abduction of small finger |
| L2 | Hip flexion |
| L3 | Knee extension |
| L4 | Dorsiflexion |
| L5 | Extension of big toe |
| S1 | Plantar flexion |

**Figure 11.1** Dermatomal map. Reproduced with permission from *Managing Obstetric Emergencies and Trauma*, Sara Paterson-Brown and Charlotte Howell. Cambridge University Press. 2014.

A LSCS requires a block to cold/pinprick to T4 bilaterally, as the peritoneum is innervated as high as T4. This corresponds to the nipple line. The arms are innervated by C5–T1 and the diaphragm by C3–5. Figure 11.1 illustrates the dermatomal nerve supply.

A high spinal can occur in a number of situations:

- The epidural catheter could be inadvertently placed into the subarachnoid (intrathecal) or subdural space. Giving a cautious test dose should enable recognition of an intrathecal catheter but not necessarily a subdural catheter.
- A correctly placed epidural catheter can migrate into the intrathecal or subdural position during labour.
- An excess dose of local anaesthetic can be given via the intrathecal or epidural route
- The patient can be positioned incorrectly, such as steep head-down positioning after administration of a hyperbaric solution.

The initial signs and symptoms usually occur within a few minutes of injection, although the onset can be delayed. They include nausea, anxiety, dysaesthesia or paralysis of upper limbs, hypotension, dyspnoea, difficulty coughing and clearing secretions and a high sensory block. Progression can lead to bradycardia, aspiration of gastric contents, cranial nerve involvement (such as a Horner's syndrome and altered speech), loss of consciousness, apnoea and cardiac arrest.

It is important to consider other potential causes and differential diagnoses. Massive thromboembolism, amniotic fluid embolism, local anaesthetic toxicity and cerebrovascular event could all present similarly and need prompt recognition and treatment.

Initial management aims to support the patient and limit the progression of the block. The patient should be reassured and the block level checked. Steep head-up positioning may help reduce further spread. Hypotension should be treated with an increase in IV fluid rate, leg elevation and boluses of vasopressor such as phenylephrine or metaraminol. Bradycardia should be treated with an anticholinergic. High-flow oxygen should be started. If the block progresses or the patient becomes compromised, a RSI should be performed. Appropriate reassurance should be given throughout and an induction agent should be used to minimize the risk of awareness. Once the airway is secure, ventilation and cardiovascular support should continue until return of adequate respiratory function can be demonstrated. This may warrant admission to ICU for ventilatory support.

# Management of epidural top-up

You are called to anaesthetize a patient for a category 2 Caesarean section. She has an epidural that the midwife says has been working well.

**How are you going to proceed?**

As with any case you need to assess the patient for yourself. Review the anaesthetic chart, history and ask about the effectiveness of the epidural.

The patient may give you a range of answers but these will fall broadly into three categories:

1. Epidural has been persistently problematic. Impression: top-up probably not going to be effective. Plan: spinal or general anaesthetic.
2. The epidural has caused concern at some point but is now working well. Plan: if the epidural was straightforward consider offering the patient a spinal anaesthetic. If regional felt to be difficult then begin top-up but if not effective quickly, offer spinal.
3. The epidural has worked well since it was sited. Impression: top-up likely to be effective. Plan: proceed with top-up.

**You decide to top up the epidural. How are you going to do this?**

Where?

The top-up can be commenced in the patient's room prior to transfer to theatre. It is essential that the patient can be monitored in the room before you give the top-up (blood pressure, heart rate and SpO$_2$) and that you remain with them once you have started it. The alternative is to wait until arrival in theatre before administering any local anaesthetic.

How?

Start by checking the existing block; otherwise it will be difficult to know if the top-up is effective.

You should always check what the recommended top-up mixture is for your hospital. The two main options are:

1. 0.5% bupivacaine
2. 2% lidocaine – usually administered as part of a 'quick mix'.

It is generally advisable to start with a 3–5 ml 'test dose' of either mix in case there has been any intrathecal catheter migration. Subsequent doses will depend on the block level, the urgency of the surgery and any medical conditions in the patient (e.g. cardiac problems). Generally, doses are 3–5 ml and spaced at least 5 minutes apart but if the block is below the umbilicus and the surgery is urgent then the next dose can be 10 ml.

Lidocaine as part of a 'quick mix' has a quicker onset of action than 0.5% bupivacaine.

A suggested 'quick mix' recipe is; 19 ml 2% lidocaine, 1 ml 8.4% sodium bicarbonate (increases pH, which promotes passage of local anaesthetic across the neuronal membrane), 0.1 ml 1:1000 adrenaline (increases speed of onset, prolongs effects, reduced peak local anaesthetic blood levels).

Opiates can also be given to improve the block. Either fentanyl 100 mcg or diamorphine 3 mg. Fentanyl acts quicker but diamorphine lasts longer. If the block is adequate then generally wait until after delivery and give diamorphine because of the hypothetical risk of respiratory depression on the neonate.

The block should be checked after each top-up to help guide further doses. It is important to check for sensory and motor block. Sensory block is generally assessed with cold and/or light touch. A level of T4 to cold and T5 to light touch is required for Caesarean section.

Motor block can be assessed using the Bromage score (see Table 11.2).

An epidural top-up may provide adequate anaesthesia without the complete motor block seen with a spinal anaesthetic.

**Table 11.2** The Bromage Motor Block Scale

| Degree of motor block | Criteria | Score |
| --- | --- | --- |
| No block | Full flexion knees and feet | 0 |
| Partial block | Just able to flex knees plus full flexion feet | 1 |
| Almost complete | Unable to flex knees, some flexion feet | 2 |
| Complete block | Unable to move legs or feet | 3 |

## Further reading

Hillyard S. G., Bate T. E., Corcoran T. B., Paech M. J., O'Sullivan G. Extending epidural analgesia for emergency Caesarean section: a meta-analysis. *Br J Anaesth* 2011; 107: 668–78.

Malhotra S., Yentis S. M., Lucas N. Extending epidural analgesia for emergency Caesarean section. *Br J Anaesth* 2012; 108(5): 879–80.

# Complications of obstetric regional anaesthesia: management of post-dural puncture headache

A 32-year-old primiparous lady had a very difficult insertion of spinal anaesthetic for trial of forceps delivery 3 days ago. She is still complaining of a headache in the frontal region, worse on sitting up, especially in the evenings. She has been taking regular paracetamol, codeine phosphate and ibuprofen in addition to three cups of coffee per day for the past 2 days.

**What would you do next?**

a) Prescribe oral theophylline
b) Arrange for CT head scan to exclude other intracranial pathology

c) Offer an autologous epidural blood patch one space lower than the spinal injection
d) Administer a 5-HT$_1$ agonist

Answer: c)

There are many causes of headaches in newly postnatal women, and it is important to take a very careful history and examination. The 2014 Saving Mothers' Lives report highlights the importance of including subdural haematoma and cerebral venous sinus thrombosis in the differential. Other differentials are: non-specific/tension headache; migraine (unusual as a first presentation); hypertension/pre-eclampsia; posterior reversible leucoencephalopathy syndrome; subarachnoid haemorrhage; space occupying lesions; cerebral infarction or ischaemia; sinusitis and meningitis.

From the history given post-dural puncture headache (PDPH) is the most likely cause. A CT head scan to exclude other intracranial pathology is beneficial if the diagnosis of PDPH is less certain. Treatment options are conservative, pharmacological or epidural blood patch (EBP).

The natural course of PDPH is that it usually resolves over 7–14 days. However, it may take weeks, and the demands of being a new mother often mean that women are keen to be treated sooner. Simple treatments should be encouraged: paracetamol, dihydrocodeine (with laxatives), NSAIDs, bed rest and hydration. Caffeine may help via its cerebral vasoconstrictor effects, but there is no strong evidence for this. The recommended dose is 300 mg per day (a cup of coffee contains about 100 mg).

Epidural blood patch is the most effective treatment (supported by a Cochrane review) and it should be performed 24–48 hours after the dural puncture with conservative management in the interim. Higher failure rates are reported when performed within 24 hours. Contraindications to EBP include sepsis (check that the patient is afebrile first), coagulopathy and patient refusal. An experienced anaesthetist should perform the EBP at the same space or space below, and the venepuncturist must maintain full aseptic conditions. Ten to thirty millilitres (usually 20 ml) of blood is used and you should stop injecting when the patient complains of pain or radicular symptoms, or you have given 30 ml. The success rate for first-time blood patch is reported to be at least 50%. The patient may experience backache after EBP and should rest for 1–2 hours before resuming non-strenuous activities.

Subcutaneous 5-HT$_1$ agonists (e.g. sumatriptan) and oral theophylline both cause cerebral vasoconstriction and have been used but with less success than an EBP. Synthetic ACTH (Synacthen) has also been reported to be effective for treating PDPH. There is no convincing evidence from randomized controlled trials to support these.

However the PDPH is managed, the MBRRACE report recommends that 'best practice…should include outpatient follow up and notification of the woman's GP'. The Royal College of Anaesthetists (RCoA) and Obstetric Anaesthetists Association (OAA) have produced a patient information leaflet for PDPH.

## Further reading

Boonmak P., Boonmak S. Epidural blood patch for preventing and treating post-dural puncture headache. *Cochrane Database Syst Rev.* 2010; (1): CD001791.

MBRRACE-UK. Saving Lives, Improving Mothers' Care. 2014. pp. 65–6 https://www.npeu.ox.ac.uk/mbrrace-uk/reports (accessed 10 March 2015).

RCoA and OAA patient information leaflet for PDPH. Available at http://www.rcoa.ac.uk/system/files/PI-HESA-COL-2012.pdf (accessed 2 January 2016).

Sabharwal A., Stocks G.M. Postpartum headache: diagnosis and management. *Contin Educ Anaesth Crit Care Pain* 2011; 11(5): 181–5.

# Obstetric emergencies: massive obstetric haemorrhage

A 32/40 pregnant multiparous woman presents with a painful antepartum haemorrhage of approximately 1000 ml. The cardiotocograph (CTG) indicates fetal distress and the decision is made to perform emergency Caesarean section under general anaesthesia. Shortly after delivery, the patient's pulse increases to 160 bpm and blood pressure drops from 95/50 mmHg to 60/30 mmHg, despite administration of 5 units of intravenous oxytocin and 500 mcg of intramuscular ergometrine. The amount of blood in the suction trap is 2000 ml, including approximately 500 ml of amniotic fluid.

**What are the therapeutic goals that should be aimed for in terms of haemoglobin, platelet count, clotting profile and fibrinogen?**

Answer: haemoglobin >80 g/l, platelet count >75 × $10^9$/l, PT and APTT < 1.5 × mean control, fibrinogen >1.0 g/l

This case of massive obstetric haemorrhage (MOH) is caused by placental abruption and uterine atony. Causes of post-partum haemorrhage are known as the four Ts: Tone; Tissue (retained products); Trauma (tears) and Thrombin (coagulopathy). As with any case of MOH your management priorities here are:

- ABC approach. Get help early.
- Adequate intravenous fluid resuscitation via two large-bore cannulae (at least 16G).
- Correct blood product replacement (see Table 11.3) guided by laboratory results and haematology advice.
- Administration of uterotonic drugs.
- Surgical control of uterine atony/trauma.

MOH is defined as >2500 ml, a greater than 5 unit transfusion or treatment for coagulopathy. Remember that blood loss is often underestimated. Management of MOH should

**Table 11.3** Suggested blood product replacement in massive obstetric haemorrhage

| Fluid | Volume | Notes |
|---|---|---|
| Crystalloid | Up to 2 litres of Hartmanns | Warmed |
| Colloid | Up to 1–2 litres | Warmed, until blood arrives |
| Blood | As indicated. Be wary of falsely reassuring early Hb level. Cross-matched if possible | Target >80 g/l owing to risk of rebleeding |
| FFP | 4 units for every 6 units of red cells 12–15 ml/kg or total 1 l (about 4 units) | Give if PT/APTT >1.5 × mean control (associated with increased surgical bleeding). Takes 30 minutes to thaw |
| Platelets | 1 or 2 pools are usually sufficient | If count <50 × $10^9$/l |
| Cryoprecipitate | 1–2 pools (5 units per pool) | Fibrinogen <0.5 g/l associated with microvascular bleeding. Takes 30 minutes to thaw |

involve senior anaesthetists, obstetricians, midwives, and early discussion with a consultant haematologist. When communicating with team members it is useful to state whether the MOH is 'controlled' or 'ongoing'.

**What other pharmacological agents can be administered to help treat the ongoing haemorrhage?**

Other uterotonic drugs that could be used include:

- Carboprost 250 mcg by intramuscular or intrauterine injection, repeated at 15-minute intervals to a maximum of 2 mg (contraindicated in asthmatics).
- Oxytocin infusion 40 units in 40 ml of 0.9% saline at 10 ml/h.
- Misoprostol 1000 mcg rectally.
- Tranexamic acid (an antifibrinolytic) is not currently recommended but is being investigated by the WOMAN trial (1 g IV as soon as possible and a further 1 g if bleeding persists after 30 minutes or recurs with 24 hours).

N.B. Ergometrine is contraindicated in hypertensive patients or those with cardiac disease.

## Further reading

MBRRACE-UK. Saving Lives, Improving Mothers' Care. 2014. pp. 45–52. https://www.npeu.ox.ac .uk/mbrrace-uk/reports (accessed 10 March 2015).
Royal College of Obstetricians and Gynaecologists. Postpartum Haemorrhage, Prevention and Management. RCOG Green-top guideline 52, May 2009. Available at www.rcog.org.uk/guidelines (accessed 10 March 2015, update due in 2016).
http://www.thewomantrial.lshtm.ac.uk (accessed 2 January 2016).

## Obstetric emergencies: eclampsia

A primigravida who is 32/40 weeks' gestation has been admitted to the delivery suite with a blood pressure of 170/120 mmHg, proteinuria 3+ on dipstick, and severe headache with visual disturbance. Within 30 minutes of arrival she has a grand mal seizure.

**What is your immediate management?**

The immediate treatment of eclampsia includes attention to airway, breathing and circulation with establishment of basic monitoring, although she will need an arterial line as soon as you are able to insert one. Experienced obstetricians, midwives and obstetric anaesthetists should be in attendance. The woman should be placed in the left lateral position and high-flow oxygen should be administered. A bolus of 4 g magnesium sulphate should be administered over 5–10 minutes, followed by a magnesium sulphate infusion at 1 g/h.

Since magnesium has been introduced as the first-line anticonvulsant, the use of phenytoin and benzodiazepines has reduced. Magnesium is thought to cause smooth muscle relaxation and treat cerebral vasospasm. Generally, seizures are short-lived, so usually intubation is not required; the airway should be supported using basic adjuncts. At the same time as commencing magnesium sulphate, control of blood pressure should be initiated, and blood tests for full blood count, clotting and biochemistry should be sent urgently. In this situation, options for control of blood pressure include intravenous labetalol or hydralazine (consider a 500 ml crystalloid bolus with hydralazine if given antenatally). In a different situation where oral agents were suitable then labetalol or nifedipine could be considered.

You should target a systolic blood pressure <150 mmHg and a diastolic between 80 and 100 mmHg.

**What should you do if seizures recur?**

Recurrent seizures should be treated with an additional 2 g bolus of magnesium and the infusion should be increased to 1.5–2 g/h. The risk of magnesium toxicity is unlikely with these doses, and levels for monitoring should only be sent if there are clinical signs of toxicity including loss of deep tendon reflexes, muscle weakness or drop in conscious level. The ideal therapeutic range for pre-eclamptic toxaemia (PET)/eclampsia is 2–4 mmol/l, and loss of deep tendon reflexes generally occurs above 5 mmol/l. Intubation may become necessary for airway protection if there are persistent seizures, and transfer to an appropriate critical care area should be arranged. Magnesium sulphate infusion should be continued for at least 24 hours after the last fit. Remember that up to 50% of eclamptic seizures occur in the post-partum period.

**When should you consider delivery?**

Delivery should be as soon as possible after cessation of seizure activity to minimize the risk of harm to both the fetus and mother. This is likely to be long before blood pressure is stabilized.

## Further reading

National Institute for Health and Care Excellence. Clinical guideline 107: Hypertension in pregnancy. 2010. Available at http://www.nice.org.uk/guidance/cg107 (accessed 10 March, 2015).

## Assessment of the critically ill parturient: puerperal sepsis

A 34-year-old with diabetes and a BMI of 40 had a normal vaginal delivery 4 days previously. You are asked to review her on the ward. She is pyrexial at 38.0 °C. Her blood pressure (BP) is 110/60 mmHg, heart rate (HR) 98 bpm and respiratory rate (RR) 20 breaths/min.

**What is the likely diagnosis? Why is a high index of suspicion required?**

Sepsis remains an important cause of direct maternal death. The most recent MBRRACE-UK report indicated that 20 women died as a result of genital tract sepsis, with 18 of these attributable to Group A *Streptococcus* or coliforms. However, sepsis as a cause of death has, once again, fallen below that of thromboembolic disease. Puerperal sepsis (PS) is defined as bacterial sepsis developing during the puerperium, i.e. birth to 6 weeks post-partum. Multiple risk factors have been identified; obesity and diabetes being among them. Symptoms of sepsis may be less distinctive in this population because of immune system modulation and as most parturients are young and fit, they may compensate physiologically for some time. Disease progression when it occurs can therefore be rapid; prompt senior review is required.

**Describe your initial assessment and management of this patient.**

Regular observations (HR, BP, RR and temperature) should be recorded on a modified early obstetric warning score (MEOWS) chart. Abnormal parameters require prompt action. A full history and examination are needed to help identify the likely source of sepsis. This may be a site distant from the genital tract, e.g. mastitis. The Surviving Sepsis Campaign lists a number of actions and timeframes as well as resuscitation targets; blood cultures and other relevant samples, e.g. breastmilk, should ideally be obtained prior to antibiotic administration. If severe sepsis is suspected, serum lactate must be measured within 3 hours. Imaging must be performed promptly. Broad-spectrum antibiotics (following local guidelines) must be administered within an hour of suspicion of severe sepsis. If the patient is hypotensive or if lactate is >4 mmol/l, an initial crystalloid bolus of 20 ml/kg should be administered. Vasopressors may be required following fluid resuscitation. Targets are mean arterial pressure (MAP) >65 mmHg and central venous pressure (CVP) of >8 cmH$_2$O. IV immunoglobulin may be considered.

**Who should be involved in this patient's care and where should this be provided?**

A multidisciplinary approach is needed with prompt senior anaesthetic, obstetric and microbiology input. Transfer to HDU or ICU level care may be required.

## Further reading

Acosta C., Knight M. Sepsis and maternal mortality. *Curr Opin Obstet Gynecol* 2013; 25: 109–16.

Dellinger R. P., Carlet J. M., Bion J. et al. Surviving Sepsis Campaign: international guidelines for management of severe sepsis and septic shock: 2008. *Crit Care Med* 2008; 36: 296–327.

MBRRACE-UK. Saving Lives, Improving Mothers' Care. 2014. Available at https://www.npeu.ox.ac.uk/mbrrace-uk (accessed 2 January 2016).

Royal College of Obstetricians and Gynaecologists. Green-top guideline no. 64b. Bacterial sepsis following pregnancy 2012. Available at https://www.rcog.org.uk/globalassets/documents/guidelines/gtg_64b.pdf (accessed 2 January 2016).

## Neonatal resuscitation

You are the anaesthetic registrar on the delivery suite when the neonatal emergency alarm sounds. A baby has just been born by spontaneous vaginal delivery at 39/40 gestation; the mother was not monitored continuously because she was deemed low risk. The baby is pale and floppy, and is not breathing. The neonatal registrar is delayed and you are asked to help.

**Put the following actions in the correct order:**

a) Assess breathing and circulation
b) Give five inflation breaths using air
c) Start the clock
d) Dry and wrap the baby
e) Open and inspect the airway
f) If the heart rate is less than 60 or undetectable then start chest compressions at a ratio of 3:1

Answer: c) d) a) e) b) f)

The basic approach to neonatal resuscitation is similar to all other types of resuscitation but with some key differences. One of the most crucial of these is keeping the baby warm. First dry and wrap the baby using towels (remembering to discard the damp ones) and use an overhead heater. Preterm babies should be placed in a plastic bag to minimize evaporative losses. Then assess the neonate by looking at its respiration (airway and breathing), heart rate (auscultate the cardiac apex), colour (pink, blue or pale/white) and tone.

Most healthy babies are blue initially and will generally cry within a few seconds of being born. A normal heart rate for a healthy neonate is >100 bpm. If, after gentle stimulation, the baby is gasping or is apnoeic, open the airway and give five inflation breaths using air. The head should be maintained in a neutral position, and a support underneath the shoulders may prevent the neck from flexing. Inflation breaths should be given over 2–3 seconds at a positive pressure of 30–40 cmH$_2$O.

Effective inflation breaths should increase a slow heart rate. Remember that the chest may not rise with the inflation breaths, so reassess the heart rate after giving the first five breaths. If this has responded you can assume the chest has been inflated. If there is no response, check the airway position. Consider the use of jaw thrust plus oropharyngeal airways, and in the presence of obstruction then direct laryngoscopy and suction is needed.

Acceptable pre-ductal (right hand) saturations in a healthy baby are 60% at 2 minutes, rising to 90% at 10 minutes. The use of oxygen should ideally be guided by pulse oximetry: oxygen saturations in the low 90s are acceptable. Remember that for preterm neonates in particular, saturations >95% are associated with significant damage as a result of hyperoxaemia.

An undetectable pulse or heart rate <60 bpm mandates chest compression/ventilation at a ratio of 3:1. The hand encircling technique is most efficient. Drugs are only needed if there has been no significant cardiac output despite cardiopulmonary resuscitation. The dose of adrenaline is 10 mcg/kg intravenously. The tracheal route is not recommended. Other drugs include bicarbonate, glucose, fluids and naloxone.

## Further reading

Advanced Life Support Group edited by M. Samuels, S. Wieteska. *Advanced Paediatric Life Support: The Practical Approach*, 5th edn. London: Wiley-Blackwell, 2011.

Chapter

# Intensive care medicine

**12**

*Whether or not you have regular sessions in ICU the principles of the management of critically ill patients are relevant and useful to all anaesthetists. In this chapter general topics such as sepsis, acute respiratory distress syndrome (ARDS), cardiogenic shock and inotrope management are covered in addition to some more specifically ICU-related topics such as sedation and end-of-life issues. Many references and sources of information are available in the further reading for those with an ICM interest or those who wish to prepare in greater depth.*

## Assessment of the critically ill patient: sepsis

A 43-year-old woman has been referred for ICU review by her medical team. Having been previously well, she was admitted 12 hours ago with radiologically confirmed right lower lobar pneumonia. She is on appropriate antibiotics, but has deteriorated over the last 6 hours. She is now pyrexial (38.8 °C), combative, tachycardic (heart rate 125 bpm) and has a respiratory rate of 30 breaths/min. A recent arterial blood gas shows a partially compensated metabolic acidosis, with a lactate of 3.4 mmol/l. Her blood pressure was 86/40 mmHg 2 hours ago, but is now 105/65 mmHg after 1 litre of crystalloid.

**Which of the following statements concerning her condition is most correct?**

a) Her condition should be described as SIRS
b) Her condition should be described as sepsis
c) Her condition should be described as severe sepsis
d) Her condition should be described as septic shock
e) Her condition should be described as hypovolaemic shock

Answer: c)

Although disease classification can seem pedantic, it is useful for prognostication in individual patients. It is also important for defining research cohorts, and for comparisons between individual hospitals and healthcare systems.

The systemic inflammatory response syndrome (SIRS) is a systemic inflammatory manifestation of a local or systemic disease process. It is defined as the presence of two or more of:

- Temperature >38 °C or <36 °C
- Heart rate >90 bpm

*Returning to Work in Anaesthesia*, ed. Emma Plunkett, Emily Johnson and Anna Pierson.
Published by Cambridge University Press. © Cambridge University Press 2016.

- Respiratory rate >20 breaths/min or $PaCO_2$ < 4.3 kPa (or ventilator dependence)
- White blood cell count >12 000 cells/mm$^3$, < 4000 cells/mm$^3$, or >10% band forms.

Sepsis is defined as SIRS in response to known or suspected infection. Sepsis becomes severe sepsis when there is evidence of organ dysfunction, hypoperfusion (characterized by lactataemia) or hypotension. Septic shock is present when sepsis is accompanied by hypotension or hypoperfusion, which is refractory to fluid resuscitation (large volumes may be required).

The patient described has SIRS. She meets three out of the four criteria (and bloods may show the presence of the fourth). Given the known infective process, this means that she has sepsis. However, her condition is best described as severe sepsis, as she has evidence of organ dysfunction with her combative behaviour, and hypoperfusion with her raised lactate. She does not have septic shock, as her blood pressure has normalized with a fluid bolus.

Mortality rises with the number of SIRS criteria met, and rises further with the progression from sepsis to severe sepsis to septic shock. Although the true mortality of severe sepsis is difficult to state exactly because of the presence of confounding co-morbidities, it is normally quoted as approximately 30%.

## Further reading

Bone R. C., Balk R. A., Cerra F. B. et al. Definitions for sepsis and organ failure and guidelines for the use of innovative therapies in sepsis. The ACCP/SCCM Consensus Conference Committee.
  American College of Chest Physicians/Society of Critical Care Medicine. Chest 1992; 101: 1644–55.
  http://survivingsepsis.org/ (accessed 13 April 2015).

## Assessment of the critically ill patient: drug overdose

A 30-year-old man with a history of schizophrenia is brought in to the emergency department having taken a witnessed overdose of clozapine and oral morphine solution 2 hours prior to admission. The patient is responsive to pain only, with pinpoint pupils, pyrexia, a respiratory rate of 6 breaths/min, a pulse rate of 120 bpm and a blood pressure of 80/40 mmHg.

**Mark the following statements true/false:**

1. Induced emesis should be undertaken within an hour of presentation
2. This patient should receive activated charcoal via a nasogastric tube
3. Intravenous naloxone should be administered at a dose of 40–100 mcg every 2 minutes until respiratory depression is reversed, up to a maximum of 15 mg
4. This patient is at risk of pulmonary oedema and rhabdomyolysis
5. Clozapine is an atypical antipsychotic
6. A 12-lead ECG should be performed urgently
7. Dobutamine is the agent of choice for managing hypotension in this case

Answers

1. False. Induced emesis is no longer recommended as it conveys no benefit, results in prolonged time in the emergency department and increases the risk of aspiration pneumonitis.
2. False. Activated charcoal should only be given within 1 hour of ingestion of the poison (or within 2 hours of paracetamol overdose), at a dose of 25–50 g. It is not recommended for overdose of lithium, iron, alcohol, methanol, ethylene glycol, petroleum distillates, corrosives, acids or alkalis.

3. True. Naloxone can also be administered SC, IM or via the trachea. It has a half-life of approximately 20 minutes so the IV bolus dose should be followed by an infusion. Failure to respond may necessitate tracheal intubation and ventilation.

4. True. Pulmonary oedema may be due to a number of factors including negative intrathoracic pressure due to attempted inspiration against a closed glottis and a sympathetic vasoactive response, similar in pathogenesis to neurogenic pulmonary oedema.

5. True. Other atypical antipsychotics include risperidone, olanzapine, quetiapine and amisulpride. Symptoms of overdose are usually evident within 6 hours of ingestion. Clozapine is often a preferred agent because of its absence of extrapyramidal effects.

6. True. The cardiovascular effects of atypical antipsychotics vary between agents, but clozapine can cause severe muscarinic effects and QTc prolongation (>450 ms) with subsequent torsade de pointes and, rarely, myocarditis. ECG with continuous cardiac monitoring is essential in all such overdoses. Electrolyte disturbances, in particular hypomagnesaemia and hypokalaemia, should be checked and corrected urgently.

7. False. Both morphine and clozapine contribute to the patient's hypotension. Clozapine causes alpha-1 blockade. The management of this should be with cautious intravenous fluid boluses, bearing in mind potential pulmonary oedema, and a vasopressor with alpha-1 agonist properties, such as noradrenaline or phenylephrine.

## Further reading

Boyer E. W. Management of opioid analgesic overdose. *N Engl J Med* 2012; 367(2): 146–55.
Minns A. B., Clark R. F. Toxicology and overdose of atypical antipsychotics. *J Emerg Med* 2012; 43(5): 906–13.
Ward C., Sair M. Oral poisoning: an update. *Contin Educ Anaesth Crit Care Pain* 2010; 10(1): 6–11.

# Management of ARDS

A 28-year-old man is admitted to the intensive care unit. He has been involved in a road traffic accident, sustaining a pelvic fracture and a liver laceration. A CT scan showed no other injuries. During resuscitation he received 12 units of packed red cells, 6 units of fresh frozen plasma and 6 units of platelets. He has undergone an exploratory laparotomy with packing of his liver and his pelvic fracture has been stabilized. On day 2 of his ICU stay his oxygen requirements have increased. His arterial blood gas reveals a $PaO_2$ of 6 kPa with a $FiO_2$ of 0.8. His chest x-ray shows bilateral infiltrates.

**Which of the following are true:**

a) Oxygen should be increased to achieve a $PaO_2$ of greater than 10 kPa
b) Tidal volumes of 6–8 ml/kg should be used
c) Tidal volumes should be calculated on actual body weight
d) A $PaCO_2$ of 4–4.5 kPa should be targeted
e) High frequency oscillatory ventilation should be commenced immediately

Answer: b)

The patient is now ventilated on a pressure control mode with a $FiO_2$ of 1.0. The positive end-expiratory pressure (PEEP) is set at 10 $cmH_2O$. His arterial blood gas shows a $PaO_2$ of 6.3 kPa and a $PaCO_2$ of 7.5 kPa with a pH of 7.25. He is not requiring inotropes.

**Which of the following strategies have an evidence base for improving outcome in ARDS?**

a) Increase PEEP
b) Start beta-2 agonists
c) Administer nitric oxide
d) Refer for extracorporeal membrane oxygenation (ECMO)
e) Commence prone ventilation

Answer: a), d), e)

Acute respiratory distress syndrome (ARDS) has recently been redefined. The Berlin definition states that there must be respiratory failure that has developed within 1 week of a known clinical insult. The chest radiograph must have bilateral opacities not fully explained by effusions, lobar/lung collapse or nodules. The respiratory failure cannot be fully explained by cardiac failure or volume overload. There are three categories of severity:

- Mild – $PaO_2/FiO_2$ 200–300 mmHg
- Moderate – $PaO_2/FiO_2$ 101–199 mmHg
- Severe – $PaO_2/FiO_2 < 100$ mmHg.

Causes of ARDS are multiple and include sepsis, pneumonia, gastric aspiration, major trauma, massive blood transfusion, near drowning, massive burns and pre-eclampsia.

Initial management involves respiratory and haemodynamic support with removal of the precipitating cause where possible.

Ventilatory strategies concentrate on lung protection which aims to prevent overdistension and the resultant release of inflammatory mediators which can worsen ARDS. Plateau pressures should ideally be kept under 30 cmH$_2$O.

The ARDSnet trial compared traditional tidal volumes of 12 ml/kg with 6 ml/kg of predicted body weight. The low tidal volume group had a 22% lower 28-day mortality. Many studies have reported conflicting results; however, low tidal volume ventilation is widely accepted and practised in the UK.

ARDSnet recommends aiming for oxygen saturation of 88–95% ($PaO_2$ 55–80 mmHg), setting the respiratory rate up to 35 breaths/min and setting PEEP to at least 5 cmH$_2$O.

Permissive hypercapnia is widely practised to minimize plateau pressures. The absolute value of $PaCO_2$ is not important. It is considered safe for the pH to fall to 7.20; exceptions to this include raised intracranial pressure.

In cases of refractory hypoxia many strategies have been used, most without survival benefit. Several studies have shown ARDS patients receiving higher PEEP had a trend towards survival. ARDSnet suggests values up to 24 cmH$_2$O for the most hypoxic patients.

Beta-2 agonists were shown to be harmful in ARDS in the recent BALTI study. Inhaled nitric oxide improves oxygenation but not outcome. Other strategies shown to be ineffective include prostacyclin therapy and corticosteroids.

The prone position has recently regained favour after a recent multicentre trial showed a 17% absolute risk reduction for mortality. Other ventilatory strategies that have been used include high frequency oscillatory ventilation (HFOV) and airway pressure release ventilation (APRV). HFOV intuitively appeals as a low tidal volume strategy, but recent trials have failed to show benefit. OSCILLATE was stopped early owing to increased mortality in the

HFOV group. OSCAR showed no benefit by using HFOV as first line in ARDS, but it could still be considered as rescue therapy. APRV may improve oxygenation, but no study to date has shown survival benefit over conventional ventilation.

ECMO is becoming more common following the CESAR trial, which showed a survival benefit in those referred to ECMO centres. Referral should be considered in severe refractory hypoxia.

## Further reading

Acute Respiratory Distress Network. Ventilation with lower tidal volumes as compared with traditional tidal volumes for acute lung injury and the acute respiratory distress syndrome. *N Engl J Med* 2000; 342: 1301–8.

ARDS Definition Task Force. Acute respiratory distress syndrome. The Berlin definition. *JAMA* 2012; 307: 2526–33.

Ferguson N., Cook M., Gordon H. et al. High frequency oscillation in early acute respiratory distress syndrome. *N Engl J Med* 2013; 368(9): 795–805.

Guerin C., Reignier J., Richard J. et al. Prone position in severe acute respiratory distress syndrome. *N Engl J Med* 2013; 36: 2159–68.

Peek G., Elbourne D., Mugford M. et al. CESAR trial collaboration. Efficacy and economic assessment of conventional ventilator support versus extracorporeal membrane oxygenation for severe adult respiratory failure (CESAR): a multicentre randomised controlled trial. *Lancet* 2009; 374(9698): 1351–63.

Smith F., Perkins G., Lamb S. et al. Effect of intravenous B2 agonist treatment on clinical outcomes in acute respiratory distress syndrome. *Lancet* 2012; 379: 229–35.

Young D., Lamb S., Shah S. et al. High frequency oscillation for acute respiratory distress syndrome. *N Engl J Med* 2013; 368: 806–13.

## Surviving sepsis

You are asked to review a 43-year-old man receiving chemotherapy for acute myeloid leukaemia. He presents to the emergency department feeling short of breath and generally unwell. On arrival his oxygen saturation was recorded as 88% on 15 l/min $O_2$. His blood pressure was initially 63/40 mmHg (mean arterial pressure (MAP) 48) and his pulse 125 bpm. He has received 2 litres of fluid and his blood pressure is now 74/50 mmHg (MAP 58). His oxygen saturations remain the same.

**Would you:**

a) Administer hydrocortisone immediately
b) Administer 500 ml of hydroxyethyl starch
c) Start peripheral dopamine whilst inserting a central venous catheter
d) Perform blood cultures before administering antibiotics
e) Target a mean arterial blood pressure of 75 mmHg

Answer: d)

The patient had been transferred to the intensive care unit. It is 3 hours since his admission to the hospital. His mean arterial blood pressure is 50 mmHg despite a further 1000 ml of intravenous fluid. A central venous catheter has been inserted. A lactate measurement is 7 mmol/l.

**Which of the following statements is true:**

a) Piperacillin/tazobactam would be sufficient antimicrobial treatment for presumed chest sepsis
b) Adrenaline would be the inotrope of choice
c) Vasopressin should be used as first-line vasopressor in severe hypotension
d) Intravenous immunoglobulins should be considered
e) Enteral nutrition should be started within 48 hours

Answer: e)

Severe sepsis can be defined as acute organ dysfunction secondary to documented or suspected infection. Septic shock is severe sepsis plus hypotension not reversed with fluid resuscitation. Severe sepsis and septic shock kill a quarter of those affected and the incidence is rising. Timely and appropriate management in the initial phases is likely to influence outcome.

The surviving sepsis guidelines were developed in 2002 as part of a commitment to reduce mortality from severe sepsis and septic shock worldwide.

The guidelines are divided into two bundles: one to be completed within 3 hours and one to be completed within 6 hours.

Within 3 hours:

1. Measure blood lactate.
2. Obtain blood cultures prior to antibiotic administration (provided delay no longer than 45 minutes).
3. Administer broad-spectrum antibiotics.
4. Administer 30 ml/kg of crystalloid for hypotension or lactate >4 mmol/l.

Within 6 hours:

1. Apply vasopressors (for hypotension that does not respond to fluid resuscitation) to maintain a MAP > 65 mmHg.
2. In the event of persistent arterial hypotension despite volume resuscitation or initial lactate >4 mmol/l, maintain adequate central venous pressure and adequate central venous oxygen saturation.
3. Re-measure lactate if initial lactate was high.

Crystalloids are the fluid of choice and starches should be avoided. Albumin can be considered if large volumes of crystalloid are being used. Blood transfusion should generally be avoided in most cases unless haemoglobin is less than 70 g/l.

Noradrenaline is the first-line vasopressor. Adrenaline may be considered as an additional agent to maintain MAP. Vasopressin may be added to noradrenaline to increase MAP or decrease noradrenaline dose. Vasopressin is not recommended as a single initial vasopressor. Dobutamine can be used in patients with an adequate MAP, with evidence of myocardial dysfunction or ongoing hypoperfusion. Dopamine may be considered in selected patients, those at low risk of a tachyarrhythmia and with an absolute or relative bradycardia.

Corticosteroids may be used if haemodynamic instability is not restored with fluid and vasopressor therapy.

Administration of antibiotics within the first hour should be a therapy goal. Empirical broad-spectrum antibiotics should be started and de-escalation to appropriate monotherapy should occur as soon as the susceptibility profile is known. Combination therapy should be instituted for neutropenic patients and those with multi-drug resistant pathogens such as acinetobacter and pseudomonas.

Activated protein C, immunoglobulins and selenium are not recommended. Supportive therapies such as lung protective ventilation, glucose control, deep venous thrombosis prophylaxis and early enteral nutrition should be instituted.

## Further reading

Dellinger R. P., Levy M. M., Rhodes A. et al. Surviving Sepsis Campaign: international guidelines for the management of severe sepsis and septic shock: 2012. *Crit Care Med.* 2013; 41: 580–637.

# Cardiogenic shock

A 65-year-old man with known ischaemic heart disease, essential hypertension and severe chronic obstructive pulmonary disease requiring home nebulizers, presents with a 4-hour history of central chest pain. He is cold, diaphoretic and confused. ECG shows an acute anterolateral myocardial infarction.

**Consider whether the following five statements are true or false.**

1. This patient has a 40% chance of developing cardiogenic shock.
2. The patient should be referred urgently for consideration of coronary revascularization.

The patient undergoes emergency percutaneous coronary intervention (PCI) and is transferred to the intensive care unit as his systolic blood pressure (SBP) remains below 90 mmHg and his urine output is 10 ml/h. A pulmonary artery flotation catheter is inserted and records the following:

- Mean arterial pressure (MAP) 50 mmHg
- Cardiac index (CI) 1.4 l/min/m$^2$
- Left ventricular end-diastolic pressure (LVEDP) 25 mmHg
- Right ventricular end-diastolic pressure (RVEDP) 12 mmHg
- Pulmonary artery occlusion pressure (PAOP) 25 mmHg

3. These cardiac indices are consistent with a diagnosis of cardiogenic shock.
4. Noradrenaline is the first-line agent of choice in this scenario.
5. Mechanical circulatory support is contraindicated for this patient.

Answers

1. False. Cardiogenic shock occurs as a complication of approximately 5–10% of cases of acute myocardial infarction.
2. True. The SHOCK (Should we emergently revascularize occluded coronary arteries for cardiogenic shock) trial demonstrated a significant decrease in mortality at 1 and 6 years following early PCI or coronary artery bypass grafting within 18 hours of onset of shock, compared with medical stabilization or delayed revascularization.
3. True. The haemodynamic criteria include persistent hypotension (SBP < 90 mmHg or MAP 30 mmHg lower than baseline) with a CI < 1.8 l/min/m$^2$ without inotropic or mechanical circulatory support (<2.0–2.2 l/min/m$^2$ with inotropes) and normal or elevated filling pressures (LVEDP > 18 mmHg, RVEDP > 10–15 mmHg) and a PAOP > 15 mmHg.

4. False. Current clinical practice supports the initiation of inotropic support, followed by a vasopressor in the event of refractory hypotension, although high quality evidence to support this practice is lacking. Agents of choice include dobutamine, adrenaline, noradrenaline, dopamine (high and low dose), phenylephrine and vasopressin. Adjunctive agents include phosphodiesterase inhibitors, e.g. milrinone, calcium sensitizers, e.g. levosimendan, and diuretics.
5. True. Mechanical support includes intra-aortic balloon pumps, left ventricular assist devices and extracorporeal membrane oxygenators. Contraindications to such devices are:

- Prolonged cardiopulmonary resuscitation with inadequate perfusion
- Advanced age
- Advanced malignancy
- Existing organ dysfunction
  - Advanced chronic obstructive pulmonary disease
  - Interstitial lung disease
  - Liver cirrhosis
- Previous stroke with significant disability
- Dementia
- End-stage renal failure (relative)
- Contraindication to anticoagulation (relative)
- Contraindication to transplant (relative)
- Severe aortic regurgitation or other aortopathies (intra-arterial blood pressure only).

## Further reading

Cove M. E., MacLaren G. Clinical review: mechanical circulatory support for cardiogenic shock complicating acute myocardial infarction. *Crit Care* 2010; 14(5): 235.
Nativi-Nicolau J., Selzman C. H., Fang J. C., Stehlik J. Pharmacologic therapies for acute cardiogenic shock. *Curr Opin Cardiol* 2014; 29(3): 250–7.
Van Herck J. L., Claeys M. J., De Paep R. et al. Management of cardiogenic shock complicating acute myocardial infarction. *Eur Heart J Acute Cardiovasc Care* 2015; 4(3): 278–97.

## Organ support: renal replacement therapy (RRT)

A 67-year-old man is admitted to the intensive care unit following emergency repair of a ruptured abdominal aortic aneurysm. On day 3 of his stay he is ventilated, with a $FiO_2$ of 0.5. He is receiving noradrenaline to maintain a mean arterial pressure (MAP) of 70 mmHg. His urine output is 10–20 ml/h. His creatinine is 331 µmol/l and his urea 25 mmol/l. His pH is 7.1 with a base deficit of −11 mEq/l. His $K^+$ is 5.9 mmol/l. His international normalized ratio (INR) is 4.5.

**Which of the following are true:**

a) Haemofiltration should be started on the basis of his urea and creatinine
b) Haemofiltration should be started on the basis of his urine output
c) Subclavian vein is the preferred site for vascular access for renal replacement therapy
d) A starting ultrafiltration rate of 20 ml/kg/h should be used
e) Anticoagulation will not be required for this patient

Answer: e)

Acute kidney injury can be defined as a sudden decline in kidney function resulting in electrolyte, fluid and acid–base dysregulation. It occurs in 13–18% of people admitted to hospital and between 4% and 25% of patients admitted to intensive care. Mortality is high in ICU patients with acute renal failure. Requirement for RRT is an independent risk factor for mortality.

Common causes of acute renal failure in the ICU include sepsis, major surgery, low cardiac output and hypovolaemia. Other causes include hepatorenal syndrome, trauma, cardiopulmonary bypass, abdominal compartment syndrome, obstruction and rhabdomyolysis.

Basic management includes treating the precipitating cause, ensuring adequate hydration and maintaining mean arterial blood pressure. Nephrotoxic drugs such as NSAIDs and ACE inhibitors should be stopped. Medical management should be used to treat complications such as hyperkalaemia and fluid overload.

However, patients should be considered for RRT if any of the following are not responding to medical management:

- Hyperkalaemia
- Metabolic acidosis
- Fluid overload including pulmonary oedema
- Complications of uraemia (e.g. pericarditis, encephalopathy)
- Drug toxicity of specific drugs (e.g. salicylates, methanol, ethylene glycol, barbiturates and lithium).

The decision to start RRT is usually based on the overall condition of the patient, rather than a single indication. Continuous methods of RRT are of benefit in the critically ill as they afford greater haemodynamic stability. Several modalities are available, including continuous veno-venous haemofiltration (CVVH), continuous veno-venous haemodiafiltration (CVVHDF), and continuous veno-venous haemodialysis (CVVHD). There is no evidence to favour any one in particular.

An ultrafiltrate rate of around 35 ml/kg/h is generally used. There has been interest in higher rates, particularly in sepsis, but no survival benefit has been found.

Vascular access is via a double lumen catheter placed in a central vein. The subclavian route is not the first choice, because of bleeding complications and a high rate of subclavian stenosis. This is particularly important for those who may need an arterio-venous fistula for long-term haemodialysis.

Anticoagulation is often required as the blood is in constant contact with the circuit and filter, triggering the clotting cascade. Clotting of the filter results in ineffective dialysis and increased cost. Heparin, prostacyclin or citrate may be used. In practice, anticoagulation may not be required in the critically ill owing to coexistent coagulopathy.

## Further reading

Dennen P., Douglas I. S., Anderson R. Acute kidney injury in the intensive care unit: an update for the intensivist. *Crit Care Med* 2010; 38(1): 261–75.

The RENAL Replacement Therapy Study Investigators. Intensity of continuous renal-replacement therapy in critically ill patients. *N Engl J Med* 2009; 361: 1627–38.

## Organ support: inotrope management

A good understanding of inotropes, vasopressors and their appropriate usage is a fundamental part of anaesthetic and ICU practice.

**Consider the following true/false questions:**
**Question 1**

a) Noradrenaline would be an adequate treatment for a high SVR
b) A $SvO_2$ of 61% implies a high output state
c) A fluid challenge would be first-line treatment in a patient with a SVV of 6
d) Dobutamine has vasopressor activity
e) Vasopressin is a vasopressor

**Question 2**

a) Patients can suffer from more than one cause of shock simultaneously
b) GTN has negative vasopressor activity
c) Enoximone has positive vasopressor activity
d) Milrinone has positive inotropic activity
e) Digoxin is a positive inotrope

Answers: FFFFT; TTFTT

Tables 12.1 and 12.2 are reminders of the basic physiology underlying the management of inotropes.

**Table 12.1** Adrenoceptor effects

| Adrenoceptor subtype | Clinical effect of stimulation |
|---|---|
| $\alpha_1$ | EXCITATORY: vasoconstriction, gut smooth muscle relaxation, saliva secretion, hepatic glycogenolysis |
| $\alpha_2$ (presynaptic) | INHIBITORY: inhibition of neurotransmitter release (noradrenaline and acetylcholine), stimulation of platelet aggregation |
| $\beta_1$ | EXCITATORY: increased heart rate (chronotropy), increased myocardial contractility (inotropy), gut smooth muscle relaxation, lipolysis |
| $\beta_2$ | INHIBITORY: vasodilatation, bronchodilation, visceral smooth muscle relaxation, hepatic glycogenolysis |
| $\beta_3$ | Lipolysis, thermogenesis |

Fundamentally, a decision must be made as to whether the hypotensive patient requires fluid, inotropy, chronotropy or vasoconstriction. Diastolic function is also important and diastolic dysfunction can be an independent cause of heart failure. Ventricular compliance and optimal filling are dependent on efficient myocardial relaxation (lusitropy). Lusitropy is an active process and can be improved by beta-adrenergic stimulation.

Central venous saturations can be monitored in critically ill patients and offer an indication of oxygen delivery ($SvO_2 = [SaO_2 - VO_2/CO][1/Hb \times 1.34]$). A requirement for increased systemic oxygen utilization ($VO_2$) will be compensated for by increased cardiac output (CO). If oxygen demand is not met, elevated oxygen extraction occurs in the peripheral tissues and $SvO_2$ falls. The normal range is 65–75%. Low $SvO_2$ is predictive of a poor outcome. However, a normal or high $SvO_2$ does not guarantee adequate tissue oxygenation, as in the case of shunting or cell death; here, the tissues fail to extract oxygen and $SvO_2$ may be high despite ongoing cellular hypoxia.

When faced with a hypotensive patient, acceptable practice is to administer an initial fluid challenge. Patients may respond with a blood pressure that increases and remains elevated. A systematic approach to hypotension management is key and in many cases more formal

**Table 12.2** Summary of commonly used inotropes

| Inotrope | Site of action | Major clinical effect |
|---|---|---|
| Adrenaline | $\beta_2, \beta_1, \alpha_1$ | Inotropy, chronotropy, increased systemic vascular resistance (SVR) and increased glucose |
| Noradrenaline | $\alpha_1$ | Vasoconstriction |
| Dopamine | $DA_1$ (at low dose) $\beta_1$ (at moderate dose) $\alpha_1$ (at high dose) | Reno-splanchnic dilatation Inotropy Increased SVR |
| Dobutamine | $\beta_2, \beta_1$ | Inotropy, chronotropy, decreased SVR |
| Dopexamine | $DA_1, \beta_2$ | Reno-splanchnic dilatation, chronotropy |
| Isoprenaline | $\beta_1, \beta_2$ | Chronotropy, decreased SVR |
| Enoximone | Phosphodiesterase inhibitor | Inotropy, decreased SVR and decreased pulmonary vascular resistance (PVR) |
| Levosimendan | Calcium sensitizer | Inotropy, decreased SVR |
| Vasopressin | $V_1$ | Increased SVR |

cardiac output monitoring is required (see Chapter 10). Most causes of hypotension can be considered as a problem with one of the following: preload, contractility and afterload. Typically, the clinical history may suggest a contribution from all three; therefore, a more objective method of assessment is required. This may include:

- Stroke volume variation (SVV) – a high SVV suggests decreased preload. Fluids are most likely to be required here.
- Systemic vascular resistance (SVR) – a low SVR suggests vasodilatation +/− vasoplegia. Common causes for this are sepsis and drugs. Many anaesthetic and sedative agents are implicated here, including central neuraxial blockade. Treatment is with a vasopressor such as noradrenaline or vasopressin. Adrenaline also has vasopressor activity, although would not be a first-line agent because of its potent beta activity.
- Cardiac index – a low cardiac index implies that the cardiac output is insufficient for the body surface area. This may be due to a low heart rate or stroke volume. Bradycardias are easily diagnosed and treated. If a low stroke volume is not the result of a reduced preload, the treatment is with an inotrope. Examples include adrenaline and dobutamine. Incidentally, an extreme tachycardia can also cause hypotension by means of a reduction in stroke volume (as a result of a low left ventricular end-diastolic volume due to a reduced filling time). Milrinone and enoximone are also inotropes. They increase the stroke volume for a given preload. However, they do not increase the afterload. Dobutamine is a commonly used inotrope in the intensive care unit, which also increases contractility but can also decrease SVR.

## Further reading

Brookes Z. L. S. Pharmacological modulation of cardiac function and blood vessel calibre. *Anaesth Intensive Care Med* 2013; 14(1): 27–31.

Trinh J., Palmer K. Inotropes. *Anaesth Intensive Care Med* 2012; 13(10): 492–8.

van Beest P., Wietasch G., Scheeren T., Spronk P., Kuiper M. Clinical review: use of venous oxygen saturations as a goal – a yet unfinished puzzle. *Crit Care* 2011; 15(5): 232. Available at http://ccforum.com/content/15/5/232 (accessed 30 August 2015).

# Sedation in the intensive care unit

Sedation is the reduction of stress, anxiety, irritability or excitement by administration of a sedative agent or drug. A combination of pharmacological and non-pharmacological therapies are commonly adopted on intensive care units (ICUs). Sedation is required to facilitate certain procedures within the unit and maximize successful patient outcome.

Consider the following true/false questions:

a) Benzodiazepines are related to a higher rate of ICU delirium
b) When used as an infusion, alfentanil has been shown to reduce length of stay when compared to fentanyl
c) Remifentanil produces tachyphylaxis
d) Clonidine and dexmedetomidine are both alpha-2 agonists
e) Under-sedation has been shown to produce higher rates of ICU delirium

Answers: TTTTF

Over-sedation is a major problem, and maintenance of lighter sedation in patients who are otherwise stable has been shown to reduce length of stay, whilst decreasing mortality and morbidity. Sedation should be titrated so that the patient receives the minimum effective dose that ensures safety and comfort. ICU delirium has been associated with higher sedation levels.

There are different tools available to measure the depth of sedation on the ICU, and no tool has been shown to be superior. However, it makes sense that units adopt a single scoring tool to avoid confusion between patients and staff. Some of the sedation scores you may encounter are:

• Sedation-Agitation Scale (Riker)
• The Ramsay Sedation Scale
• The Richmond Agitation-Sedation Scale (RASS)
• The Motor Activity Assessment Scale.

The RASS has been demonstrated to be simple to perform and reproduce. Patients are scored from −5, which is unresponsive to physical stimulus, through 0, which is alert and calm, to +4, which is combative and an immediate danger to staff. Appropriate levels (when neuromuscular blockade is not required) are −2 to +1. The RASS score makes up part of the Confusion Assessment Method for the ICU (CAM-ICU) delirium screen.

Delirium is defined as an acute confusional state and includes:

• Disturbance of consciousness
• Change in cognition
• Development over a short time period
• Evidence there is a pathophysiological cause related to a general medical or surgical condition.

There are three subtypes: hyperactive, hypoactive and mixed, where the state fluctuates between the former two. The incidence is somewhere between 22% and 81% in intensive care patients and it is associated with significantly higher mortality and increased length of stay.

Table 12.3 shows some of the advantages and disadvantages of commonly used drugs in providing sedation and treating delirium.

**Table 12.3** Drugs commonly used to provide sedation or treat delirium

| Drug | Advantages | Disadvantage |
|------|-----------|-------------|
| Propofol | Infusion easy to titrate, antiemetic | Hypotension, respiratory depression, hyperlipidaemia and metabolic acidosis – propofol infusion syndrome |
| Opioids (morphine, fentanyl, alfentanil, remifentanil) | Potent analgesia, cough suppression | Reduced blood pressure in hypovolaemia, respiratory depression, gastric stasis, nausea and vomiting, constipation |
| Benzodiazepines (midazolam, lorazepam, diazepam) | Anxiolysis, cardiovascular system stable | May promote delirium, active metabolites |
| Ketamine | Potent analgesia, airway reflexes intact, maintains blood pressure, bronchodilation | Sympathetic stimulation, hypersalivation, hallucinations |
| Alpha-2 agonists (clonidine, dexmedetomidine) | Analgesia and anxiolysis, minimal respiratory depression | Bradycardia, hypotension, decreased clearance in hepatic failure (dexmedetomidine) |
| Atypical antipsychotics (risperidone, quetiapine) | Reduced extrapyramidal side effects | Hypotension (orthostatic), sedation |
| Thiopentone | Anticonvulsant, reduces intracranial pressure and cerebral metabolic rate | Decreased cardiac output, respiratory depression, infusion – long context sensitive half-life, intra-arterial injection – distal limb ischaemia |
| Dopamine antagonists (haloperidol, levomepromazine) | Antiemetic, useful in palliative care | Akathisia, anticholinergic effects, may cause neuroleptic malignant syndrome |

Some drugs have been shown to have additional superior qualities to others in providing sedation and treating delirium:

- Benzodiazepines have been shown to result in a higher rate of ICU delirium.
- Propofol has been shown to produce shorter lengths of stay.
- Fentanyl has been shown to have an increased length of stay due to a context sensitivity-related prolonged half-life.

Dexmedetomidine has been used successfully outside the United Kingdom for many years; however, the cost has prohibited its use thus far in the UK.

There are a number of validated non-pharmacological interventions that can help reduce anxiety and pain. These include reduction in noise levels, ensuring adequate uninterrupted natural sleep, normalizing the diurnal pattern, continuous orientation of the patient in terms of time, place and person, room temperature and cognitive stimulation.

# Further reading

Porter R., McClure J. Sedation and delirium in the intensive care unit. *Anaesth Intensive Care Med* 2013; 14(1): 22–6.

Riker R. R., Fraser G. L. Altering intensive care sedation paradigms to improve patient outcomes. *Anesthesiol Clin* 2011; 29: 663–74.

Rowe K., Fletcher S. Sedation in the intensive care unit. *Contin Educ Anaesth Crit Care Pain*. 2008; 8(2):50–5.

Salluh J. I., Soares M., Teles J. M. et al. Delirium epidemiology in critical care (DECCA): an international study. *Crit Care* 2010; 14: R210.

# End-of-life issues and donation after brainstem death (DBD)

A 19-year-old male is diagnosed as brainstem dead on your intensive care unit following a road traffic collision. His family are keen for organ donation and he is a suitable candidate. While the retrieval teams are being organized you notice he is becoming hypotensive and polyuric.

**The most appropriate course of action is:**

a) These are the pathophysiological changes associated with brainstem death, and as such treatment should be withdrawn
b) Inotropic support should not be escalated, as it will damage the organs suitable for retrieval
c) Vasopressin should be considered and DDAVP used if the polyuria continues
d) Plasma and urine electrolytes and osmolalities should be sent and a 5% dextrose infusion started
e) Cancel the retrieval team and inform the family, as the organs will no longer be suitable for retrieval

Answer: c)

Once brainstem death has been confirmed, the emphasis of treatment changes from that of preservation of brain function to optimization of the transplantable organs. By maintaining haemodynamic, respiratory and endocrine stability with prompt treatment, transplantable organ function will hopefully be maintained, and even improved. This ultimately leads to a greater chance of transplantation success.

General intensive care measures should continue with ongoing nutritional support, maintenance of tight glycaemic control, continuation of antibiotics and physiotherapy. Methylprednisolone (15 mg/kg IV) should be given as soon as possible. Donor organ goals should be set with respect to cardiovascular, respiratory and endocrine support, and may be easier to achieve than those set for brain function preservation previously.

Cardiovascular changes are common. Initially there may be a Cushing's response with a subsequent 'sympathetic storm' of varying intensity (hypertensive episodes, tachycardia and vasoconstriction). Tachycardia may need to be treated with short-acting beta blockade. Following this there is usually marked vasodilatation and relative hypovolaemia (approximately 80% of patients will develop this). This should be treated with fluid resuscitation, but the most effective first intervention may in fact be restoration of vascular tone using vasopressin (4 mcg bolus followed by a 3 mcg/h infusion).

'Lung-protective' strategies for ventilation should be continued with the aim of keeping $SpO_2$ at 92–95% and $PaO_2 > 8$ kPa, using the lowest possible inspired oxygen concentration. Head-up positioning and regular turning should continue, and recruitment manoeuvres should be used as necessary.

Diabetes insipidus (DI) occurs in approximately 65% of patients. The resulting polyuria will lead to electrolyte and water losses and exacerbate the vasodilator hypotension. If there has been a sudden unexplained rise in urine output, treatment should be commenced even before receiving confirmation, which is obtained by urinary and plasma electrolytes and osmolality. Vasopressin infusions may often treat DI, but a 1–2 mcg bolus of desmopressin (DDAVP) may also be needed. This can be repeated as required.

## Further reading

McKeown D. W., Bonser R. S., Kellum J. A. Management of the heart-beating brain dead donor. *Br J Anaesth* 2012; 108(Suppl 1): i96–107.

NHS Institute for Innovation and Improvement. *Map of Medicine.* Medicine/Organ donation/ Donation after brain-stem death, Adult. Available at http://mapofmedicine.com/supporting-organ-donation-development-programme (accessed 9 January 2016).

Waldmann C., Soni N., Rhodes A. The potential heart-beating organ donor. In *Oxford Desk Reference: Critical Care.* Oxford: Oxford University Press, 2008, pp. 534–6.

# End-of-life issues and donation after cardiac death (DCD)

A patient on ICU has his treatment withdrawn and suffers a cardiac arrest. His kidneys are suitable for non-heart-beating organ donation. The transplant coordinator is asking for death to be confirmed quickly so that he can be moved to theatre where the retrieval team is waiting. During your examination he takes a few shallow breaths.

**The best course of action is:**

a) If there is no ECG activity, confirm death so that he can be moved to theatre promptly
b) Stop the examination and observe for a further 5 minutes from the next point of cardiorespiratory arrest
c) Start CPR as he has shown signs of life
d) Continue to examine him and confirm death as soon as he stops breathing again
e) Tell the transplant coordinator to cancel the retrieval team as he is still breathing

Answer: b)

The current position in law is that there is no statutory definition of death in the UK. Subsequent to the proposal of the 'brain death criteria' by the Conference of Medical Royal Colleges in 1976, the courts in England and Northern Ireland have adopted these criteria as part of the law for the diagnosis of death.

For people suffering cardiorespiratory arrest, death can be diagnosed when a registered medical practitioner, or other appropriately trained and qualified individual, confirms the irreversible cessation of neurological (pupil), cardiac and respiratory activity. Diagnosing death in this situation requires confirmation that there has been irreversible damage to the vital centres in the brainstem, due to the length of time in which the circulation to the brain has been absent.

The individual should be observed by the person responsible for confirming death for a minimum of 5 minutes to establish that irreversible cardiorespiratory arrest has occurred. The absence of mechanical cardiac function is normally confirmed using a combination of the absence of a central pulse on palpation and absence of heart sounds on auscultation.

These criteria will normally suffice in the primary care setting. However, their use can be supplemented in the hospital setting by one or more of the following: asystole on a continuous ECG display, absence of pulsatile flow using direct intra-arterial pressure monitoring or absence of contractile activity using echocardiography.

Any spontaneous return of cardiac or respiratory activity during this period of observation should prompt a further 5 minutes of observation from the next point of cardiorespiratory arrest. After 5 minutes of continued cardiorespiratory arrest, the absence of the pupillary responses to light, or the corneal reflexes, and of any motor response to supra-orbital pressure should be confirmed. The time of death is recorded as the time at which these criteria are fulfilled.

## Further reading

Academy of Medical Royal Colleges. *A Code of Practice for the Diagnosis and Confirmation of Death*. London: the Academy, 2008. Available at www.aomrc.org.uk/publications/reports-a-guidance?lang=en&limit=100&start=100 (accessed 9 January 2016).

# Paediatrics

*Encountering a sick child or even dealing electively with healthy children is an area that you may feel particularly anxious about on returning to work. This chapter covers practical points for dealing with children including fluid management, sedation and intraosseous access. Some paediatric emergencies are also covered including management of the stridulous child, asthma and shock. In addition there are chapters on paediatric physiology and equipment (Chapter 28), paediatric resuscitation algorithms (Chapter 30) and the joint Association of Paediatric Anaesthetists (APA) and Difficult Airway Society (DAS) guidelines for management of the difficult paediatric airway (Chapter 33). Using these sections together should help you to feel more confident approaching paediatric cases on your return to work.*

## Paediatric fluids in sepsis

A 6-year-old child presents with a 4-day history of right iliac fossa pain and vomiting. She has signs of peritonism. The surgical team is concerned she has a perforated appendix and wish to take her to theatre immediately. You review her on the admissions unit. She is lying quietly following some analgesia and appears pale. Her observations reveal a tachypnoea and tachycardia although she is normotensive. You are asked for your advice on preoperative fluid management by the foundation doctor on the ward.

**What will your initial approach to her fluid management be, including fluid choice, volume and speed of administration?**

- She is showing signs of shock. Hypotension in children is a very late sign.
- Fluid resuscitation with bolus of 10–20 ml/kg as per APLS protocol.
- Isotonic crystalloid (0.9% sodium chloride/Hartmann's solution) or albumin over 5–10 minutes.
- Reassess after each bolus.
- The development of crackles or hepatomegaly indicate fluid overload.

**At what point would you consider her shock to be resistant to fluid therapy and what would be your course of action?**

- After administration of 40 ml/kg it is suggested that intubation and ventilation are considered if shock is not improving.
- After 60 ml/kg consider the need for inotropes.

---

*Returning to Work in Anaesthesia*, ed. Emma Plunkett, Emily Johnson and Anna Pierson.
Published by Cambridge University Press. © Cambridge University Press 2016.

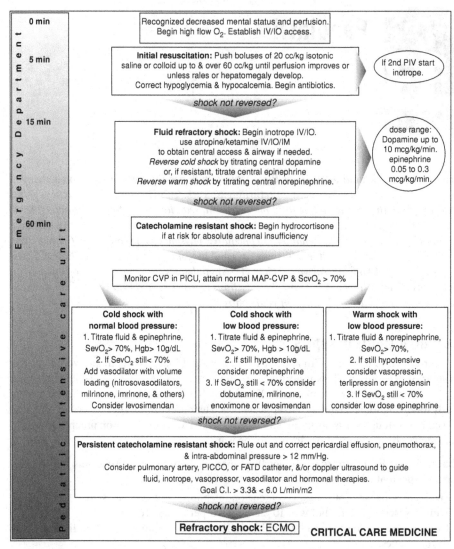

**Figure 13.1** Algorithm for Management of Paediatric Sepsis. Reproduced with permission Brierly J., Carcillo J. A., Choong K., et al. Clinical Practice Parameters for hemodynamic support of pediatric and neonatal septic shock: 2007 update from the American College of Critical Care Medicine. *Crit Care Med* 2009; 37(2): 666–99. Copyright © 2009 by the Society of Critical Care Medicine and Lippincott Williams & Wilkins.

- If signs of fluid overload develop prior to this, diuretics and inotropes should be considered at this point.
- For the management of refractory shock see Figure 13.1.

**Once you feel any signs of shock are adequately reversed what other aspects of fluid therapy must be covered?**

- Correction of dehydration.
- Maintenance fluid.
- Replacement of ongoing losses.

# Further reading

Advanced Life Support Group edited by M. Samuels, S. Wieteska. *Advanced Paediatric Life Support: The Practical Approach*, 5th edn. London: Wiley-Blackwell, 2011.

APA Consensus Guideline on Perioperative Fluid Management in Children. V1.1 September 2007. AAGBI. Available at http://www.apagbi.org.uk/sites/default/files/Perioperative_Fluid_Management_2007.pdf (accessed 2 January 2016).

Brierley J., Carcillo J. A., Choong K. et al. Clinical practice parameters for hemodynamic support of pediatric and neonatal septic shock: 2007 update from the American College of Critical Care Medicine. *Crit Care Med* 2009; 37: 666–88.

Dellinger R. P., Levy M. M., Rhodes A., et al. Surviving Sepsis Campaign: international guidelines for management of severe sepsis and septic shock: 2012. *Crit Care Med* 2013; 41: 580–637.

# Practical differences between adult and paediatric anaesthesia

You are asked to anaesthetize a 4-year-old child for an open reduction and internal fixation of her forearm. She is usually fit and well. She is fasted. She weighs 17 kg.

**Consider the following true/false questions:**

1. Premedication with 500 mg of oral paracetamol is suitable
2. Oral midazolam 0.5 mg/kg can be administered 60 minutes preoperatively
3. The starvation time for formula milk is 6 hours
4. A T-piece circuit should be used
5. A size 3 laryngeal mask airway (LMA) could be used
6. A size 5 uncuffed endotracheal tube could be used
7. The minimum alveolar concentration (MAC) of sevoflurane is lower in infants than in adults
8. Maintenance fluid requirements are 54 ml/h
9. The maintenance fluid of choice is sodium chloride 0.18% with glucose 4%
10. Codeine phosphate at 1 mg/kg is a suitable post-operative medication

Answers: FFTTFTFTFF

The practical differences between anaesthetizing adults and children include differences in preoperative management, equipment, drug dosing and fluids. During the preoperative assessment the child will be seen alongside his or her parents and, age permitting, have their questions and anxieties addressed. The planned approach to induction should be explained to the child and parent. Analgesic options should be discussed and consent for suppositories obtained if planned.

Starvation times are identical to adults except breast milk, which can be allowed up to 4 hours preoperatively. Starvation should be minimized for comfort and to reduce risk of nausea and vomiting.

The child should be weighed to allow drug dosing. Premedication may include sedative agents, analgesics and topical local anaesthetic cream.

Sedatives may often fail and timing of administration is important. Options include:

- Midazolam 0.5 mg/kg given 15–30 minutes preoperatively.
- Ketamine 3–8 mg/kg orally can be used 30–60 minutes before surgery.
- Chloral hydrate 50 mg/kg orally.

Equipment should be prepared and a range of airways in different sizes should be available. A laryngoscope with a straight blade may be preferable in babies and infants, changing to a curved blade in the older age group. Endotracheal tube size can be calculated using the formula age/4 + 4. Generally uncuffed tubes are used until the age of 8 years. However, there has been a recent move to using cuffed tubes in a younger age group in emergencies, for those at risk of aspiration or those with low lung compliance.

Laryngeal masks are available in the sizes shown in Table 13.1.

A T-piece circuit can be used in children less than 20 kg as it has less dead space but a paediatric circle is also available.

Similar induction agents to adults may be used but a gas induction may be preferred by some children. For maintenance of anaesthesia MAC is higher in infants than adults. Propofol infusions should be avoided in children under 16 years of age as propofol infusion syndrome is more common in children.

During maintenance of anaesthesia attention to temperature management is important. Radiation is the main source of heat loss and babies and infants have a higher thermo-neutral environmental temperature than older children. Exposure should be minimized and babies' heads covered. Overhead heaters, warming mattresses and forced air warming systems can be used.

Intravenous fluids are not usually required for short procedures.

The Holliday–Segar formula can be used for maintenance calculations, shown in Table 13.2.

Children above 1 month of age should receive isotonic fluid. Less than 1 month of age or at risk of hypoglycaemia should receive dextrose-containing solutions or have blood glucose checked regularly.

Shocked children should receive fluid boluses of 10–20 ml/kg titrated to response.

Intra and post-operative analgesia can include:

- Paracetamol at 15 mg/kg maximum 4 hourly, 4 times a day. If being administered intravenously the dose should be reduced to 7.5 mg/kg for children under 10 kg.
- Ibuprofen 5–10 mg/kg 3–4 times a day. (Maximum 30 mg/kg/day.)
- Oral morphine 200–400 mcg/kg 4 hourly.

Codeine should now be avoided in children under 12 years and any child with a history of sleep apnoea. This is because of the unreliable metabolism and risk of apnoea.

**Table 13.1** LMA sizes by weight

| LMA size | 1 | 1.5 | 2 | 2.5 | 3 |
|----------|---|-----|---|-----|---|
| Weight | Up to 5 kg | 5–10 kg | 10–20 kg | 20–30 kg | 30–50 kg |

**Table 13.2** Holliday–Segar formula for paediatric maintenance fluid calculation

| Body weight | Daily fluid requirement |
|-------------|-------------------------|
| 0–10 kg | 4 ml/kg/h |
| 10–20 kg | 40 ml/h + 2 ml/kg/h above 10 kg |
| >20 kg | 60 ml/h + 1 ml/kg/h above 20 kg |

# Further reading

APA Consensus Guidelines on Perioperative Fluid Management in Children. V1.1 September 2007. APAGBI. Available at http://www.apagbi.org.uk/sites/default/files/Perioperative_Fluid_Management_2007.pdf (accessed 2 January 2016).

# Intraosseous access

A 6-year-old child presents to the emergency department, moribund. Intravenous access is proving impossible and so intraosseous access (IO) is suggested to facilitate ongoing resuscitation.

**Which sites would you choose for your first access attempt?**

Intraosseous access is popular in paediatric resuscitation. It provides a non-collapsible compartment in which to infuse drugs and fluids in a population who not only require rapid intervention but also can have very difficult venous access. It should be attempted in a resuscitation setting if intravenous access is not achieved within 90 seconds. It is increasingly popular owing to its ease of insertion and low risk of complications.

A number of sites of insertion have been described, with the proximal tibia (2–3 cm below the anterior tuberosity) or distal femur (3 cm above the lateral condyle) being the preferred sites for resuscitation as they leave access to the airway and chest.

**What other sites can be used?**

Other sites you might consider are the proximal humerus (older children) or distal tibia.

**What are the contraindications for insertion?**

These include ipsilateral fracture, previous placement in the same limb, osteopetrosis and osteogenesis imperfecta (risk of fracture), coagulopathy and overlying skin infection (a relative contraindication).

**What kit is available?**

Paediatric patients have the benefit of thin, easily penetrable cortical bone which facilitates the use of hand-held needles. For the paediatric age group most people will be familiar with the Cook IO needle. This device consists of a needle and stylet with a shaped handle which is contoured for the palm of the hand. This allows firm pressure to be applied to pierce the bone cortex. In neonatal patients spinal needles may be used for IO access.

The extension of IO access into adult practice has necessitated the introduction of powered devices. These devices are increasingly popular in paediatrics. The EZ-IO has a battery-powered driver with several choices of needle size. The size of the needle is determined by the weight of the patient and the depth is set by the operator prior to insertion. A give is felt as the bone cortex is breached.

Complications of IO insertion include fracture, embolism, extravasation, compartment syndrome, haematoma formation and infection.

**What blood tests can be done on samples taken?**

Full blood count, biochemistry, cross-matching and cultures can be done on blood samples but you need to inform the laboratory of the sample site. In some hospitals, a bedside glucose test can also be done. It is reported that venous blood gas analysis can be performed on marrow samples but in practice you should check first: the sample will clog up some machines.

**What drugs and fluids can be given via the intraosseous route?**

All resuscitation drugs and fluids (including blood products) can be administered via the IO route.

IO access is usually removed when IV access is established, usually by 6–12 hours. It may be left in place for longer (up to 96 hours) but the risk of infection and dislodgement increases.

## Further reading

Eslami P. Pediatric intraosseous access. *Medscape Reference* 2014. Available at http://emedicine .medscape.com/article/940993-overview (accessed 5 April 2015).
Intraosseous infusion. *Patient Plus*. Available at http://www.patient.co.uk/doctor/intraosseous-infusion (accessed 5 April 2015).

## Intravenous fluid replacement

You see a 17-month-old weighing 10 kg who is listed for orchidopexy. His mother tells you that he has not had anything to eat or drink since 20:00. It is now 11:00 and the patient is third on the list and expected to go to theatre at 15:00. You give the child a drink now (150 ml).

**What will his fluid deficit be at induction?**

a) 190 ml
b) 240 ml
c) 550 ml
d) 610 ml
e) 760 ml

Answer: d)

Maintenance fluid requirements, and therefore fluid deficit in starved patients, can be calculated using the formula of Holliday and Segar shown in Table 13.2.

This child's maintenance fluid requirements are estimated at 40 ml/h. Without the drink, the deficit when he arrives in theatre will be 40 ml × 19 = 760 ml. The drink reduces this to 610 ml, which equates to 10% of total body water (TBW). The child described in this scenario should have been given his usual breakfast at 07:00 and ideally a clear fluid drink at 11:00. He would then have a fluid deficit of only (40 × 7) – 200 = 80 ml (approx. 1% TBW).

It is important to note that even the gross error of a 15-hour fast as opposed to a 2-hour fast for clear fluid is unlikely to make a physiologically significant impact on the cardiovascular status of the child, or necessitate a different anaesthetic technique for an otherwise fit child. However, it may give you a very unhappy and uncooperative child! General principles of paediatric fluid management require consideration of the following three issues:

1. Fluid deficit
2. Maintenance requirements
3. Losses due to surgery.

Isotonic fluid should be given in theatre to replace these losses. This should contain dextrose if the child is:

- less than 1 month of age
- less than the 3rd centile for weight
- requiring parenteral nutrition
- requiring a dextrose-containing drip before theatre

- having prolonged surgery (>3 hours)
- having extensive regional anaesthesia.

Blood loss can be replaced with crystalloid or colloid initially, and with blood when the haematocrit has fallen to less than 25%. In practice, if sensible fasting guidance is followed (6 hours for food, 2 hours for clear fluids), a fluid bolus of 10 ml/kg can be given, followed with maintenance fluid at a rate determined using the Holliday–Segar formula.

## Further reading

APA Consensus Guideline on Perioperative Fluid Management in Children. V1.1 September 2007. APAGBI. Available at http://www.apagbi.org.uk/sites/default/files/Perioperative_Fluid_Management_2007.pdf (accessed 5 April2015).

## Use of codeine: post-tonsillectomy analgesia

An 8-year-old in a District General Hospital is to undergo tonsillectomy for recurrent tonsillitis. They have a diagnosis of mild asthma.

**When considering post-operative analgesia are the following statements true or false:**

a) A non-steroidal anti-inflammatory drug (NSAID) cannot be given
b) Discharging them with a higher dose of paracetamol (90 mg/kg/day) would be appropriate
c) Codeine is a suitable option as they do not have a history of obstructive sleep apnoea
d) Dexamethasone may help

Answers: FFFT

a) Although leukotriene production as a result of NSAID use may exacerbate asthma, this is rare with 2% potentially being sensitive to aspirin and only 5% of those to other NSAIDs. Unless there is a documented history of sensitivity, children should not be denied a trial, especially in the controlled setting of a hospital.
b) It used to be suggested that doses up to 90 mg/kg/day could be used safely; however, there is evidence that doses greater than 75 mg/kg/day for at least 2 days may cause liver damage but with minimal analgesic benefit.
c) The Medicines and Healthcare Products Regulatory Agency released a drug safety update in July 2013 stating that codeine should only be used to relieve acute moderate pain in children over 12 years of age (18 years if they are undergoing tonsillectomy or adenoidectomy and have obstructive sleep apnoea). The inability to know the extent of conversion to morphine given the genetic variability of the CYP2D6 enzyme makes both analgesia and the risk of side effects, such as respiratory depression, unpredictable. If paracetamol and a NSAID are insufficient, the Association of Paediatric Anaesthetists suggest alternative agents are oral morphine, oxycodone and tramadol but that each has its own considerations, and as such you should refer to local guidelines or discuss it with the local tertiary centre.
d) In combination with intraoperative opioids and regular NSAID and/or paracetamol, dexamethasone is recommended by the Association of Paediatric Anaesthetists. It has the added benefit of antiemetic properties.

# Further reading

Anderson B., Woollard G. A., Holford N. H. A model for size and age in the pharmacokinetics of paracetamol in neonates, infants and children. *Br J Clin Pharmacol* 2000; 50(2): 125–34.

Association of Paediatric Anaesthetists. Codeine and Paracetamol in Paediatric use. 2013. Available at http://www.apagbi.org.uk/news/2013/ codeine-and-paracetamol-use-children-new-advice-october-2013 (accessed January 2016).

Association of Paediatric Anaesthetists and Royal College of Paediatrics and Child Health. Guidance for the administration of codeine and alternative opioid analgesics in children. 2013. http://www .apagbi.org.uk/sites/default/files/images/Codeine_Nov2013.pdf (accessed January 2016).

Association of Paediatric Anaesthetists of Great Britain and Ireland. Good practice in postoperative and procedural pain management, 2nd edition, 2012. *Paediatr Anaesth* 2012; 22 Suppl 1: 1–79. Available at http://www.apagbi.org.uk/publications/apa-guidelines.pdf (accessed 2 January 2016).

Kozer E., Greenberg R., Zimmerman D. R., Berkovitch M. Repeated supratherapeutic doses of paracetamol in children a literature review and suggested clinical approach. *Acta Paediatr* 2006; 95: 1165–71.

Medicines and Healthcare Regulatory Agency. UK Public Assessment Report. Liquid paracetamol for children: revised UK dosing instructions have been introduced. 2011. Available at http://www .mhra.gov.uk/home/groups/s-par/documents/websiteresources/con134921.pdf (accessed 2 January 2016).

Medicines and Healthcare Regulatory Agency. *Drug Safety Update* 2013; 6(12): A1.

# Sedation in paediatrics: premedication

A 7-year-old, 20 kg child presents for orthopaedic surgery. He is very anxious and does not want to cooperate with examination. His parents say that he had a traumatic experience with a previous anaesthetic and they would rather he had a sedative premedication this time. The case is scheduled second on a busy list. You expect it will be about an hour before this patient is called for.

**Which of the following would you choose as a pre-med?**

a) Oral clonidine 60 mcg, 30 minutes before anaesthetic
b) Intranasal ketamine 20 mg, 30 minutes before anaesthetic
c) Oral chloral hydrate 600 mg, 45 minutes before anaesthetic
d) Oral midazolam 10 mg, 30 minutes before anaesthetic

Answer: d)

Appropriate use of sedative premedication in paediatric practice can turn a traumatic experience into a tolerable one. Inappropriate use is counterproductive. Timing and dosage are critical.

All of the doses listed here are correct. Clonidine may be used as an oral sedative, and the dose of 3–4 mcg/kg is appropriate but it takes slightly longer to work; at least 45 minutes. The dose of chloral hydrate is 30–50 mg/kg, 45–60 minutes prior to the procedure (maximum dose of 1 g). Chloral hydrate is more commonly used to sedate younger children for imaging investigations. It has an unpleasant taste so needs to be diluted with water or juice.

Midazolam is probably the most commonly used preoperative sedative. The dose of 0.5 mg/kg is appropriate for oral dosing up to a maximum of 20 mg. It has a rapid onset of action (20–30 minutes for peak effect) and a faster recovery than other benzodiazepines. Its bitter taste also needs disguising – Calpol© is sometimes used for this.

There is evidence for the efficacy of intranasal agents in this situation and ketamine (6 mg/kg) has been used successfully. Intranasal diamorphine (0.1 mg/kg) is sometimes given in the emergency department to treat acute pain in children, but the BNFc states that there is limited safety and efficacy data to support this.

## Further reading

British National Formulary for Children. March 2015. 15.1.4 Sedative and analgesic perioperative drugs.

## The shocked neonate

A 10-day-old neonate presents to the emergency department of a District General Hospital with irritability and difficulty feeding following an uneventful pregnancy and delivery. On examination the infant's heart rate is 200 bpm, respiratory rate 80 breaths/min and capillary refill time is 4 seconds.

**How would you recognize shock in a neonate?**

Prompt diagnosis of neonatal shock is vital as early recognition and aggressive resuscitation improves outcome.

**Table 13.3** Signs suggestive of neonatal shock

| | |
|---|---|
| Heart rate | <100 or >180 bpm |
| Respiratory rate | >60/min |
| Systolic blood pressure (late sign) | <65 mmHg (if under 1 week)<br><75 mmHg (if 1 week to 1 month) |
| Capillary refill time | >3 seconds |
| Lethargy or Glasgow Coma Score (GCS) | <12/15 (irritable, responding only to pain or unresponsive) |

**What would your initial management of this infant be?**

If working in a hospital without paediatric intensive care facilities, early communication with the regional paediatric retrieval service will enable support to be provided during resuscitation whilst the team is mobilized.

Your 'ABC' approach to the initial assessment should involve:

Airway and breathing: apply 100% oxygen initially. Positive end-expiratory pressure will reduce the work of breathing. Ventilation will be required if there is respiratory failure or a reduced conscious level.

Circulation: rapidly secure intravenous access (ideally two). If difficult, site an intraosseous needle and give an initial bolus of 20 ml/kg fluid. Ongoing signs of shock after three fluid boluses (60 ml/kg) or development of fluid overload (hepatomegaly, worsening respiratory function) requires inotropes and ventilation. Inotropes (usually

**Table 13.4** Drugs and equipment used during resuscitation of the shocked neonate

| | |
|---|---|
| ETT size | 3.0–3.5 mm (site orogastric tube in ventilated neonates) |
| Intraosseous site | 2–3 cm below the tibial tuberosity or distal tibia |
| Fluid resuscitation | 20 ml/kg boluses of crystalloid or 4.5% human albumin solution |
| Induction drugs | Ketamine 1–2 mg/kg<br>Fentanyl 2–5 mcg/kg<br>Suxamethonium 1–2 mg/kg |
| Sedative infusions:<br>• Morphine (10–40 mcg/kg/h)<br>• Midazolam (1–4 mcg/kg/min) | Morphine: 1 mg/kg in 50 ml 5% dextrose (1 ml/h = 20 mcg/kg/h)<br>Midazolam: 3 mg/kg in 50 ml 5% dextrose (1 ml/h = 1 mcg/kg/min) |
| Correction of hypoglycaemia | 2 ml/kg of 10% dextrose |
| Inotrope infusions:<br>• Dopamine (2.5–20 mcg/kg/min)<br>• Adrenaline (0.1–4 mcg/kg/min) | Dopamine: 15 mg/kg in 50 ml 5% dextrose (1 ml/h = 5 mcg/kg/h)<br>Adrenaline: 0.3 mg/kg in 50 ml 5% dextrose (1 ml/h = 0.1 mcg/kg/min) |
| Dinoprostone infusion<br>(5–10 ng/kg/min) | 15 mcg/kg body weight made up to total volume of 50 ml 5% dextrose<br>1ml/h = 5 ng/kg/min |

dopamine or adrenaline in the first instance) may be run peripherally until central access is secured.

Initial investigations: blood cultures and blood glucose are a priority.

**What is the differential diagnosis?**

• Sepsis: micro-organisms isolated from neonates are usually acquired from the maternal genital tract during birth. Antibiotics to cover group B strep and *Escherichia coli* are first-line treatment.

• Duct-dependent congenital cardiac lesions: these may present in the neonatal period with cyanosis, heart failure or cardiogenic shock (weak femoral pulses, severe hypoxia). An infusion of prostaglandin $E_2$ (dinoprostone) will reopen/maintain ductal patency.

• Inborn errors of metabolism: clues are hypoglycaemia, vomiting, congestive cardiac failure, jaundice, hepatosplenomegaly and seizures. Supportive management of hypovolaemia, hypoglycaemia and seizures, and urgent discussion with a metabolic specialist are required.

• Non-accidental injury: a high index of suspicion is necessary. Neonates can lose a large proportion of their blood volume into their abdomen or skull, causing hypovolaemic shock.

# Further reading

Barker C. L. Practical management of the shocked neonate. *Emerg Med Australas* 2013; 25: 83–6.

Children's Acute Transport Service. Septic Shock. Available at http://site.cats.nhs.uk/wp-content/uploads/2013/12/cats_sepsis_2013.pdf (accessed 4 May 2015).

Children's Acute Transport Service. Duct dependent congenital heart disease. Available at http://site.cats.nhs.uk/wp-content/uploads/2013/12/cats_chd_2013.pdf (accessed 5 April 2015).

Children's Acute Transport Service. Metabolic emergencies. Available at http://site.cats.nhs.uk/wp-content/uploads/2013/12/cats_metabolic_2013.pdf (accessed 5 April 2015).

# Child with stridor

A 2-year-old presents to the emergency department in respiratory distress with stridor.

**Are the following statements true or false?**

a) Croup is the most likely cause
b) You should always make a visual inspection of the pharynx
c) Exact diagnosis is unlikely to alter your immediate management
d) If the patient requires ventilating an inhalational induction is the most appropriate method of induction

Answers: TFTT

a) Responsible for 80% of paediatric cases of acute stridor, laryngotracheobronchitis (croup) is viral in origin. The history will aid in diagnosis. Differentials include those shown in Table 13.5.

**Table 13.5** The differential diagnosis of stridor in a child

| Diagnosis | Clinical features |
|---|---|
| **Pharynx** | |
| Retropharyngeal and peritonsillar abscess | Neck pain and swelling, fever, drooling, dysphagia, trismus, limited neck movement |
| **Larynx** | |
| Croup | Coryzal, barking cough, mild pyrexia |
| Epiglottitis | Drooling, hoarse voice, septic |
| Foreign body | Sudden onset, history of choking |
| Oedema (e.g. anaphylaxis) | Facial swelling, rash, wheeze, cardiovascular signs |
| **Trachea** | |
| Bacterial tracheitis | Coryzal, copious secretions upon coughing, retrosternal pain, |
| External compression | hoarse voice, NO drooling |

Whilst a poor vaccination history may make you more likely to consider epiglottitis or tracheitis, they should still be ruled out in those who are fully vaccinated as they can still occur.

The type of stridor may help indicate the level of the problem: inspiratory stridor suggests a supraglottic lesion, expiratory stridor indicates the lower trachea and biphasic stridor is likely to originate from the glottic or subglottic regions. Increasing volume of the stridor does not indicate severity although a decrease may do as consciousness is lost.

b) Upsetting the child will increase respiratory effort and could precipitate complete airway obstruction. They should be left in the position that they are most comfortable and any distressing procedures, such as cannulation, avoided. Examination should include an assessment of the work of breathing. Pulse oximetry may be tolerated.

c) Your immediate management should consist of the following:

- Consider the need for senior anaesthetic and ENT help early.
- Oxygen (parents are best placed to hold the mask).
- Adrenaline nebulizer (5 ml 1:1000) may temporarily improve the situation whilst creating a definitive plan.
- Consider the need for steroid (especially in croup) or antibiotics.

d) Sevoflurane is the most common inhalational agent of choice.

## Further reading

Advanced Life Support Group edited by M. Samuels, S. Wieteska. *Advanced Paediatric Life Support: The Practical Approach*, 5th edn. London: Wiley-Blackwell, 2011.

Leung A., Cho H. Diagnosis of stridor in children. *Am Fam Physician* 1999; 60(8): 2289–96.

Maloney E., Meakin G. Acute stridor in children. *Contin Educ Anaesth Crit Care Pain* 2007; 7(6): 183–6.

## Caudal analgesia

A 1-year-old 8 kg boy is having a routine circumcision as a day case under regional anaesthesia. He is otherwise fit and well. He has just begun to crawl but is unable to pull himself up to standing.

**What are the best options for post-operative analgesia?**

a) Paracetamol 15 mg/kg qds
b) Ibuprofen 10 mg/kg tds
c) Oral morphine 0.1 mg/kg
d) Penile block with up to 6 ml of 0.25% bupivacaine
e) Caudal block with 6 ml of 0.25% bupivacaine
f) Local infiltration by surgeons with 1% lidocaine

Answer: a) + b) + e)

Planning the post-operative analgesia of young children is important so that you can prepare the child and parents adequately. Simple analgesia as an adjunct to a regional technique is the preferred combination here and many people would choose to do a caudal. A penile block is also acceptable but local infiltration alone has been shown to provide inferior analgesia and 1% lidocaine is too short-acting. Oral morphine is not usually required.

If you are planning to perform a caudal, you should counsel the parents about the side effects/risks: motor and sensory block, urinary retention, hypotension, headache, intravascular injection and failure of analgesia. Complications are rare but the side effect of a motor block is not. This child is not very mobile, so this is unlikely to be a significant issue. However, in older children weakness can be distressing and cause injury if the child falls.

To perform the block, position the patient on their side with their legs flexed. Aseptic technique should be used with hat, gloves, mask and chlorhexidine spray as a minimum. Do not be tempted to just use the glove packet for your equipment: use a dressing pack with a sterile field. The landmark technique is often used to identify the caudal space, but ultrasound-guided blocks are increasingly used, especially if a catheter is threaded (not indicated here).

The sacral hiatus is found at the apex of an equilateral triangle with the posterior superior iliac spines at the other two corners. Identify this and insert a 22G cannula at 60 degree angle. After you feel a 'give', indicating that you have pierced the sacro-coccygeal membrane, flatten the cannula off and advance it. Remove the needle and wait. A good tip is to leave the drawing up of your local anaesthetic until now, as this removes the temptation to rush. Aspirate gently and inject: it should inject easily.

The dose of local anaesthetic in children is sometimes quoted as 1 ml/kg of 0.25% bupivacaine (or levobupivacaine with its more favourable side effect profile). However, the maximum dose is 2 mg/kg. A solution of 0.25% bupivacaine contains 2.5 mg/ml so a 1 ml/kg dose is excessive: use 0.8 ml/kg. If a larger volume is required then the local anaesthetic will need diluting.

One of the major limitations of the single-injection technique is a relatively short duration of post-operative analgesia (4–6 hours). The use of opioids or clonidine as adjuncts results in clinically relevant prolongation of post-operative analgesia. The recommended doses are morphine 50 mcg/kg and clonidine 1–2 mcg/kg. Morphine is associated with post-operative urinary retention and sedation occurs with higher doses of clonidine. Preservative-free ketamine is no longer used due to concerns over potential increased neuronal apoptosi.

## Further reading

Berg S. Paediatric and neonatal anaesthesia. In: K. G. Allman, I. H. Wilson, eds. *Oxford Handbook of Anaesthesia*, 3rd edn. Oxford: Oxford University Press, 2011, pp. 799–860.
Gandhi M., Vashisht R. Anaesthesia for paediatric urology. *Contin Educ Anaesth Crit Care Pain* 2010; 10: 152–5.

## Acute severe asthma

You are called to the emergency department to see a 6-year-old asthmatic child. He is too breathless to complete a sentence and his respiratory rate is 45 breaths/min. His saturations are 93% on oxygen and his heart rate is 150 bpm. He has received three back-to-back salbutamol nebulizers.

**Answer the following true or false:**

1. He has acute severe asthma
2. Ipratropium bromide nebulizers can be added
3. Intravenous magnesium sulphate can be used
4. Nebulized magnesium sulphate can be used
5. 10 mg prednisolone is suitable for this age group

Answers: TTTTF

**Regarding acute severe asthma in children aged 2 and under the following are true or false:**

1. Wheezing attacks are more likely to be viral in origin than due to asthma
2. Inhaled ipratropium bromide may not be used
3. 10 mg prednisolone is suitable for this age group
4. Tracheomalacia should be considered as an alternative diagnosis
5. This age group has a consistent response to asthma treatment

Answers: TFTTF

The management of acute severe asthma in children can be divided into under and over 2 years old. Below the age of 2 the assessment of asthma can be difficult. Many other conditions can present with wheezing, including viral infections and bronchiolitis, pneumonia, aspiration pneumonitis and tracheomalacia. Prematurity and low birth weight are risk factors for recurrent wheezing and underlying conditions such as cystic fibrosis may present in this way. Under 2s may have a variable response to asthma treatment particularly if the wheeze is viral in origin.

Treatment includes inhaled beta-2 agonists with the addition of inhaled ipratropium bromide for severe symptoms. The steroid dose in this age group is 10 mg prednisolone.

The management of acute severe asthma in the over 2s age group includes recognition of severity and treatment.

Acute severe asthma is defined as:

- $SpO_2$ < 92%; peak expiratory flow (PEF) 33–50% predicted
- Unable to complete sentences or too breathless to talk/feed
- Heart rate >125/min (>5 years) or >140 (2–5 years)
- Respiratory rate >30 breaths/min (>5 years) or >40 (2–5 years).

Life-threatening asthma is defined as:

- $SpO_2$ < 92%; PEF < 33% predicted
- Silent chest
- Cyanosis
- Poor respiratory effort
- Hypotension
- Exhaustion
- Confusion.

Treatment should commence with oxygen followed by inhaled beta-2 agonists. For symptoms refractory to initial treatment, nebulized ipratropium bromide can be added. In children presenting with oxygen saturations of less than 92%, 150 mg magnesium sulphate can be added to each salbutamol/ipratropium nebulizer in the first hour.

Steroid doses in this age group are 20 mg for 2–5 years old and 30–40 mg for children >5 years.

Second-line treatment of acute severe asthma includes a bolus dose of intravenous salbutamol (15 mcg/kg). Aminophylline should not be used in mild or moderate acute asthma but can be considered in severe asthma where there is poor response to beta-2 agonists and steroids. Intravenous magnesium sulphate is considered a safe treatment although its use in paediatric asthma has not been established.

## Further reading

British Thoracic Society. British guideline on management of asthma. 2014. Available at https://www .brit-thoracic.org.uk/guidelines-and-quality-standards/asthma-guideline/ (accessed 9 January 2016).

**Chapter**

# Pain medicine

**14**

*This chapter includes commonly encountered pain issues, including assessment of pain in children, management of perioperative pain including in opioid-tolerant cases, use of ketamine as an analgesic and the basics of chronic pain assessment. Analgesic ladders are included in Chapter 32. Together these sections aim to refresh your pain assessment and management skills.*

## Paediatric pain assessment tools

You are required to assess a 2-year-old child 1 hour after a paraumbilical hernia repair as the nurses are concerned that they are in pain.

**Which of the following pain assessment tools would be the most appropriate?**

a)  Autonomic responses to pain
b)  The FLACC (face, legs, activity, cry, consolability) pain scale
c)  The Wong–Baker faces pain rating scale
d)  A visual analogue scale
e)  The child's own report

Answer: b)

Studies have demonstrated that pain is under-assessed and poorly documented in children and this can result in poor pain management. There are three approaches to pain assessment in children:

1.  Self-reporting
2.  Observational/behavioural
3.  Physiological.

The most appropriate approach will depend upon the age of the child and whenever possible, self-reporting should be regarded as the most reliable assessment. However, in the case of young children, this is not possible. It is therefore necessary to look for physiological, behavioural and/or observational clues, and there are many pain scales available for children within each of these categories.

The appropriate age ranges for the scales overlap. In general, a child below 2 years old is unable to rate pain intensity, and the FLACC scale is most appropriate. This scale involves a score of 0, 1 or 2 for each element, based on observation. The maximum score is therefore

*Returning to Work in Anaesthesia*, ed. Emma Plunkett, Emily Johnson and Anna Pierson.
Published by Cambridge University Press. © Cambridge University Press 2016.

10, with zero indicating absence of pain. The FLACC scale has been validated up to the age of 18 years.

The Wong–Baker faces scale is valid for 4- to 12-year-olds. It involves the child choosing from five face diagrams with varying expressions to describe the pain. Visual analogue and numerical scales are useful over the age of 8 years.

The COMFORT scale is frequently used for infants through to adults in the critical care setting. It encompasses scores for alertness, calmness/agitation, respiratory response, physical movement, blood pressure, heart rate, muscle tone and facial tension. Other pain scales in use include Pieces of Hurt (3–8 years) and the Multiple Size Poker Chip Tool (MSPCT: 4–6 years).

The use of physiological approaches alone has been shown to be unreliable and should not be used.

## Further reading

Association of Paediatric Anaesthetists of Great Britain and Ireland. Good practice in postoperative and procedural pain management, 2nd edition, 2012. *Paediatr Anaesth* 2012; 22 Suppl 1: 1–79. Available at http://www.apagbi.org.uk/publications/apa-guidelines (accessed 2 January 2016).

## Management of acute post-operative pain

A 50-year-old woman is in recovery following bilateral mastectomy. She has a history of type 2 diabetes, obstructive sleep apnoea requiring overnight continuous positive airway pressure (CPAP) and CKD (chronic kidney disease) stage 3. Previously she has had post-operative vomiting due to opioids. She has received 1 g paracetamol, 50 mg tramadol and 10 mg morphine. Her pain score is 8/10.

**Which of the following would be most suitable for managing her pain and why?**

a) Further boluses of intravenous morphine, up to 30 mg until comfortable and then morphine PCA with 1.5 mg boluses and 5-minute lockout period
b) Further bolus of 10 mg intramuscular morphine now with as-required or oral morphine 5–10 mg every 4 hours
c) Further 200 mg intravenous tramadol now, and then morphine PCA with 1 mg boluses and 5-minute lockout period
d) Boluses of intravenous oxycodone, up to 10 mg now until comfortable, and then oxycodone PCA with 1 mg boluses and 5-minute lockout period
e) Boluses of intravenous fentanyl up to 100 mcg now, and then fentanyl PCA with 20 mcg boluses and 5-minute lockout period

Answer: e)

This lady is at risk of post-operative respiratory failure, which could be worsened by excessive opioid administration. She is also at risk of nausea and vomiting. Fentanyl is a good choice as it is short-acting and considered to be the safest opioid for use in renal impairment. Oxycodone may have a better side-effect profile than morphine but should be used with caution in patients with renal impairment.

Opioids are frequently used in large doses for acute post-operative pain. The side effects of opioids must be considered carefully, and often it is a balance between two or three conflicting problems.

Obese patients are often more challenging to manage. Higher doses are required, but the weight used for any calculations is as yet undefined and will vary greatly between patients. In addition these patients are more at risk of obstructive sleep apnoea, and consequently the sedative effects of opioids are more profound. In general it is better to use opioids with shorter half-lives. Fentanyl is a good choice, although the short half-life is due to distribution, meaning that as compartments become saturated the pharmacokinetics alter greatly. Morphine has a longer half-life and is even more unpredictable when administered intramuscularly or subcutaneously. Post-operative nausea and vomiting is problematic and will increase pain and reduce mobility.

Opioids are associated with nausea and vomiting through a variety of mechanisms. There is some evidence to suggest that the emetic side effects of oxycodone are less than those of morphine, although most studies have been performed in patients receiving opioids for chronic cancer pain.

The use of morphine must be carefully considered in patients with renal disease. This patient will have a risk of post-operative acute kidney injury in addition to the chronic disease. Morphine-6-glucuronide is a metabolite of morphine and is 13 times more potent. Like morphine, it is renally excreted, and will therefore accumulate quickly in patients with renal failure. For this reason fentanyl is the analgesic of choice.

## Further reading

UK Medicines Information (UKMi) Pharmacists. Which opioids can be used in renal impairment? Q&A 402.2 30 September 2014 (accessed via the NHS evidence website www.evidence.nhs.uk on 23 March 2015).

## Advanced management of perioperative pain

A 70-year-old patient with metastatic breast carcinoma undergoes prophylactic intramedullary nailing of a lytic lesion in her femur. She regularly takes paracetamol 1 g 6 hourly, morphine sulphate 30 mg 12 hourly, tramadol 100 mg 6 hourly, with the addition of oramorph 10 mg for breakthrough pain. She is in severe pain in recovery, despite having received her regular analgesia and 20 mg intravenous morphine.

### What would be the most appropriate agent to administer for her acute pain?

a) Diclofenac 50 mg orally
b) Morphine 10–20 mg intravenously titrated to pain
c) Oral morphine 10 mg
d) Codeine phosphate 60 mg orally
e) Clonidine 50–100 mcg titrated to pain

Answer: e (with b)

This patient is likely to have developed significant tolerance to opioids. Therefore, the 20 mg of morphine intravenously that would be expected to provide adequate post-operative analgesia in the vast majority of opioid-naive patients is unlikely to be sufficient here. NSAIDs are effective for metastatic bone pain but diclofenac is unlikely to control this acute pain sufficiently. Oral morphine and codeine are not indicated for severe pain in this setting. Further increased doses of morphine should provide analgesia but you may wish to consider trying an opioid-sparing agent in preference. Clonidine is an example of an opioid-sparing agent and may be used as a rescue agent in recovery.

The analgesic effects of clonidine are mediated by the activation of alpha-2 adrenoreceptors in the dorsal horn of the spinal cord in addition to augmentation of spinal endogenous opioid release. When clonidine is administered via the intravenous route it can cause significant hypotension and bradycardia, and it should therefore only be administered to patients with full monitoring. Intravascular volume should be restored/adequate before administration. Clonidine also causes sedation, therefore increased drowsiness may be a problem if administered to a patient in the recovery room emerging from a general anaesthetic.

Successful management of these patients requires a multidisciplinary approach involving the chronic pain and palliative care teams. Daily opioid intake should be established and formulation of a perioperative plan should occur. A post-operative baseline opioid requirement will be necessary to address physical dependence and prevent withdrawal symptoms.

## Further reading

Lewis N., Williams J. Acute pain management in patients receiving opioids for chronic and cancer pain. *Contin Educ Anaesth Crit Care Pain* 2005; 5(4): 127–9.
Sasada M., Smith S. *Drugs in Anaesthesia and Intensive Care*, 3rd edn. Oxford: Oxford University Press, 2003, pp. 320–1.

# Ketamine

You are working with a consultant anaesthetist on an Upper GI list. Your first patient is a 60-year-old female who is scheduled to undergo an open gastrectomy for gastric adenocarcinoma. She tells you that she suffered from severe post-operative nausea and vomiting (PONV) associated with the use of a morphine PCA following an open cholecystectomy last year. She is very concerned that this might happen again. She also asks about the risks of developing chronic postsurgical pain. You discuss the use of adjuvant analgesic agents with her. Your consultant colleague prefers to use ketamine in addition to morphine PCA.

**Consider the following single best answer questions**

Current evidence suggests that ketamine:

a) Is effective in reducing total opioid requirements and delaying time to first analgesic dose
b) Is most effective in patients with low–moderate pain scores post-operatively
c) Has fewer side effects when used in addition to a morphine PCA compared to using a morphine PCA alone
d) Increases the incidence of PONV when used in addition to a morphine PCA, compared to that when using a morphine PCA alone

Answer: a)

Ketamine reduces the incidence of PONV, whilst it seems to increase the incidence of neuropsychiatric side effects. Therefore, its use must be considered carefully. It is most effective when used in anticipation of severe pain. It has repeatedly been shown to reduce the total dose of opioid administered in the perioperative period and hence, the burden of opioid-related side effects. It is particularly beneficial for patients undergoing abdominal and thoracic procedures.

Ketamine, as a perioperative analgesic adjunct to morphine, should be administered:

a) As a single preoperative bolus (1 mg/kg)
b) As a continuous low dose infusion (<1 mg/kg/h)
c) As a PCA
d) As either a, b or c

Answer: d)

There is no current evidence to support the use of one dosing regime over another. There is no evidence of pre-emptive effect, despite the theoretical advantage of preventing wind up. Ketamine is equally efficacious if administered pre or post incision. Low dose ketamine infusion appears to be as effective as higher dose infusions (>1 mg/kg).

Current evidence supports the use of the following in the perioperative period to prevent chronic postsurgical pain (CPSP):

a) Amitriptyline, pregabalin and ketamine
b) Amitriptyline, magnesium and pregabalin
c) Clonidine, pregabalin and ketamine
d) Amitriptyline, ketamine and lidocaine

Answer: c)

Whilst antidepressants, anticonvulsants, membrane stabilizers and alpha-2 agonists are used to treat neuropathic pain, current evidence does not support the use of magnesium or antidepressants for the prevention of CPSP. There is some evidence for the use of ketamine, gabapentinoids, alpha-2 agonists and intravenous lidocaine.

## Further reading

Jouguelet Lacoste J., La Colla L., Schilling D., Chelly J. E. The use of intravenous infusion or single dose of low-dose ketamine for postoperative analgesia: a review of the current literature. *Pain Med* 2015; 16: 383–403.

Laskowski K., Stirling A., McKay W. P., Lim H. J. A systematic review of intravenous ketamine for postoperative analgesia. *Can J Anesth* 2011; 58(10): 911–23.

Ramaswamy S., Wilson J. A., Colvin L. Non-opioid-based adjuvant analgesia in perioperative care. *Contin Educ Anaesth Crit Care Pain* 2013; 13(5): 152–7.

## Basic assessment of chronic pain

A 75-year-old man is referred to the pain clinic. He has a 3-year history of post-herpetic neuralgia in the T6 dermatome. He cannot allow even cool water to touch the affected area when washing; he feels the area is being scalded, resulting in unbearable pain.

**Which one of the following terms most accurately describes his symptoms?**

a) Hyperalgesia
b) Allodynia
c) Hyperpathia

d) Central pain
e) Hyperaesthesia

Answer: b)

This patient is describing allodynia, which is defined as 'pain which is due to a stimulus which does not normally provoke pain'. In this case, a non-painful thermal stimulus provokes an unexpected pain response, thermal allodynia. Tactile allodynia may be suggested by the patient who is unable to allow bed sheets or clothing to touch the skin of a painful limb affected by a neuropathic pain syndrome.

The International Association for the Study of Pain (IASP) Task Force on Taxonomy has defined the following terms:

- *Hyperalgesia* is 'increased pain from a stimulus that normally provokes pain'. On sensory neurological examination using pinprick testing on the affected area the patient will be much more sensitive, showing a marked response to the sharp sensation in comparison to other areas on the body.
- *Allodynia* involves a change in the quality of a sensation, whereby a stimulus that is not usually painful results in an unexpected painful response. By contrast, hyperalgesia represents an augmented pain response to a painful stimulus.
- *Hyperaesthesia* describes 'increased sensitivity to stimulation, excluding the special senses'. It is a broad term encompassing both hyperalgesia and allodynia.
- *Hyperpathia* is an increased painful reaction to a stimulus (especially a repetitive stimulus) as well as an increased threshold before that stimulus evokes a response. When eventually the stimulus is recognized, the pain reaction is often explosive in character. The stimulus may or may not normally be perceived as painful.
- *Central pain* is a neuropathic pain syndrome caused by a primary lesion or dysfunction of the central nervous system. Examples of central pain may be seen in denervated limbs following a stroke or spinal cord injury.

## Further reading

International Association for the Study of Pain (IASP). *IASP Taxonomy*. Available at http://www .iasp-pain.org/Education/Content.aspx?ItemNumber=1698&navItemNumber=576 (accessed 23 March 2015).

**Chapter**

# 15

# Regional anaesthesia

*Regional anaesthesia is a rapidly developing area and keeping refreshed requires considerable effort even for those with regular commitment to its provision. This chapter includes some of the major issues involved in this area to refresh background knowledge. These include consent, safe use of nerve stimulators, transversus abdominis plane (TAP) blocks and serious complications including local anaesthetic toxicity and management of suspected epidural haematoma. Central neuraxial blockade and other relevant materials are covered in Chapter 29, Practical procedures. In addition the NAP3 results are summarized in Chapter 34 and management of local anaesthetic toxicity in Chapter 25. For more detailed updates on specific blocks there are numerous online resources; some of the more useful are included under further reading at the end of the chapter.*

## Regional anaesthesia: consent

You are planning a femoral nerve block for a patient having an elective knee replacement.

**Which one of the following statements regarding his consent is true?**

a) A separate written consent form should be completed for the block
b) It is only necessary to discuss life-changing or life-threatening risks
c) The anaesthetic room is a suitable place to obtain consent
d) Permanent nerve damage is very rare
e) Failure of the block to provide adequate analgesia is very rare

Answer: d)

Consent must be obtained for any investigation or treatment in patients who are deemed to have capacity. This includes any regional analgesic techniques such as a peripheral nerve block or epidural. It should include details of the potential benefits to the patient as well as the significant, foreseeable risks and what the consequences of these risks might be. Consent should be gained at the preoperative visit, and ideally, written information (such as patient information leaflets produced by the Royal College of Anaesthetists (RCoA)) should have been given out prior to this. More general information about consent and capacity can be found in Chapter 24.

Consent for a peripheral nerve block or catheter will vary according to the block required, individual patient factors and the individual practitioner. The benefits will usually be

*Returning to Work in Anaesthesia*, ed. Emma Plunkett, Emily Johnson and Anna Pierson.
Published by Cambridge University Press. © Cambridge University Press 2016.

avoiding or reducing the amount of general anaesthetic required, provision of post-operative analgesia and minimizing side effects related to systemic analgesics.

Common risks of a peripheral nerve block include failure, bruising and temporary nerve damage. Less common risks include infection and damage to adjacent structures, which will be block dependent. Rare risks include permanent nerve damage, local anaesthetic toxicity and anaphylaxis.

Nerve damage can be caused by direct trauma, chemical irritation by local anaesthetics, haematoma formation, infection and ischaemia. Risk of short-term nerve damage can be quoted as less than 1 in 10 and permanent nerve damage between 1 in 2000 and 1 in 5000.

In addition to these general risks, each block will have its own side effects or risks, such as phrenic nerve palsy or Horner's syndrome with an interscalene block.

Consent for an epidural should include the intended benefits (intra- and post-operative analgesia, attenuation of stress response, avoidance of opioids, etc.) and risks. Very common side effects and risks include motor block, hypotension, nausea, shivering, bruising over site, urinary retention and failure to provide adequate analgesia (1 in 10). Uncommon risks include post-dural puncture headache (risk of 1 in 100 to 1 in 500) and temporary nerve damage.

Rare but serious risks include permanent nerve damage, epidural abscess, epidural haematoma, meningitis, high block, local anaesthetic toxicity, and anaphylaxis. The 3rd National Audit Project (NAP3) has provided us with a better knowledge of the risk of perioperative epidurals. Permanent harm (including death) can be quoted as being between 1 in 6000 and 1 in 12 000, and paraplegia or death between 1 in 16 000 and 1 in 100 000 (see Chapter 34).

## Further reading

Counsell D. Complications after perioperative CNB. NAP3. The Third National Audit Project of the Royal College of Anaesthetists: Major Complications of Central Neuraxial Block in the United Kingdom. Report and Findings, January 2009, pp. 101–11.

## Principles of performing local, regional and neuraxial techniques: TAP blocks

When performing a transversus abdominis plane (TAP) block, the aim is to deposit local anaesthetic in between which of the following muscles?

a) External oblique and internal oblique
b) Internal oblique and transversus abdominis
c) External oblique and transversus abdominis
d) Internal oblique and latissimus dorsi
e) External oblique and latissimus dorsi

Answer: b)

Transversus abdominis plane (TAP) blocks can be performed either by using a landmark technique or with the aid of ultrasound. The aim is to place a large volume of local anaesthetic in the fascial plane between the internal oblique and transversus abdominis, which contains the nerves from T7 to L1.

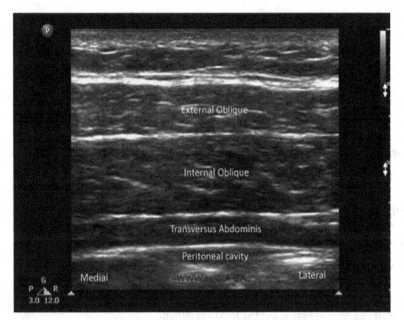

**Figure 15.1** Muscular layers of the anterolateral abdominal wall. Reproduced with permission from Ultrasound for Regional Anaesthesia: TAP block (http://usra.ca/tapscan.php).

The block was originally described using a landmark technique. The TAP is accessed from the lumbar 'triangle of Petit', bounded anteriorly by the external oblique, posteriorly by the latissimus dorsi, and inferiorly by the iliac crest. A blunt-tipped, short-bevelled needle is placed perpendicular to the skin immediately cephalad to the iliac crest. The needle is advanced through the external oblique and a first 'pop' sensation is felt when the needle enters the plane between the external oblique and internal oblique. Further advancement of the needle results in a second 'pop' after it passes through the internal oblique fascia into the TAP. At this point, after careful aspiration, 20 mL of long-acting local anaesthetic is injected in 5 mL aliquots. For incisions at or crossing the midline, a bilateral TAP block is indicated.

Ultrasound can also be used to identify the muscle layers and ensure accurate placement of local anaesthetic. The ultrasound probe is placed transversely between the 12th rib and the iliac crest in the mid-axillary line. The TAP can easily be observed, and using a 10 cm short-bevelled needle with an 'in-plane' approach, local anaesthetic spread distending the plane between the transversus abdominis and internal oblique can be seen in real time.

The TAP block provides analgesia for the abdominal wall but not for the visceral contents, and it is ideally used as part of a multimodal approach to analgesia. Good post-operative analgesia and a decrease in morphine requirements have been demonstrated. Used bilaterally, it provides a simple alternative in patients for whom an epidural is not possible. It may not provide equivalent analgesia, but there may be a lower risk of systemic side effects.

Complications include block failure, intravascular injection or injection into the peritoneal cavity, with associated risks of damage to bowel and other abdominal viscera.

## Further reading

Townsley P., French J. Transversus Abdominis Plane Block. WFSA Tutorial of the Week. Available at http://www.aagbi.org/sites/default/files/239%20Transversus%20Abdominus%20Plane%20Block.pdf (accessed 30 January 2015).

Ultrasound for Regional Anaesthesia. TAP Block. Available at http://www.usra.ca/tapscan.php (accessed 30 January 2015).

Yarwood J., Berrill A. Nerve blocks of the anterior abdominal wall. *Contin Educ Anaesth Crit Care Pain* 2010; 10: 182–6.

# Regional anaesthesia techniques: when to inject using a nerve stimulator

You are performing a sciatic nerve block for a patient undergoing an Achilles tendon repair. You are using the posterior approach and a nerve stimulator technique. At a depth of 4 cm, you elicit twitching of the calf muscles, which gradually decreases as you reduce the current until there is no further motor response below 0.26 mA.

**What is the most appropriate course of action?**

a) Withdraw the needle completely and start the block again
b) Withdraw the needle slightly and slowly inject the local anaesthetic
c) Aspirate and, if negative, slowly inject the local anaesthetic
d) Slowly inject the local anaesthetic
e) Withdraw the needle slightly and recheck the minimum current required to obtain a motor response

Answer: c)

When using a nerve stimulator technique to perform a nerve block, it is important to have a good understanding of the anatomy of the nerve that you are planning to block, and also how to use the nerve stimulator effectively and safely. With regard to the anatomy, the sciatic nerve is large and essentially comprises two distinct nerves, the tibial and the common peroneal, of which the tibial remains medial to the common peroneal throughout its course. This knowledge is important, as it helps identify the location of the needle tip. Tibial stimulation causes plantar flexion of the foot and inversion, whereas common peroneal stimulation causes dorsiflexion and eversion.

When using a nerve stimulator technique, you should start with a current impulse of 1–2 mA, a frequency of 2 Hz and a pulse width of 100 ms. The current should be reduced to the threshold level (the minimum current to obtain a motor response). Ideally, this current should be between 0.2 and 0.5 mA. If the threshold level is below 0.2 mA, you should be suspicious of intraneural placement and therefore not inject the local anaesthetic mixture but reposition the needle. In the case here, the calf twitch suggests that the sciatic nerve is being stimulated – remember you may not see plantar flexion with this if the Achilles tendon has ruptured. The minimum current to obtain a motor response in this case is 0.26 mA, and it is therefore in the 'safe range' – and so providing aspiration is negative (making intravascular injection unlikely), it would be safe to slowly inject the local anaesthetic agent.

It is important to remember, however, that if there is a large amount of resistance or the patient complains of pain on injection, you should stop injecting and reposition the needle before continuing. Although the first and last options presented are not incorrect, they would both result in further manipulation of the needle, resulting in more pain for the patient and increasing the likelihood of damaging surrounding structures – and therefore they are not the best answers.

Although a negative aspiration does not completely rule out intravascular needle placement, it will detect some cases, and it is therefore an important step to undertake prior to injecting the local anaesthetic.

## Further reading

Jeng C. L., Torrillo T. M., Rosenblatt M. A. Complications of peripheral nerve blocks. *Br J Anaesth* 2010; 105(Suppl 1): i97–107.

Nicholls B., Conn D., Roberts A. *The Abbott Pocket Guide to Practical Peripheral Nerve Blockade.* Maidenhead: Abbott Anaesthesia, 2007, pp. 8, 74–5.

# Complications of regional anaesthesia: local anaesthetic toxicity

An 87-year-old lady (50 kg) requires debridement and skin grafting of a pretibial laceration. Because she has multiple co-morbidities, you perform a combined femoral and sciatic nerve block, injecting 30 mL of 0.25% levobupivacaine at each site. Ten minutes after performing the block the patient becomes agitated, following which she has a tonic–clonic seizure. She has a sinus bradycardia and blood pressure 75/38 mmHg.

**What is the most appropriate dose of 20% lipid emulsion?**

a)   150 ml over 1 minute and an infusion of 750 ml/h
b)   75 ml over 5 minutes and infusion of 1000 ml/h
c)   150 ml over 1 minute and an infusion of 1500 ml/h
d)   75 ml over 1 minute and an infusion of 750 ml/h
e)   100 ml over 5 minutes and an infusion of 1000 ml/h

Answer: d)

The risk of developing local anaesthetic toxicity is dependent on the total dose of local anaesthetic given and the site where the mixture is injected. Regarding the dose of local anaesthetic, there are published maximum recommended doses for each local anaesthetic agent, with the dose for bupivacaine being 2 mg/kg. As for the site of injection, the likelihood of developing local anaesthetic toxicity is closely related to the vascularity of the site. Intercostal blocks produce the highest systemic concentrations, followed by caudal blocks, epidurals, brachial plexus blocks and finally subcutaneous infiltration producing the lowest systemic concentrations when equal doses are given.

In this case, the patient is only 50 kg and has been given a dose of 3 mg/kg of levobupivacaine. Her symptoms are consistent with local anaesthetic toxicity with central nervous system and cardiovascular sequelae. The Association of Anaesthetists of Great Britain and Ireland (AAGBI) has produced guidelines for the management of such cases. The immediate management is to stop injecting the local anaesthetic, call for help and use a standard ABC approach. The airway should be secured with a tracheal tube if necessary and 100% oxygen given (hyperventilation may help by increasing the plasma pH if there is a metabolic acidosis). For further guidance and management, see Section 3, Chapter 25.

If the patient has suffered a cardiac arrest, standard ALS protocols should be followed. Where cardiac arrest has not occurred, hypotension and brady- or tachyarrhythmias should be treated by conventional therapies. Seizures should be treated with a benzodiazepine, thiopental or propofol in small incremental doses.

The guidelines state that lipid emulsion should be given in all cases of cardiac arrest induced by local anaesthetic toxicity, and considered in cases where cardiac arrest has not occurred. The dose of 20% lipid emulsion is a starting bolus of 1.5 ml/kg over 1 minute (which can be repeated up to three times, each 5 minutes apart). As well as a bolus dose, an infusion of 20% lipid emulsion should be commenced at a rate of 15 ml/kg/h, which can be doubled if cardiovascular stability has not been restored or if an adequate circulation deteriorates. Once successfully treated, the patient should be moved to a critical care unit for a period of observation, and in the United Kingdom the case should be reported to the National Patient Safety Agency (as is stated in the guidelines).

## Further reading

Association of Anaesthetists of Great Britain and Ireland (AAGBI). AAGBI Safety Guideline: Management of Severe Local Anaesthetic Toxicity. London: AAGBI, 2010. Available at www.aagbi .org/sites/default/files/la_toxicity_2010_0.pdf (accessed 1 February 2015).
Peck T. E., Hill S., Williams M. *Pharmacology for Anaesthesia and Intensive Care*, 3rd edn. Cambridge: Cambridge University Press, 2008, pp. 163–74.

# Complications of regional anaesthesia: management of suspected epidural haematoma

You are called to assess a man with a thoracic (T8/9) epidural in situ, inserted for a laparotomy 2 days previously. A standard mix of bupivacaine (0.1%) and fentanyl (2 mcg/ml) is currently being infused (unchanged over the last 6 hours) at 10 ml/h. His observations are stable and he is very comfortable but is concerned that his legs are becoming progressively weaker.

**What should you do next?**

a) Halve the epidural infusion rate and review the patient every 30 minutes to monitor recovery of motor function
b) Stop epidural infusion and review the patient every 30 minutes to monitor recovery of motor function then restart the epidural infusion at a lower dose
c) Stop the epidural and remove the epidural catheter
d) Continue infusion at 10 ml/h as the current level of analgesia is good
e) Stop the infusion and arrange urgent imaging of the spinal cord and surrounding structures

Answer: e)

Vertebral canal haematoma, abscess and spinal cord ischaemia are all complications of epidural insertion and can cause severe, permanent neurological damage. The 3rd National Audit Project (NAP3) highlighted several cases of delayed management of spinal cord compression as a result of delayed identification, review and diagnosis of patients following central neuraxial blockade with leg weakness. Of these patients, decompressive laminectomy was successful in cases of vertebral canal abscess, but less so for vertebral canal haematoma. Early imaging and definitive neurosurgical intervention are likely to improve outcome. A clear protocol should be in place describing the actions required in this situation, including informing senior anaesthetists and immediate availability of imaging and surgical expertise.

Chapter 34 summarizes the main findings from NAP3. However, the following points are of particular relevance to this case:

1. Motor function should be assessed and recorded as a baseline function in the recovery area using an appropriate scale (Bromage scale) and then every 4 hours alongside other routine monitoring.
2. Abnormal motor or sensory function during any epidural infusion should be reported to the responsible anaesthetist and the infusion stopped if deemed necessary. Regular assessment (e.g. every 30 minutes) should then be performed to ensure that motor function is returning, which should be expected within 4 hours.
3. If recovery is not observed then imaging (MRI) should be considered.
4. The use of epidural analgesia cannot be deemed as safe in circumstances where monitoring of motor block density and its recovery cannot be undertaken.
5. The epidural should only be restarted when adequate motor recovery has been observed.
6. If the epidural is restarted then increased surveillance should continue, and if abnormal neurology recurs then it is prudent to abandon the epidural.
7. When epidural analgesia is terminated it is important to remove the catheter only when it is safe to do so.
8. Neurological observation should continue for 24 hours following catheter removal in patients with abnormal neurology (and longer in patients who remain immobile after catheter removal).

When any epidural infusion is stopped it is important to prescribe alternative methods of analgesia.

Significant motor block in a thoracic epidural (Bromage score 3) is extremely uncommon and warrants immediate referral to an anaesthetist. The following are described as 'red flags' and often require immediate referral to an experienced anaesthetist and early neuroimaging:

- Significant motor block with a thoracic epidural
- Unexpectedly dense motor block, including unilateral block
- Markedly increasing motor block during epidural infusion
- Motor block that does not regress when the infusion is stopped
- Recurrent unexpected motor block after restarting an epidural infusion that was stopped because of motor block.

## Further reading

New York School of Regional Anaesthesia. http://www.nysora.com/ (accessed 2 January 2016).

Regional anaesthesia in patients taking anticoagulants. Anaesthesia UK, 2005. Available at www.frca.co.uk/Search.aspx (accessed 9 January 2016).

Royal College of Anaesthetists. *Major Complications of Central Neuraxial Block in The United Kingdom* (NAP3). London: RCA, 2009. Available at www.rcoa.ac.uk/document-store/nap3-full-report (accessed 12 April 2015).

Royal College of Anaesthetists Faculty of Pain Medicine. *Best Practice in the Management of Epidural Analgesia in the Hospital Setting*, November 2010. Available at www.aagbi.org/sites/default/files/epidural_analgesia_2011.pdf (accessed 13 April 2015).

The European Society of Regional Anaesthesia and Pain Therapy. http://esraeurope.org (accessed 2 January 2016).

Chapter

# 16

# Neuroanaesthesia

*Although the title of this chapter would seem subspecialist, the majority of the scenarios and topics discussed here are likely to be encountered by general anaesthetists or intensivists. We cover neurotrauma – both brain and spinal cord injury, acute subarachnoid haemorrhage, the management of the unstable spine and venous air embolism. There are also relevant sections in other chapters, such as the management of raised intracranial pressure (Chapter 7) and remote site anaesthesia in Chapter 23. A flow chart for management of traumatic brain injury can be found in Chapter 31.*

## Traumatic brain injury

You are called to resus. A motorcyclist has been brought in with obvious head trauma. He cannot open his eyes to pain, is groaning but shows normal flexion to stimulus.

**Which of the following statements are true regarding the severity of his head injury?**

a) GCS is 5
b) GCS is 7
c) He has a severe head injury
d) He has a moderate head injury
e) GCS is 11

Answers: FTTFF

A Glasgow Coma Score (GCS) of 7 (E1, M4, V2) is consistent with severe head injury. Head injury is graded according to GCS; 13–15 is mild, 9–12 is moderate and ≤8 is severe.

**Which of the following are indications for intubation?**

a) GCS ≤ 8
b) A decrease in motor score of ≥1 point
c) $PaCO_2$ of >4.5 kPa
d) $PaO_2$ of <13 kPa
e) Seizures

Answers: TFFTT

Intubation is required for airway protection. Ventilatory control helps prevent secondary brain injury. Decreased motor score of two or more points should prompt intubation. Low

*Returning to Work in Anaesthesia*, ed. Emma Plunkett, Emily Johnson and Anna Pierson.
Published by Cambridge University Press. © Cambridge University Press 2016.

$PaO_2$ and raised $PaCO_2$ adversely affect intracranial pressure (ICP) by increasing cerebral blood flow. The Association of Anaesthetists of Great Britain and Ireland (AAGBI) advise a $PaCO_2$ of 4.5–5.0 kPa and a $PaO_2$ of >13 kPa. Reduction of cerebral metabolic rate is important; seizures cause an increase. Transfer of the patient is also an indication for intubation.

**Regarding the intubation process:**

a) Four people may be required to intubate this patient
b) Jaw thrust and nasal airways can be used prior to a definitive airway
c) Where GCS is 3, patients can be safely intubated without drugs
d) Ketamine may be used as an induction agent
e) Achieving a mean arterial pressure (MAP) >70 mmHg helps to prevent secondary brain injury

Answers: TFFTF

Assistance is needed to stabilize the C-spine, apply cricoid pressure and give drugs during rapid sequence induction (RSI). Potentially difficult intubations (facial fractures, full stomach etc.) require preparation. Extra kit may be needed, for example an Airtraq. Perform jaw thrust but avoid nasal airways as there may be a base of skull fracture. Ketamine increases ICP but this may not be significant. Use drugs to obtund the pressor response to laryngoscopy as this raises ICP. Cerebral perfusion pressure (CPP) = MAP − ICP. Use fluids and vasopressors to achieve a MAP of 80–90 mmHg until ICP monitoring is established.

## Further reading

Association of Anaesthetists of Great Britain and Ireland (AAGBI). Recommendations for the Safe Transfer of Patients with Brain Injury. London: AAGBI, 2006. Available at http://www.aagbi.org/sites/default/files/braininjury.pdf (accessed 9 January 2016).

Bhalla T., Dewhirst E., Sawardekar A. et al. Perioperative management of the pediatric patient with traumatic brain injury. *Paediatr Anaesth* 2012; 22: 627–40.

Moppett I. K. Traumatic brain injury: assessment, resuscitation and early management. *Br J Anaesth* 2007; 99: 18–31.

Shardlow E., Jackson A. Cerebral blood flow and intracranial pressure. *Anaesth Intensive Care Med* 2011; 12: 220–3.

## Spinal cord injury

A 40-year-old woman is admitted to the emergency department following a fall from a horse. She complains of back pain and is unable to move her legs. On examination: A = maintaining own; B = $SpO_2$ 92% on 15 l, respiratory rate 18 breaths/min, equal air entry with no added sounds on auscultation; C = heart rate 60 bpm, blood pressure 80/40 mmHg; D = Glasgow Coma Score (GCS) 15/15, loss of power and sensation in lower limbs; E = T 36, BM 5, bruising to left flank, no other obvious injuries.

**Put the following steps in the most logical order:**

a) Arrange a CT abdomen to exclude intra-abdominal haemorrhage
b) Insert an arterial line
c) Immobilize her C-spine
d) Obtain IV access and give a fluid bolus

e) Insert a urinary catheter
f) Start a peripheral vasopressor infusion

Suggested answer: c) d) b) f) a) e)

Patients with acute spinal cord injury (SCI) do not always present to specialist centres, although this may be changing with the advent of major trauma centres. An understanding of how to manage these patients is important. Often the SCI is incomplete but secondary damage caused by haemorrhage, oedema or ischaemia due to neurogenic shock can worsen outcome. Prevention or reduction of secondary insults can make a dramatic difference to quality of life.

Spinal shock develops as the result of the loss of reflexes below the level of the SCI. Patients with spinal shock initially present with a flaccid areflexia and neurogenic shock. The symptoms of flaccid areflexia last for 1–2 days after the SCI with a gradual return of reflexes and development of hyperreflexia in the weeks and months following injury.

Immediately after SCI there is a massive surge in catecholamine release, causing hypertension and tachycardia, and after this phase neurogenic shock develops as a result of the loss of sympathetic nerve supply below the level of the injury. This results in vasodilation and, if the injury is above the level of the sympathetic innervation of the heart (T5), bradycardia. Remember that where there is a SCI as the result of trauma it is still important to exclude hypovolaemia as a cause for shock and treat appropriately, as well as treating the spinal shock. One-third of patients with SCI will have associated major injuries. Treatment for neurogenic shock is with vasopressors +/− inotropes; excessive fluid may result in pulmonary oedema. It can last for a period of days to weeks.

She is found to have an unstable T3 # and the spinal surgeon plans to perform a fixation. She is admitted to ICU for observation in the meantime. Despite being nursed lying flat (a more optimal position for diaphragmatic excursion), her respiratory function deteriorates.

**What drugs would you use for intubation?**

In the first 72 hours after injury it is safe to use suxamethonium. After this time the development of extra-junctional acetylcholine receptors can lead to fatal hyperkalaemia following administration of suxamethonium, this effect can persist for 6 months following injury.

Her deterioration is not unexpected, given the level of her injury. She will have partial loss of intercostal muscle function. Total loss will occur with a lesion above T1 and above T8 will result in loss of inspiratory intercostals.

## Further reading

Bonner S., Smith C. Initial management of spinal cord injury. *Contin Educ Anaesth Crit Care Pain* 2013; 13(6): 224–3.

# Interventional neuroradiology: acute subarachnoid haemorrhage

A 55-year-old lady with a Grade 1 subarachnoid haemorrhage (SAH) is listed for embolization of a ruptured intracerebral aneurysm.

**Please answer the following questions true or false**

a) The anterior communicating artery is the most common site of intracerebral aneurysms
b) The most common non-neurological causes of death are cardiovascular complications

c)  Coiling of aneurysms is associated with a better outcome than clipping
d)  Sevoflurane may be preferable to propofol TCI for maintenance of anaesthesia during coiling as it has been shown to be associated with a more rapid recovery
e)  Triple-H therapy (HHH) for vasospasm involves: haemodilution, hypervolaemia and hypertension

Answers: TFTTT

Grading of SAH: there are various grading systems for severity of SAH. The Hunt and Hess scoring system (1968) is a 5-point scale used to determine surgical risk but is somewhat subjective. The World Federation of Neurosurgeons (WFNS) grading (Table 16.1) is more objective and used for prognostication of morbidity and mortality and also to aid decision making regarding timing of intervention (early vs. late). The Fisher scale is a radiological grading system based on CT appearance.

**Table 16.1** WFNS grading of acute subarachnoid haemorrhage

| Grade | GCS | Motor deficit |
| --- | --- | --- |
| 1 | 15 | Absent |
| 2 | 13–14 | Absent |
| 3 | 13–14 | Present |
| 4 | 7–12 | Present or absent |
| 5 | 3–6 | Present or absent |

Treatment of SAH: the International Subarachnoid Aneurysm Trial (ISAT) published in 2002 was a multicentre randomized controlled trial investigating outcome after surgical clipping or endovascular coiling (Grade 1 or 2 aneurysms). The results showed an improved disability-free survival with coiling although a higher risk of needing re-treatment and a slightly increased risk of rebleeding. Some aneurysms are not amenable to coiling so clipping still occurs occasionally.

Anaesthetizing for coiling: points to remember include:

- You are likely to be in a remote site and should have appropriate support (please see Chapter 23 for a recap of guidance on anaesthetizing in a remote site).
- SAH can have cardiovascular, respiratory and metabolic consequences (as well as neurological ones). Catecholamine surges can lead to arrhythmias, ECG abnormalities, left ventricular dysfunction and pulmonary oedema. Patients with SAH are often smokers, and a reduced level of consciousness and supine position also increases their risk of atelectasis and pneumonia. Respiratory complications are the most common non-neurological causes of death. Dehydration and electrolyte disturbance may also be present.
- The patient should be on nimodipine and prophylactic phenytoin may also be indicated.
- Good control of glucose is important (poor control is associated with a worse outcome).
- The patient will be heparinized after femoral arterial cannulation and so consider the timing of central line insertion (useful for HHH).
- Large-bore peripheral access and invasive arterial pressure monitoring is essential. If problematic, the femoral arterial catheter can be transduced.
- Intraoperative priorities are to have a still (i.e. no coughing) and cardiovascularly stable patient. This includes induction and emergence. Various techniques are possible but

high concentrations of volatile anaesthetic are best avoided, as is nitrous oxide. Remember that the procedure itself is not stimulating and vasopressor support may be needed to offset the effects of the anaesthetic agents.

- The procedure is usually lengthy so monitor temperature and using warming devices.
- Intraoperative complications can be divided into haemorrhagic (rupture or rebleeding) and occlusive (various causes, including vasospasm).
- Vasospasm can be treated with nimodipine, which may be administered intra-arterially during the procedure, and HHH.

The risk of rebleeding is 30% in the first 2 weeks; the highest risk is in the first 24 hours. Vasospasm peaks at 3–4 days and can result in delayed neurological deficit. Other later complications include obstructive hydrocephalus, seizures and cerebral oedema.

## Further reading
Dorairaj I. L., Hancock S. M. Anaesthesia for interventional neuroradiology. *Contin Educ Anaesth Crit Care Pain* 2008; 8(3): 86–9.

Luoma A., Reddy U. Acute management of aneurysmal subarachnoid haemorrhage. *Contin Educ Anaesth Crit Care Pain* 2013; 13(2): 52–8.

Manara A., Shinde S. Anaesthesia for vascular lesions. In: K. G. Allman, I. H. Wilson. *Oxford Handbook of Anaesthesia*, 2nd edn. Oxford: Oxford University Press, 2006, pp. 410–11.

# Management of the unstable spine

A 65-year-old man is listed for Anterior Cervical Discectomy and Fusion (ACDF) following a fall at home yesterday resulting in an unstable fracture at C4. He has no neurological deficit. He has a history of hypertension but is otherwise fit and well. He takes amlodipine and ramipril and has no known drug allergies. He has had a previously uneventful anaesthetic for inguinal hernia repair 3 years ago. On examination he is lying flat in bed in a hard collar.

**How would you assess this gentleman's airway?**

You should perform your normal airway assessment, including Mallampati view, jaw subluxation and mouth opening. An assessment of neck movement is clearly not possible. In addition, look at the imaging for soft-tissue swelling, which may be visible on the CT.

**What will your approach to airway management be?**

Preparation: careful preparation and assistance is key. There should normally be two anaesthetists plus one person (ideally the surgeon) to maintain manual in-line stabilization and an anaesthetic assistant. Ensure you have all the equipment you require: fibre-optic laryngoscope, Mackintosh laryngoscopes, alternative airway devices such as video laryngoscopes that you are familiar with, LMAs, and emergency front-of-neck airway access devices. Discuss your airways plans with your team and explain the procedure carefully to the patient.

Cervical spine stabilization: after applying manual in-line stabilization, the front of the hard collar and blocks can be removed. Carefully pre-oxygenate the patient to prevent hypoxia.

Options for intubation: there are a number of safe intubation options.

- Awake nasal or oral fibre-optic intubation. Nasal is usually preferred. Spinal immobilization should be maintained.

- Asleep fibre-optic intubation following IV induction with manual in-line stabilization.
- Asleep direct laryngoscopy following IV induction with manual in-line stabilization.

The choice of induction agent and airway management technique will depend on your experience and the individual patient. Awake fibre-optic nasal intubation is commonly used, but the most important point is to avoid hypoxia and use a technique with which you are familiar. Manual in-line stabilization worsens view at direct laryngoscopy and may be associated with more neck movement. However, as long as care is taken with the precautions mentioned above, then neurological injury is unlikely to result. Following intubation the hard collar and blocks should be reapplied.

## Further reading

Bonner S., Smith C. Initial management of spinal cord injury. *Contin Educ Anaesth Crit Care Pain* 2013; 13(6): 224–31.
Griffiths R., Leighton R. Anaesthesia for repair of cervical spine fracture. In: K. G. Allman, I. H. Wilson. *Oxford Handbook of Anaesthesia*, 2nd edn. Oxford: Oxford University Press, 2006, pp. 486–7.

## Venous air embolism

You are anaesthetizing an otherwise healthy 40-year-old man for removal of a posterior fossa tumour in the sitting position, with Trendelenburg tilt and leg elevation. Anaesthesia and surgery have been proceeding uneventfully. You have an arterial line, a RIJ CVP line, and peripheral intravenous access and are using a total intravenous anaesthesia (TIVA) technique. Midway through the surgery, you notice a drop in saturations, associated with a reduction in blood pressure. You increase the $FiO_2$ and give a bolus of metaraminol. Observations improve transiently but a few minutes later the same thing happens, this time associated with a drop in end-tidal $CO_2$ ($EtCO_2$). You suspect a venous air embolism (VAE).

**What should you do?**

- Inform the surgeons and ask them to cover the surgical field with saline-soaked gauze to prevent further entrainment.
- Use an ABC approach to resuscitation.
- Increase the $FiO_2$ to 1.0. (You were not using nitrous oxide, but in another situation you should discontinue this as it will diffuse into the venous air embolism, increasing its size.)
- Give IV crystalloids to increase venous pressure.
- Administer vasopressors $+/-$ inotropes as necessary.
- Aspirate the CVP line for air (there are special air aspiration lines available that are often used in this situation).

Other considerations

- Consider moving the patient to be supine or head down (practically easier) or left lateral if possible (harder logistically).
- Consider compression of the jugular vein to elevate cerebral venous pressure and reduce venous return from the site of entrainment. However, this increases intracranial pressure

and can also result in compression of the carotid artery and reduce cerebral blood flow.

- If cardiac arrest occurs perform CPR as per ALS guidelines.

Confirming the diagnosis

VAE is a clinical diagnosis but there are some methods of monitoring to detect it. These include:

- Transoesophageal echocardiography. Most sensitive but practically difficult and has complications.
- Precordial Doppler (placed in the right parasternal region). This can detect small quantities of intra-cardiac air.
- Measurement of end-tidal nitrogen. It will increase as the air in the embolus is expelled.

Other methods include an oesophageal stethoscope (now out-dated) and a pulmonary artery catheter (not routinely used for this purpose).

**What is the pathophysiology of a VAE?**

Small volumes of gas are absorbed from the circulation usually producing no clinical manifestations. Moderate volumes cause microvascular occlusion of the pulmonary vessels leading to ventilation-perfusion mismatch and vascular injury, resulting in pulmonary hypertension and pulmonary oedema. When large volumes of gas are involved the embolism can get trapped in the right atrium, creating an 'air lock', obstructing the right ventricular outflow tract and reducing cardiac output.

**How does a VAE present?**

The clinical picture is variable, and depends on both the volume of gas and rate of entrainment. An awake patient may complain of chest pain, may become agitated, may have a 'sense of impending doom' or a reduced Glasgow Coma Score (GCS). It is important to remember that signs are often late and can be very non-specific.

The lethal volume of gas is not exactly known, and varies with rate of entrainment, but is thought to be around 3–5 ml/kg.

**Table 16.2** Cardiovascular and respiratory signs of venous air embolism. They are listed in an approximate order of them occurring, but this is not absolute

| Cardiovascular | Respiratory |
| --- | --- |
| Increased PAP, then CVP | Reduced oxygen saturations |
| Tachycardia, hypotension | Reduced EtCO$_2$ |
| ECG changes: tachyarrhythmia, AV block, right ventricular strain, ST and T wave changes | Tachypnoea 'Gasp reflex' |
| Classic 'mill wheel' murmur | Pulmonary oedema |

CVP = central venous pressure; PAP = pulmonary artery pressure.

**What other clinical situations are associated with VAE?**

For a VAE to occur there must be a gas source, a communication with the venous circulation and a pressure gradient favouring transfer of gas into the circulation.

**Table 16.3** Causes of venous air embolism

| Surgery | Neurosurgery | Where surgical site is above the heart, creating a pressure gradient favouring the passage of air into the circulation |
| --- | --- | --- |
| | Head and neck | Including LASER procedures |
| | Orthopaedics | Arthroscopy, arthroplasty |
| | Laparoscopic | (Release pneumoperitoneum immediately) |
| | Obstetrics | C-section, termination of pregnancy |
| Trauma | Penetrating trauma to head, neck, thorax, abdomen | |
| Intravascular catheterization | Air in IV giving sets | |
| | During central venous access, disconnection or removal | |
| Barotrauma | Positive-pressure ventilation | |

# Further reading

Jagannathan S., Krovvidi H. Anaesthetic considerations for posterior fossa surgery. *Contin Educ Anaesth Crit Care Pain* 2014; 14(5): 202–6.

Shaikh N., Ummunisa F. Acute management of vascular air embolism. *J Emerg Trauma Shock* 2009; 2: 180–5.

Webber S., Andrzejowski J., Francis G. Gas embolism in anaesthesia. *Contin Educ Anaesth Crit Care Pain* 2002; 2(2): 53–7.

# Chapter 17

# General, urological and gynaecological surgery

*This chapter provides a refresher of some common clinical scenarios facing anaesthetists for general surgical, urological and gynaecological lists. It also includes a question on Enhanced Recovery Protocols which are well established for general surgical patients, but expanding into other specialties and another which discusses information from the organizational report from the National Emergency Laparotomy Audit. Whilst the national data will be published in due course, your hospital's data can help to shape your local systems and it will be something worth finding out about if relevant to your area of practice.*

## General: epidural analgesia for laparotomy

Consider the following general surgical patients. In which patient(s) would you consider siting an epidural? What would be your analgesic plan for the other(s)?

a) 51-year-old, emergency laparotomy for bowel perforation, systemically well, no significant past medical history
b) 80-year-old, emergency laparotomy for bowel perforation, systemic inflammatory response syndrome (SIRS), pyrexial 39 °C, WBC $22 \times 10^9/l$
c) 74-year-old, elective open hemicolectomy, significant IHD and chronic obstructive pulmonary disease (COPD)
d) 35-year-old, emergency laparotomy for Crohn's abscess, previously intolerant of opioids

Answer: Both c) and d) are suitable candidates for an epidural as the benefits are likely to outweigh the risks. An epidural is contraindicated in b) because of the risk of sepsis. An alternative regional technique may be more suitable in a).

Advantages: epidural analgesia for major abdominal surgery has traditionally been seen as gold-standard care. An epidural can provide superior analgesia and patient satisfaction when compared with alternatives such as opioid PCAs. However, few studies have compared more modern multimodal approaches with epidurals. Good analgesia allows for early mobilization (providing that lines, monitors etc. allow for this) and avoids opioid-related side effects.

Epidurals are known to obtund the stress response to surgery although the theoretical benefits to patients have not been consistently proven. The incidence and duration of

*Returning to Work in Anaesthesia*, ed. Emma Plunkett, Emily Johnson and Anna Pierson.
Published by Cambridge University Press. © Cambridge University Press 2016.

post-operative ileus is reduced, and return of normal gastrointestinal function is faster. It is widely accepted that epidural analgesia reduces pulmonary complications in high-risk patients; the effects on cardiovascular complications are less conclusive.

Disadvantages: These include hypotension (which can lead to excess fluid administration and additional complications if managed inadequately) and motor block, both of which may cause reduced mobility.

The risks of an epidural are not insignificant and should be considered in view of the likely benefits. Severe complications include vertebral canal haematomas, spinal cord ischaemia, vertebral canal abscess and other neurological injury. NAP3 identified the risk of permanent damage of between 1 in 24 000 and 1 in 54 000 cases. Contraindications to siting an epidural include systemic sepsis and those with an increased risk of bleeding, whether pharmacological or pathological. Careful multidisciplinary team management is vital in order to reduce risks, identify potential complications and maximize benefits.

Alternatives: There are a number of regional alternatives to epidural analgesia; these include transversus abdominis plane (TAP) blocks, rectus sheath blocks and local anaesthetic infiltration. These can be single shot or an infusion or bolus regimen via a catheter. Systemic analgesics should be optimized, including consideration of NSAIDs and alternative analgesics such as ketamine, clonidine, pregabalin and IV lidocaine infusions.

In conclusion, most experts agree that there is still a role for well-managed epidural analgesia in major abdominal surgery, provided that the risks and benefits have been carefully considered on an individual basis. Examples where an epidural may be favoured include the high-risk, co-morbid patient undergoing high-risk surgery and patients in whom opioids need to be avoided. In patients outside of these categories, an alternative regional technique should be considered as part of a multimodal regime.

## Further reading

Counsell D. Complications after perioperative CNB. NAP3. The Third National Audit Project of the Royal College of Anaesthetists: Major Complications of Central Neuraxial Block in the United Kingdom. Report and Findings, January 2009, pp. 101–11.

## General: laparoscopic bowel surgery

You have anaesthetized a 50-year-old female who is currently in the Trendelenburg position undergoing a laparoscopic hemicolectomy. The surgeon has insufflated the abdomen with gas and is midway through the operation when you notice that the patient has become bradycardic with a heart rate of 30 bpm. The gas insufflation pressures are >30 mmHg.

**What is the most likely cause of her bradycardia?**

The bradycardia is most likely to be secondary to vagal stimulation from peritoneal distension.

**What are safe insufflation pressures for establishing a pneumoperitoneum?**

The pneumoperitoneum is established by insufflating the abdomen with gas at pressures of 15 to 20 mmHg. A pressure of >30 mmHg is excessive: decompression of the abdomen is indicated.

**What are the complications associated with laparoscopic surgery?**

Problems associated with gas insufflation

  i) Reduced cardiac output. Compression of the inferior vena cava reduces preload and may lead to a decrease in cardiac output and subsequent decrease in arterial pressure, particularly if the patient is hypovolaemic. As intra-abdominal pressure increases, systemic vascular resistance is increased owing to both mechanical compression of the abdominal aorta and production of neuro-humoral factors such as vasopressin and activation of the renin–angiotensin–aldosterone axis.
 ii) Bradycardia secondary to vagal stimulation from peritoneal distension.
iii) Gas embolism secondary to high insufflation pressures or inadvertent direct injection of gas into a vessel leading to circulatory collapse.
 iv) Abdominal distension resulting in diaphragmatic splinting and increased intrathoracic pressure. This leads to a reduction in pulmonary compliance and functional residual capacity. The end result is V/Q mismatching and hypoxaemia.
  v) $CO_2$ absorption resulting in a gradual rise in $EtCO_2$.
 vi) Surgical emphysema and pneumothorax.
vii) Shoulder tip pain secondary to diaphragmatic irritation from intra-abdominal gas.

Trauma associated with instruments

  i) Puncture of a viscus such as stomach or bowel. The stomach is especially at risk if it has been distended after bag and mask ventilation.
 ii) Vascular trauma involving the abdominal aorta, inferior vena cava and other great vessels.

Problems associated with positioning

  i) Reverse Trendelenburg position (head up) can lead to hypotension and cerebral hypoperfusion.
 ii) Trendelenburg position (head down) can result in cerebral oedema, vocal cord oedema and retinal detachment after prolonged operations.
iii) Compartment syndrome can result from impaired arterial perfusion to raised lower limbs, compression of veins by leg supports and reduced femoral drainage secondary to the pneumo-peritoneum.

# Further reading

Bricker S. *Short Answer Questions in Anaesthesia*. Cambridge: Cambridge University Press, 2005.
Hayden P., Cowman S. Anaesthesia for laparoscopic surgery. *Contin Educ Anaesth Crit Care Pain* 2011; 11(5): 177–80.

# General: emergency laparotomy

Approximately 30 000 patients undergo an emergency laparotomy each year in England and Wales. Several studies in recent years have shown that post-operative complications and even death are common, with 15% of all patients dying within a month of having an emergency laparotomy.

**What measures could lead to the improved management of this group of patients?**

Improving the quality of care of patients undergoing emergency laparotomy is the focus of the National Emergency Laparotomy Audit (NELA). At the time of writing, the organizational report has been published and the first patient audit results are due. The following list includes common themes which would lead to the improvement of care of patients undergoing emergency laparotomy.

- Prioritization of resources towards emergency care.
- The timely review by a senior surgeon following admission.
- The ready availability of diagnostic investigations.
- Consultant led perioperative care for both surgery and anaesthesia.
- A formal assessment of preoperative risk.
- A pathway of defined perioperative care.
- The early involvement of critical care, even before surgery if necessary.
- The prompt administration of antibiotics.
- Patients should be optimally resuscitated before emergency surgery; this may involve resuscitation in the anaesthetic room depending on the urgency of surgery.
- Prompt access to an operating theatre.
- The admission of high-risk patients to a critical care unit following surgery.
- Routine daily input from elderly medicine should be available to elderly patients undergoing emergency laparotomy.
- Multidisciplinary reviews of processes and patient outcomes (morbidity and mortality meetings) should be held for all emergency laparotomy patients.
- Structured handover of care is required at all times by all clinicians treating emergency laparotomy patients.

Key facts about NELA include:

- It was initially funded for 3 years, this has been extended for a further 2 years, and is run by the National Institute of Academic Anaesthesia Health Services Research Centre (NIAA HSRC).
- Year 1 was the organizational audit (2013–2014); Years 2 and 3 are the patient audit (Year 3 began in December 2014).
- It is mandatory for trusts to collect data – it is part of the standard NHS contract with commissioners.
- All patients over 18 years of age having a general surgical (not gynaecological, vascular, urology or trauma) emergency laparotomy are included.

The audit team are keen that hospitals use local data to enhance their local processes, and it is worth engaging with the data collection process and finding out about your hospital's results.

# Further reading

National Emergency Laparotomy Audit (NELA). NELA project team. Executive Summary, first organisational report of the National Emergency Laparotomy Audit. London: RCoA, 2014.
Royal College of Anaesthetists. Guidance on the provision of anaesthesia services for emergency surgery (RCoA GPAS). London: RCoA, 2014.

## General: Enhanced Recovery Programmes

With regards to Enhanced Recovery Programmes (ERPs), which of the following statements is not true?

a) General Practitioners (GP) should check the patient's haemoglobin and if iron deficiency anaemia is noted, patients should be started on iron supplements preoperatively
b) Complex carbohydrate drinks are allowed up to 2 hours prior to surgery
c) Nasogastric tubes in the post-operative period help drain the gastric fluids and promote healing of the intestinal anastomosis
d) For open abdominal surgeries, thoracic epidural analgesia for the post-operative period should be encouraged
e) Urinary catheters should be removed within 48 hours of colorectal surgery if possible

Answer: c)

ERPs are now standard practice in colorectal surgery and the principles of management are increasingly being applied to other surgical specialities. They aim to standardize management of surgical patients through their perioperative period, ensuring they arrive for surgery in the best possible health and leave hospital as early as possible.

The process begins in primary care where pre-existing co-morbidities such as diabetes, hypertension and anaemia are treated or optimally controlled. Preoperative assessment and education aims to reduce anxiety and stress and address patients' expectations. High-risk patients should be seen by an anaesthetist and referred for cardiopulmonary exercise testing for risk stratification and planning of post-operative care. Where practical, patients should be admitted on the day of surgery and encouraged to drink up to 2 hours prior to surgery, preferably carbohydrate drinks to improve hydration and reduce duration of fasting. This may help to reduce anxiety and the surgical stress response. (Diabetic patients on insulin should not be given high carbohydrate drinks.)

Mode of anaesthesia is also addressed in ERPs. Balanced multimodal analgesia with regional techniques and wound catheters should be used to reduce the amount of long-acting opioid required. Identifying and treating patients with high risk of post-operative nausea and vomiting (PONV) and/or modification of the anaesthetic technique should be considered, for example use of total intravenous anaesthesia (TIVA). Over-hydration and hypothermia should be prevented as these are thought to impair wound healing. Goal-directed intraoperative fluid therapy and patient warming techniques can be used to address these.

Minimally invasive surgical techniques should be employed wherever possible. Nasogastric tubes delay gastric emptying and surgical drains reduce patient mobility and so both should be avoided if possible.

Post-operative rehabilitation should focus on early nutrition and mobilization and a discharge plan with social care support if needed.

## Further reading

Kitching A., O'Neill S. S. Fast-track surgery and anaesthesia. *Contin Educ Anaesth Crit Care Pain* 2009; 9(2): 39–43.

Delivering enhanced recovery: Helping patients to get better sooner after surgery. 2010. Available at http://webarchive.nationalarchives.gov.uk/20130107105354/ http://www.dh.gov.uk/prod_consum_dh/groups/dh_digitalassets/@dh/@en/@ps/documents/digitalasset/dh_115156.pdf (accessed 2 January 2016).

Guidelines for patients undergoing surgery as part of an Enhanced Recovery Programme (ERP). 2012. Available at http://www.rcoa.ac.uk/system/files/CSQ-ERP-Guide2012.pdf (accessed 2 January 2016).

## Urology: transurethral resection of prostate

You have performed a spinal anaesthetic on a patient undergoing a transurethral resection of the prostate (TURP). After around 60 minutes of surgery you notice the patient is becoming restless. On questioning he seems confused and complains of a headache and difficulty in breathing. His systolic blood pressure has dropped to 60 mmHg.

**Which of the following is the most likely diagnosis?**

a) Anaphylaxis
b) Sepsis
c) Total spinal anaesthetic
d) TUR syndrome
e) Bladder perforation

Answer: d)

All of the above diagnoses are possible, but this is most likely to be TUR syndrome based on the symptoms and timing of events. This is a clinical diagnosis based upon a collection of symptoms and signs caused by excessive absorption of irrigation fluid into the circulation. It comprises acute changes in intravascular volume, plasma solute concentrations, and osmolality, and direct effects of the irrigation fluid used. The effects are proportional to the volume of irrigating solution absorbed. The presentation is not always uniform, and milder cases may be unrecognized.

Mild to moderate TUR syndrome may occur in 1–8% of patients undergoing TURP. The overall mortality is 0.2–0.8%. It may present as early as 15 minutes after resection starts or as late as 24 hours after operation. Severe TUR syndrome is rare; however, it carries a mortality of up to 25%. When glycine is used as the irrigation fluid, early features of this syndrome include restlessness, headache, and tachypnoea, or a burning sensation in the face and hands. Visual disturbance including transient blindness may be reported. Features of increasing severity include respiratory distress, hypoxia, pulmonary oedema, nausea, vomiting, confusion, convulsions and coma. Acute volume changes predominantly affect the cardiovascular system. The rapid absorption of a large volume of irrigation fluid can cause hypertension with reflex bradycardia, and can precipitate acute cardiac failure and pulmonary oedema. The magnitude of the hypertension is not related to the volume of fluid absorbed. Rapid equilibration of hypotonic fluid with the extracellular fluid compartment may precipitate sudden hypotension in association with hypovolaemia. Hypotension and hypovolaemia may be compounded by the sympathetic block of spinal anaesthesia. Acute changes in plasma sodium concentration and osmolality predominantly affect the central nervous system. Acute hyponatraemia is produced initially by the dilutional effect of a large volume of absorbed irrigation fluid, but later is caused by natriuresis, and may cause headache, altered level of consciousness, nausea and vomiting, seizures, coma and death.

**What would be your immediate management?**

If TUR syndrome is suspected, surgery must be abandoned as soon as possible and intravenous fluids stopped. Treatment should involve supporting breathing (with intubation if necessary) and the circulation. Bradycardia and hypotension should be treated with atropine, adrenergic drugs and calcium. Anticonvulsants (e.g. diazepam or lorazepam) should be used to control seizures, and magnesium therapy considered if seizures prove difficult to control. Blood should be obtained and checked for sodium, osmolality and haemoglobin. Diuretic therapy is only recommended to treat acute pulmonary oedema, as it may worsen the hyponatraemia. Hypertonic saline (3%) is indicated to correct severe hyponatraemia, if serum sodium <120 mmol/l or if severe symptoms develop. Further management is likely to include insertion of central line, invasive monitoring and admission to the HDU or ICU.

## Further reading

O'Donnell A., Foo I. Anaesthesia for transurethral resection of the prostate. *Contin Educ Anaesth Crit Care Pain* 2009; 9: 92–6.

## Urology: renal transplant

A 58-year-old woman is undergoing cadaveric renal transplant. Her medical history includes end-stage renal failure secondary to glomerulonephritis, and hypertension. She was dialysed 2 days prior to the operation. During the operation, her blood pressure falls to 86/49 mmHg, with heart rate 88 bpm and central venous pressure (CVP) 5 mmHg.

**What would be the most appropriate course of action to manage this blood pressure?**

a) Give an alpha-adrenoreceptor agonist, e.g. phenylephrine
b) Give a $D_2$ receptor agonist, e.g. dopamine
c) Give intravenous fluid
d) Give a beta-adrenoreceptor agonist, e.g. dobutamine
e) Allow this level of hypotension

Answer: c)

In patients with end-stage renal failure undergoing surgery, intravenous fluids are usually minimized to avoid fluid overload. The exception to this rule is with renal transplant surgery. Following removal of the vascular clamps, good perfusion of the transplanted kidney is needed to increase the chance of it functioning. The primary anaesthetic goal is an adequate intravascular volume, with a target central venous pressure (CVP) of 10–12 mmHg, or if a pulmonary artery catheter is in situ, a pulmonary capillary wedge pressure of approximately 15 mmHg. This may, on occasion, require administration of several litres of intravenous fluid. Recent dialysis in the preoperative period can contribute to intravascular depletion.

If hypotension persists despite reaching these goals, the next step would be inotropic support with either low dose dopamine or a beta-adrenoreceptor agonist. The aim is to avoid the use of sole alpha-adrenoreceptor agonists, as this may reduce perfusion of the new kidney.

Most centres have their own recipe for drugs to be administered during the transplant procedure once the graft is perfused, to improve survival. These may include steroids and diuretics. It is worth checking with your surgical team at the WHO briefing what they would like and when.

## Further reading

Rabey P. G. Anaesthesia for renal transplantation. *BJA CEPD Rev* 2001; 1: 24–7. Available at
http://ceaccp.oxfordjournals.org/content/1/1/24 (accessed 12 April 2015).

Schmid S., Jungwirth B. Anaesthesia for renal transplant surgery: an update. *Eur J Anaesthesiol* 2012;
29: 552–8. Available at http://journals.lww.com/ejanaesthesiology/Fulltext/2012/12000/
Anaesthesia_for_renal_transplant_surgery_an.3.aspx (accessed 2 January 2016).

# Gynaecology: airway management for laparoscopic surgery

The first patient on your gynaecology list is scheduled to have a diagnostic laparoscopy. She
has been seen at the preoperative assessment clinic and her body mass index was recorded
as 35. She also gives a history of occasional reflux after eating certain foods.

**What are the relevant issues to consider when planning airway management for this case?**

Intra-abdominal laparoscopic surgery requires the generation of a pneumoperitoneum to
allow visualization of the intra-abdominal organs to enable surgery to be performed. The
physiological effects that this causes are described in a previous question and in a patient
with a high BMI these effects are even more pronounced.

The most common technique for airway management for laparoscopic surgery is endotracheal intubation and ventilation. This protects against gastric acid aspiration, allows optimal control of $CO_2$ and facilitates surgical access. Ideally, mask ventilation before intubation
should be minimized to avoid gastric distension. If this occurs then insertion of a nasogastric tube may be required to deflate the stomach and minimize the risk of gastric injury on
trochar insertion and to improve the surgical view.

The use of the classic laryngeal mask airway (LMA) in laparoscopic surgery remains con-
troversial because of the increased risk of aspiration and difficulties encountered when trying to maintain effective gas transfer while delivering the higher airway pressures required
during pneumoperitoneum. However, the development of newer LMAs has addressed some
of the concerns and prompted consideration of alternatives to intubation in certain patient
groups for short laparoscopic procedures, such as in gynaecology.

There have been several randomized controlled trials comparing the use of the ProSeal
LMA with endotracheal intubation. The ProSeal LMA has a modified cuff to increase the
seal against the glottis without causing an increase in mucosal pressure. This enables the use
of positive pressure ventilation. It also has a built-in drainage tube to provide a channel for
regurgitated fluid, prevent gastric insufflation and allow insertion of a gastric decompression
tube. Data advocate that in laparoscopic surgery, the ProSeal LMA is as effective and efficient
for pulmonary ventilation as an endotracheal tube in patients of BMI < 30 without a history
of reflux.

The i-gel is a supraglottic airway device that has a soft gel-like non-inflatable cuff to provide an anatomical fit over the laryngeal inlet. Like the ProSeal LMA it too has a gastric
drainage tube. Studies show that the i-gel provides a reliable seal during anaesthesia for positive pressure ventilation and is safe to use in laparoscopic surgery.

The patient in this scenario has both a high BMI and a history of acid reflux and so the
safest means for securing the airway is with an endotracheal tube. In slim patients, with no
history of reflux, the evidence suggests it is reasonable to consider using an LMA for short
laparoscopic procedures.

# Further reading

Hayden P., Cowman S. Anaesthesia for laparoscopic surgery. *Contin Educ Anaesth Crit Care Pain* 2011; 11(5): 177–80.

Lim Y., Goel S., Brimacombe J. The ProSeal laryngeal mask airway is an effective alternative to laryngoscope-guided tracheal intubation for gynaecological laparoscopy. *Anaesth Intensive Care* 2007; 35(1): 52–6.

Sharma B., Sehgal R., Sahai C. et al. PLMA vs. i-gel: a comparative evaluation of respiratory mechanics in laparoscopic cholecystectomy. *J Anaesthesiol Clin Pharmacol* 2010; 26(4): 451–7.

# Day surgery

## 18

*More procedures of an increasingly complex nature are being performed on a day case basis. Patients attending for day surgery are evermore complex. To help to optimize efficiency of day surgery services, protocols and guidelines have been developed, some nationally and many specific to individual organizations. This chapter covers some of the relevant issues when anaesthetizing for day surgery.*

## Day surgery list management

You have been asked to cover a morning day case general surgery list. Listed are two laparoscopic cholecystectomies and one inguinal hernia repair. During your preoperative assessments you discover that one of the patients has type 1 diabetes and the patient listed for the hernia repair has severe chronic obstructive pulmonary disease (COPD), with an FVC of 1 l and markedly reduced exercise tolerance. He has been optimized as much as possible by the respiratory team.

**What are your considerations when deciding on list order?**

Communication with the operating surgeon is essential to ensure that the right patient is operated on at the right time. Although not an issue here, children should be prioritized first on the list. Patients with diabetes should also take priority, given that their glycaemic control may be impaired if fasted for prolonged periods.

There is an anaesthetic challenge on this list in the form of the patient with COPD. His pulmonary function tests and functional capacity suggest that he is unlikely to be suitable for a general anaesthetic, and a regional technique would be more appropriate. Given that this is a morning list, there is an opportunity to deliver a spinal anaesthetic whilst allowing adequate recovery time, should you feel the patient is suitable to be discharged. You have fewer grounds for cancellation as he is maximally treated.

Communication with the surgeon and theatre team at the team brief is vital – remember, other factors may influence list order, e.g. equipment availability, surgical concerns.

**What strategies could you employ to ensure both efficiency and patient comfort?**

Organizing list order allows you to be proactive in managing starvation times and analgesia particularly. Anaesthetic techniques should ensure minimum stress and maximum comfort for the patients and should take into consideration the risks and benefits of the individual techniques.

*Returning to Work in Anaesthesia*, ed. Emma Plunkett, Emily Johnson and Anna Pierson.
Published by Cambridge University Press. © Cambridge University Press 2016.

Analgesia is paramount and must be long-acting but, as morbidity such as nausea and vomiting must be minimized, the indiscriminate use of opioids is discouraged (particularly morphine). Prophylactic oral analgesics, e.g. paracetamol, along with long-acting NSAIDs should be given to all patients unless contraindicated. These should be clearly prescribed and nursing staff informed to ensure drugs are given in a timely fashion. It should be noted that NSAIDs are to be avoided in ischaemic heart disease, cerebro- and reno-vascular disease, as per Medicines and Healthcare Products Regulatory Agency (MHRA) recommendations.

For certain procedures (e.g. laparoscopic cholecystectomy) there is evidence that standardized anaesthesia protocols or techniques improve outcome. Anaesthetists should adhere to such guidelines if they exist. Information regarding this can be found in the Association of Anaesthetists of Great Britain and Ireland (AAGBI) leaflets.

The use of local/regional anaesthetic techniques also needs consideration and may also serve to minimize IV opioid use. Prilotekal (hyperbaric 2% prilocaine) is now indicated for spinal anaesthesia in adults undergoing short surgical procedures – a standard dose to achieve a block up to T10 has a duration of action lasting, on average, 100–130 minutes.

Your aim is to ensure a quick turnaround of patients, who need minimal time in recovery. In addition to the analgesic strategies above, routine use of antiemetics, modest intraoperative IV fluid administration and minimizing starvation times all enhance throughput. Do not forget: patients are permitted clear fluids up to 2 hours prior. Where possible, allow them to drink water or a carbohydrate-loading drink. This will only work if you are certain of list order.

## Obesity and day surgery

A 44-year-old female patient presents to the pre-assessment clinic for laparoscopic cholecystectomy as a day case procedure. She has a BMI of 39 kg/m$^2$ and type 2 diabetes mellitus, which is controlled with metformin 1 g BD and pioglitazone 30 mg OD. She has no abnormal cardiorespiratory symptoms.

**Select the most appropriate course of action:**

a) List for day case surgery immediately
b) List as a day case if glycosylated haemoglobin (HbA1c) is <80 mmol/mol (9.5%) with a normal ECG
c) List for an inpatient procedure; she will need a variable-rate insulin infusion on the day of surgery
d) List for day case surgery if HbA1c is ≤69 mmol/mol (8.5%) with a normal ECG, FBC, liver function tests and U&Es
e) List for day case surgery if echocardiogram, ECG, arterial blood gas (ABG), HbA1c and U&Es are all normal

Answer: d)

The patient should not be listed for immediate day case surgery, as it is necessary to establish that she has stable disease, and no obesity-related risk factors to increase her anaesthetic and surgical risk. HbA1c is used to assess glycaemic control over the preceding 2–3 months. A value ≤69 mmol/mol (8.5%) is considered to be acceptable in a diabetic patient. A value of 80 mmol/mol (9.5%) is too high and would require referral to primary care for further management.

The patient also requires investigation into possible end-organ damage and should have her renal function and electrolytes checked. The side effects of metformin include renal dysfunction, and pioglitazone can induce liver dysfunction. The BNF recommends stopping metformin and pioglitazone on the morning of surgery and restarting when the patient is able to eat and drink.

This approach fits in well with recent NHS diabetes guidance for perioperative diabetes management, which highlights the importance of involving patients in planning and managing care of their diabetes in the perioperative period. These patients should be prioritized on the operating list, and high-risk patients (with poor glycaemic control/complications of diabetes) should be identified preoperatively so that their risk can be managed appropriately.

Patients with no more than one missed meal (i.e. a short starvation period) should be managed by modification of their usual diabetes regime. Patients who miss more than one meal should receive a variable-rate intravenous insulin infusion (VRIII – the new term for insulin sliding scale). Admitting the patient prior to the planned procedure is an option, but this does not fit in with AAGBI/NHS Diabetes guidance, which aims to allow patients to take control of their diabetes while in hospital – which they are generally very good at doing.

The AAGBI guideline on obesity suggests that risk factors for cardiorespiratory compromise should be sought, as these would put the patient in a higher risk group. Any metabolic syndrome should be assessed by looking for end-organ damage and assessing control. The guidance also suggests that patients with BMI $> 40$ kg/m$^2$ should be reviewed by a bariatric anaesthetist, but this should not preclude the patient being listed for day surgery. There is no reason to perform echocardiogram or ABG on all obese patients unless there is an indication to do so, for example suspicion of obstructive sleep apnoea. The AAGBI recommends eliciting the history and measuring SpO$_2$ as a screening tool.

## Discharge criteria following day surgery

A 25-year-old female has attended for a day case hysteroscopy. She has recovered from her general anaesthetic and is well enough to be discharged from hospital.

**Which of the following statements is true regarding current discharge criteria from a day case facility after a general anaesthetic?**

a) All patients should receive verbal and written instructions on discharge
b) The patient must be able to tolerate oral fluids before being discharged
c) The patient must have passed urine before discharge
d) Advice should be given not to drink alcohol, operate machinery or drive for 48 hours after a general anaesthetic
e) All patients should be discharged with a supply of appropriate analgesics and antiemetics

Answer: a)

Advances in anaesthetic and surgical techniques have led to an increased number of operations being performed on a day case basis. The AAGBI in association with the British Association of Day Surgery (BADS) have produced concise guidelines on the delivery of day case and short stay surgery.

Effective preoperative assessment and preparation with protocol-driven, nurse-led discharge are fundamental to safe and effective day and short stay surgery. In 2000, The

Department of Health published an NHS plan which set a target that 75% of elective surgery should be performed on a day case basis. The complexity of procedures has increased with a wider range of patients now considered suitable for day surgery. In addition, the advancement of minimally invasive surgery is allowing more procedures to be performed on a day case basis.

Some of the traditional discharge criteria such as tolerating fluids and passing urine are no longer enforced. Mandatory oral intake is not necessary and may provoke nausea and vomiting and delay discharge. Voiding is also not always required, although it is important to identify and retain patients who are at particular risk of developing later problems, such as those who have experienced prolonged instrumentation or manipulation of the bladder.

All patients should receive verbal and written instructions on discharge and be warned of any symptoms that might be experienced. Wherever possible, these instructions should be given in the presence of the responsible person who is to escort and care for the patient at home. Advice should be given not to drink alcohol, operate machinery or drive for 24 hours after a general anaesthetic.

All patients should be discharged with a supply of appropriate analgesics and instructions in their use. It is not essential to provide a supply of antiemetics although the patient should obviously be free from nausea and vomiting before being discharged.

## Further reading

Association of Anaesthetists of Great Britain and Ireland (AAGBI). Perioperative Management of the Morbidly Obese. London: AAGBI, 2007. Available at http://www.aagbi.org/sites/default/files/Obesity07.pdf (accessed 4th February 2015).

Association of Anaesthetists of Great Britain and Ireland (AAGBI) and British Association of Day Surgery. Day Case and Short Stay Surgery. London: AAGBI, 2011. Available at http://www.aagbi.org/sites/default/files/Day%20Case%20for%20web.pdf (accessed 6 June 2015).

Association of Surgeons of Great Britain and Ireland (ASGBI). The Peri-operative Management of the Adult Patient with Diabetes. London: ASGBI, 2012. Available at www.asgbi.org.uk (accessed 14 April 2015).

NHS Diabetes. Management of adults with diabetes undergoing surgery and elective procedures: improving standards. Available at http://www.diabetes.nhs.uk/areas_of_care/emergency_and_inpatient/perioperative_management (accessed 14 April 2015).

# Trauma and orthopaedics

**19**

*The first half of this chapter covers topics relevant to those dealing with patients with trauma: burns, recent developments in major trauma and how to optimally manage the increasing numbers of patients with fractured hips. The second half covers common issues applicable to those anaesthetizing for orthopaedic lists: cementing, compartment syndrome and tourniquets. They may seem rather surgical topics but, as key members of the theatre team, anaesthetists should be aware of these issues and how to manage them.*

## Initial assessment and resuscitation of burns

You are called to A+E where a 25-year-old man has just arrived. He has been involved in a warehouse fire and has extensive burns to his face, neck, chest and arms.

**What are the key considerations in your initial assessment of this patient?**

As with any trauma patient there should be an ABC approach. In addition to the standard assessment, consider the following points specific to burns patients.

Airway (with C-spine control): assess for signs of current or potential airway compromise. Immediate tracheal intubation may be required.

Breathing: blast injuries can be associated with tension pneumothoraces. Full-thickness circumferential burns to the chest wall may necessitate escharotomies to prevent restriction to ventilation. Perform an arterial blood gas to assess for hypoxia, hypercarbia and CO poisoning (pulse oximetry cannot differentiate between $HbO_2$ and $HbCO$).

Circulation: insert cannulae through intact skin where possible. Non-invasive BP measurement can be difficult if limbs are injured, an arterial line may be required. If clinically hypovolaemic look for other injuries, burns are an unlikely cause at this early stage.

Exposure: Estimate the extent and thickness of burns, look for other injuries and keep the patient warm.

Obtain as much history as possible, it can provide valuable information about likely injuries sustained, i.e. history of confinement within a burning building makes inhalational injury more likely.

**What features would make you consider immediate intubation and how would you do this?**

*Returning to Work in Anaesthesia*, ed. Emma Plunkett, Emily Johnson and Anna Pierson.
Published by Cambridge University Press. © Cambridge University Press 2016.

Signs suggestive of inhalational injury include: stridor or hoarse voice; respiratory distress; soot in sputum; burnt nasal hair or eyebrows; oropharyngeal oedema and a raised carboxyhaemoglobin level. Other indications include full-thickness neck burns and a Glasgow Coma Score (GCS) < 8.

Intubation should be performed using a rapid sequence induction (RSI) or modified RSI technique. Within 24 hours of the burn suxamethonium can be used (after this do not use for 2 years as risk of precipitating hyperkalaemia). An uncut endotracheal tube should be inserted as facial swelling may occur, and use at least a size 8.0 where possible to allow bronchoscopy to be performed.

**How would you calculate the extent of the burn injury?**

The 'rule of nines' can be used for adult patients. The body is divided into anatomical zones representing 9% or multiples of 9%. Alternatively the Lund–Browder chart can be used for adults and children.

**How would you calculate the patient's fluid requirements?**

The Parkland formula is used to predict the fluid requirements for the first 24 hours:

$$\text{Volume required (ml)} = 4 \times \text{Wt(Kg)} \times \%\text{burn}$$

Administer half the fluid in the first 8 hours following the injury, and the other half over the next 16 hours. IV fluids already administered should be deducted from the calculation. A urinary catheter should be inserted to guide fluid resuscitation, aim for a minimum urine output of 0.5 ml/kg/h in adults.

## Further reading

Allman K. G., Wilson I. H. (eds.) *Oxford Handbook of Anaesthesia*, 3rd edn. Oxford: Oxford University Press, 2011.
American College of Surgeons Committee on Trauma. *Advanced Trauma Life Support for Doctors. ATLS Student Course Manual*, 8th edn. Chicago: American College of Surgeons, 2008.
Bishop S., Maguire S. Anaesthesia and intensive care for major burns. *Contin Educ Anaesth Crit Care Pain* 2012; 12(3): 118–22.

# Principles of management of major trauma

**What is Damage Control Resuscitation?**

Damage Control Resuscitation (DCR), also known as haemostatic resuscitation, aims to minimize the consequential 'lethal triad' of massive haemorrhage; acidosis, coagulopathy and hypothermia. DCR is often undertaken simultaneously with Damage Control Surgery; where control of immediately life-threatening injuries and major haemorrhage are addressed with definitive surgery delayed until physiological stability is achieved. For DCR to be most effective, hypovolaemic shock needs to be recognized early and resuscitation initiated immediately.

**What are the three main principles of DCR?**

The main principles of DCR are:
1. To avoid dilution coagulopathy, tissue oedema and impaired tissue oxygen delivery by minimizing administration of IV crystalloid during early resuscitation.

2. Permissive hypotension; aiming for a systolic blood pressure (BP) of 90 mmHg, to balance adequate tissue perfusion with allowing clot stabilization.
3. Transfusion of blood products in ratios similar to whole blood, approximately 1:1:1 of red blood cells, platelets and plasma. Massive transfusion should be guided by support from the massive transfusion policy/protocol, alongside support from haematology services. Coagulopathy should be recognized early and treated aggressively guided by rapid bedside dynamic assessment of coagulation and fibrinolysis such as thromboelastography (TEG) or thromboelastometry (TEM). There is no convincing evidence that use of recombinant factor VIIa improves outcomes in this situation.

**What is the current evidence for use of tranexamic acid following significant haemorrhage due to major trauma?**

The CRASH-2 trial was a randomized controlled trial of over 20 000 patients, published in 2010, which showed that administration of tranexamic acid (TXA) within 8 hours of injury (loading dose of 1 g over 10 minutes then infusion of 1 g over 8 hours) reduced all-cause mortality (relative risk 0.91, 95% CI 0.85–0.97). However, the number needed to treat was 121 patients and mortality increased when TXA was given more than 3 hours post injury. The investigators have recommended that TXA should not be administered more than 3 hours after the injury, and only in those who have severe haemorrhagic shock, with a systolic BP < 75 mmHg and a base deficit > 5, alongside hyperfibrinolysis demonstrated by TEG or TEM.

**What is the current evidence for use of corticosteroid following head injury?**

The MRC CRASH trial, published in 2005, was a near 10000 patient double blind placebo-controlled randomized trial which showed that administration of methylprednisolone post head injury increased the likelihood of death or serious disability up to 6 months following injury (odds ratio 1.15, 95% CI 1.07–1.24).

## Further reading

Bogert J. N., Harvin J. A., Cotton B. A. Damage control resuscitation. *J Intensive Care Med* 2014; pii: 0885066614558018. [Epub ahead of print]

Edwards P., Arango M., Balica L. et al. Final results of MRC CRASH, a randomised placebo-controlled trial of intravenous corticosteroid in adults with head injury-outcomes at 6 months. *Lancet* 2005; 365(9475): 1957–9.

Williams-Johnson J. A., McDonald A. H., Strachan G. G., Williams E. W. Effects of tranexamic acid on death, vascular occlusive events, and blood transfusion in trauma patients with significant haemorrhage (CRASH-2): a randomised, placebo-controlled trial. *West Indian Med J* 2010; 59(6): 612–24.

## Management of the patient with a fractured neck of femur

An 83-year-old lady was admitted 24 hours ago, with an intracapsular fracture of the left neck of femur following a fall at home. Her co-morbidities include hypertension, atrial fibrillation (AF) and asthma for which she is taking ramipril, bisoprolol, warfarin and inhalers. On pre-operative assessment she has a Glasgow Coma Score (GCS) of 15/15, heart rate 99 bpm, blood pressure 142/89 mmHg and $SpO_2$ 95% on air with clear breath sounds but an ejection systolic murmur (ESM) (no history of angina, syncope or heart failure). There is no record of an echocardiography performed previously. The only abnormal blood results are an Hb of 103 g/dl.

**She is listed for left hemiarthroplasty on your trauma list, what is your management plan?**

a) Sedation with midazolam, spinal anaesthesia in lateral position with right side down, isobaric bupivacaine 0.5%, 2.3 ml with fentanyl 15 mcg
b) Sedation with midazolam, spinal anaesthesia in lateral position with left side down, hyperbaric bupivacaine 0.5%, 1.7 ml with fentanyl 15 mcg
c) Delay surgery until urgent echocardiography to determine the severity of possible aortic stenosis followed by cardiology review for preoptimization
d) Delay surgery until urgent echocardiography to determine the severity of possible aortic stenosis followed by general anaesthesia with intraoperative arterial pressure monitoring
e) Avoid delaying surgery, general anaesthesia with intraoperative invasive arterial pressure monitoring

Answer: b)

Hip fractures are more common in the frail elderly female population, with a 30-day mortality of 8.2%. The 2011 Association of Anaesthetists of Great Britain and Ireland (AAGBI) guidelines for management of proximal femoral fractures stressed the importance of a multidisciplinary team approach. The guidelines suggest consideration of spinal/epidural anaesthesia for all patients ideally with hyperbaric bupivacaine (a dose of <10 mg is associated with less hypotension) in the lateral position (bad side down) and fentanyl as the intrathecal opioid of choice. (Intrathecal diamorphine or morphine risks causing respiratory depression or confusion post-operatively.) If sedation is required for patient positioning, ideally midazolam or propofol should be used along with supplemental oxygen. Both ketamine and hypoxia may add to post-operative confusion. Hypotension should be avoided and nerve blocks should be considered for all patients in the perioperative period.

Although this patient has an ESM she does not have any symptoms suggestive of severe aortic stenosis. Investigations such as echocardiography should not delay the surgery as a delay of more than 48 hours has been shown to increase complications and post-operative mortality. Also, post-operative early mortality in patients with or without arterial stenosis is similar.

A lesser incidence of post-operative confusion, deep vein thrombosis, early post-operative mortality, pneumonia and hypoxia with regional anaesthesia was noted in a meta-analysis in 2010.

In 2014 the results of the Anaesthetic Sprint Audit of Practice Standards (ASAP) were published. The main recommendations were that spinal anaesthesia (SA) is associated with decreased occurrence of hypotension as compared with general anaesthesia (GA) and hence should be considered for all patients. Use of perioperative nerve blocks was limited in the audit and again should be offered to all patients. If the patient would benefit from GA over SA, then inhalational agents should be considered as these have been shown to offer greater cardiostability than intravenous agents in the ASAP audit. Concomitant GA and SA should be avoided as it showed the highest occurrence of hypotension when compared with other anaesthetic techniques.

Bone cement implantation syndrome (BCIS) causing hypoxia and hypotension occurred and patients undergoing cemented hemiarthroplasty should be assessed for BCIS routinely.

# Further reading

Association of Anaesthetists of Great Britain and Ireland (AAGBI). AAGBI Safety Guideline. Management of Proximal Femoral Fractures. London: AAGBI, 2011. Available at http://www.aagbi .org/sites/default/files/femoral%20fractures%202012_0.pdf (accessed 2 January 2016).

Luger T. J., Kammerlander C., Gosch M. et al. Neuroaxial versus general anaesthesia in geriatric patients for hip fracture surgery: does it matter? *Osteoporos Int* 2010; 21: S555–72.

Maxwell L., White S. Anaesthetic management of patients with hip fractures: an update. *Contin Educ Anaesth Crit Care Pain* 2013; 13(5): 179–83.

National Hip Fracture Database. Anaesthesia sprint audit of practice (ASAP). www.hqip.org.uk/ resources/national-hip-fracture-database-anaesthesia-sprint-audit-of-practice-asap/ (accessed 2 January 2016).

# Cementing

An 80-year-old gentleman is listed to have a cemented hemiarthroplasty fixation for a hip fracture. He was admitted yesterday following a simple mechanical fall at home. He has a history of stable ischaemic heart disease and lives independently with his wife.

**What is bone cement implantation syndrome (BCIS)?**

The use of cemented prostheses for hip fracture surgery increases the likelihood of pain-free mobility, reduces the risk of re-operation and is associated with a lower mortality rate at 30 days. BCIS occurs around the time of cementing, insertion of prosthesis or reduction of the hip, and is characterized by hypoxia, hypotension, loss of consciousness or cardiac arrest. It has been highlighted as a particular risk in frail patients undergoing cemented prosthesis following hip fracture.

**Table 19.1** Incidence of adverse effects during cemented hip fracture surgery

| Grade 1 BCIS | Arterial saturation <94% or >20% fall in systolic blood pressure | c. 21% |
| --- | --- | --- |
| Grade 2 BCIS | Arterial saturation <88% or >40% fall in systolic blood pressure or loss of consciousness | c. 5% |
| Grade 3 BCIS | Cardiopulmonary resuscitation required | c. 1.7% |

**Which patients are at highest risk of developing BCIS?**

Risk factors associated with severe cardiovascular events during cemented hip fracture surgery are high ASA grade, chronic obstructive pulmonary disease and use of diuretic or warfarin medication.

**How would you minimize the risks of BCIS in this patient?**

All hip fracture surgery should be undertaken or directly supervised by appropriately experienced anaesthetists and surgeons, ideally on planned trauma lists. A multidisciplinary three-stage process is recommended to minimize the risk of BCIS:

1. Identification of patients at high risk of cardiorespiratory compromise (using the risk factors listed above).
2. Preparation of team and identification of roles in case of severe reaction (one example of role allocation in the event of cardiovascular collapse is described in the Coventry Cement Curfew):

a. Preoperative multidisciplinary discussion when appropriate.

b. Pre-list briefing and World Health Organization Safe Surgery checklist 'time-out'.

3. Specific intraoperative roles:

Surgeon:

a. Inform anaesthetist when you are about to insert cement.

b. Wash and dry femoral canal.

c. Apply cement retrogradely using the cement gun with a suction catheter and intramedullary plug in the femoral shaft.

d. Avoid excessive pressurization.

Anaesthetist:

a. Ensure adequate resuscitation pre- and intraoperatively.

b. Confirm to surgeon that you are aware they are about to prepare/apply cement.

c. Maintain vigilance for signs of cardiorespiratory compromise using either an arterial line or non-invasive blood pressure monitoring set on 'stat' mode during/shortly after application of cement. During general anaesthesia a sudden drop in end-tidal $CO_2$ may indicate right heart failure and/or catastrophic reduction in cardiac output.

d. Aim for a systolic blood pressure within 20% of pre-induction value.

e. Prepare vasopressors in case of cardiovascular collapse.

## Further reading

Griffiths R., Parker M. Bone cement implantation syndrome and proximal femoral fracture. *Br J Anaesth* 2015; 114: 6–7.

Griffiths R., White S. M., Moppett I. K. et al. Safety guideline: reducing the risk from cemented arthroplasty for hip fracture 2015. *Anaesthesia* 2015; 70: 623–6.

Olsen F., Kotyra M., Houltz E., Ricksten S.-E. Bone cement implantation syndrome in cemented hemiarthroplasty for femoral neck fracture: incidence, risk factors and effect on outcome. *Br J Anaesth* 2014; 113: 800–6.

Scase A. Coventry 'Cement Curfew': team training for crisis. *Anaesthesia News*, October 2014; 327: 8–9.

## Compartment syndrome

You are asked to review a 70-year-old male on the High Dependency Unit. The patient is 12 hours post radical cystectomy. He is complaining of severe pain in his right lower leg despite having an epidural in situ for analgesia. You examine his right calf and feel that it is tense. You inspect his anaesthetic chart and note that he had been in the lithotomy position intraoperatively. You suspect that he has developed a compartment syndrome of his right calf.

**Which of the following are risk factors for the development of compartment syndrome?**

a) Intraoperative hypotension

b) Peripheral vascular disease

c) Prolonged operative time >4 hours

d) Muscular calves

e) Trendelenburg position

Answer: all are true

The lithotomy position is commonly used to access the pelvis and perineum during urological, colorectal, and gynaecological surgery. Compartment syndrome of the lower leg occurs when increased osteofascial compartmental pressure leads to decreased tissue perfusion to the leg. It can develop after prolonged elevation of the lower limbs during surgical procedures in the lithotomy position. When a patient is in this position, lower leg compartment systolic blood pressure falls. If this decrease in systolic pressure falls below the perfusion pressure, tissue ischaemia occurs. This effect is increased by the Trendelenburg position (putting the patient in a head-down position). Ischaemia may be followed by reperfusion with subsequent capillary leakage and tissue oedema. A vicious circle of tissue oedema and further impairment of perfusion then occurs. Once compartment pressure rises above 50 mmHg for more than 4 hours irreversible neuromuscular damage will occur although damage is reversible up to 2–3 hours.

Lower limb compartment syndrome typically presents post-operatively with leg pain out of proportion to the clinical findings. The classic findings of calf swelling, paraesthesia, weakness of toe flexion and pain during passive toe extension are late and may suggest an established compartment syndrome. The presence of foot pulses does not necessarily show that the compartment is well perfused.

The definitive diagnosis of a compartment syndrome is made by a direct measurement of intra-compartmental pressure. The normal range of compartment pressure is between 0 mmHg and 10 mmHg. The decision to operate should be made in conjunction with clinical findings although a value of 30 mmHg usually shows that surgical decompression is needed. Once the decision has been made to intervene, urgent fasciotomy of all lower limb muscle compartments is usually an effective treatment.

## Further reading

Simms M. S., Terry T. R. Well leg compartment syndrome after pelvic and perineal surgery in the lithotomy position. *Postgrad Med J* 2005; 81: 534–6.

## Use of tourniquets

You have performed an axillary nerve block on a frail, 55 kg 78-year-old lady with multiple co-morbidities for exploratory surgery on her hand following a fall. Her blood pressure is 110/40. You have decided that general anaesthesia will not be required. The limb has been exsanguinated, and you have been asked to inflate the tourniquet.

**Which of the following statements are true?**

a) Tourniquet-related injury can be prevented by limiting inflation pressure to 250 mmHg, and avoiding inflation for more than 60 minutes
b) When performing awake surgery, tourniquet pain can be minimized by intercostobrachial nerve block
c) Sedation or intravenous analgesia may be required
d) Lower limbs are at higher risk of tourniquet injury than upper limbs

Answer: FTTF

Tourniquets are generally applied to reduce intraoperative blood loss, and provide a bloodless field for operating, although may also be used in special circumstances such as intravenous regional limb blockade (Bier's block). Morbidity associated with tourniquet application can be minimized by an understanding of potential risks and adherence to good practice. Risks can be divided into those associated with inappropriate tourniquet application or mal-position, and those associated with chosen cuff pressure or duration. Responsibility for the avoidance of cuff-related morbidity is shared between the operating surgeon and anaesthetist.

### Inappropriate application

Tourniquets should be correctly sized for the limb type and girth, and applied by a trained practitioner. An adequate seal must be made between the tourniquet and the operative site to prevent seepage of surgical preparation fluid under the cuff where chemical skin damage can occur.

### Cuff pressure and duration

Cuff inflation pressure should ideally not be standardized for all patients, as this leads to unnecessary risk. Ideally, the limb occlusion pressure (LOP) should be measured (the pressure at which peripheral arterial Doppler measurement is no longer measureable), and the inflation pressure applied at this plus a 40–100 mmHg safety margin. The higher safety margins are required for relatively high LOPs, for patients in which there is a likelihood of significant arterial pressure swings intraoperatively, and for Bier's block. There is no clear cut rule to define safe duration of tourniquet inflation, and safe duration must be modified based on patient characteristics – increased risks of injury in limbs with pre-existing compromise, those with little tissue to protect neurovascular structures, increased risk for upper limbs, and individuals requiring higher cuff inflation pressures. Generally, the surgeon should be alerted to inflation duration at 1 hour, and 90 minutes should not be exceeded without releasing the tourniquet for a period. Should this be required, the operating site should be covered, and the limb elevated to facilitate reperfusion and venous drainage for around 15 minutes before re-exsanguination.

## Further reading

Noordin S., McEwen J. A., Kragh J. F. Jr, Eisen A., Masri B. A. Surgical tourniquets in orthopaedics. *J Bone Joint Surg Am* 2009; 91(12): 2958–67.

# Subspecialty anaesthesia

*This chapter is a mixed bag of questions covering a number of different subspecialties. We have chosen topics within those specialties that are either common clinical scenarios (we remind you of the basics) or less common but more challenging situations (where we discuss the options). Some of these are the classic difficult situations, such as the bleeding tonsil, and you may have your preferred method of managing such cases. Hopefully the questions will prompt you to remember your own recipes or otherwise remind you of the key points to consider.*

## ENT, maxillo-facial and dental: inhaled foreign body

A previously well 2-year-old child is brought to the emergency department with a 1-hour history of wheeze and shortness of breath associated with a sudden onset of coughing while eating. On arrival, the child is distressed and coughing intermittently. The respiratory rate is 45 breaths/min with intercostal recession. No stridor is observed.

**Regarding immediate management of this patient, which one of the following is most correct?**

a) A chest x-ray is a useful investigation in this situation
b) If tracheal obstruction is suspected, positive-pressure ventilation is contraindicated
c) If the child develops complete airway obstruction in the emergency department, the child should be anaesthetized immediately for bronchoscopic foreign body removal
d) Anaesthesia should be delayed until the child is adequately fasted
e) A modified rapid sequence induction is generally accepted as the most appropriate induction technique

Answer: b)

The history of sudden onset of distress followed by coughing and wheezing should raise suspicion of an inhaled foreign body. Foreign body (FB) aspiration is one of the leading causes of death in young children. An FB in the upper airways may present as an emergency airway obstruction. Obstruction of the lower airways may present later with a history of persistent cough and signs of lower respiratory chest infection. A chest x-ray may aid the diagnosis in the stable child, but the majority of inhaled FBs are organic and therefore will not be visible on x-ray. Therefore, a chest x-ray may appear normal, especially if taken early in the clinical course. Other frequent radiological findings include gas trapping (due to ball-valve effect),

*Returning to Work in Anaesthesia*, ed. Emma Plunkett, Emily Johnson and Anna Pierson.
Published by Cambridge University Press. © Cambridge University Press 2016.

atelectasis and lobar collapse. This child is unstable; therefore an x-ray is not an appropriate investigation.

Immediate management involves assessment as per the choking child algorithm included in Advanced Paediatric Life Support. In the child with an effective cough, gold-standard management is FB removal using a rigid open tube bronchoscope. Ideally, anaesthesia would be delayed until the child is adequately fasted. However, this decision is dependent on the clinical state of the child.

Inhalational induction allows the maintenance of spontaneous ventilation (despite the potential full stomach). Rapid sequence induction presents problems with pre-oxygenation of the distressed child, pre-induction intravenous access and the potential for a 'can't intubate, can't ventilate' scenario. In this situation, most anaesthetists would favour an inhalational induction.

Maintenance of anaesthesia may be difficult owing to the issue of shared access. Usually, spontaneous ventilation is maintained throughout with the bronchoscope connected to an Ayre's T-piece. If tracheal or ball-valve obstruction is suspected, positive-pressure ventilation is contraindicated, as this may lead to further distal movement of the FB. A common time for serious intraoperative compromise is during removal of the FB, as it may become dislodged, leading to severe/complete airway obstruction.

## Further reading

Allman K. G., Wilson I. H. *Oxford Handbook of Anaesthesia*, 2nd edn. Oxford: Oxford University Press, 2007; p. 808.

Resuscitation Council (UK). Paediatric basic life support. Resuscitation Guidelines 2010. Available at www.resus.org.uk/pages/guide.htm (accessed 24 January 2015).

Skinner A. Inhaled foreign body in children. WFSA Tutorial of the Week, 8 July 2008. Available at www.wfsahq.org/components/com_virtual_library/media/befa3502e385e9012680cd35432f1614-b9ce6b5dcb00b2397d392d8ecd6f60ab-99-Inhaled-foreign-body-in-children.pdf (accessed 9 January 2016).

Wang K., Harnden A., Thomson A. Foreign body inhalation in children. *BMJ* 2010; 341: c3924. Available at http://www.bmj.com/content/341/bmj.c3924 (accessed 4 January 2016).

## ENT, maxillo-facial and dental: bleeding tonsil

You have been asked to review a 5-year-old child who underwent a tonsillectomy 6 hours ago; she has been spitting blood since returning from theatre and has now started vomiting blood. The observations available are heart rate 130 bpm and blood pressure 90/40 mmHg.

**What are the potential issues with this case that would immediately come to mind?**

- Hypovolaemia secondary to blood loss.
- Full stomach due to swallowed blood and any post-op oral intake.
- Difficult intubation due to blood in the airway and post-op airway oedema.
- A second general anaesthetic within a short time period.
- Scared and anxious child and parents.
- The need for senior anaesthetic support.

**How would you assess this child?**

You would use an 'ABC' approach paying particular attention for signs of hypovolaemic shock such as tachycardia, hypotension (late sign), prolonged capillary refill time, pallor, peripheral cyanosis, core/peripheral temperature difference (>2 °C is an important sign of shock), tachypnoea, reduced urine output (<1 ml/kg/h) and reduced conscious level (late sign). It is important to remember that actual blood loss is difficult to measure as much is swallowed, and is often underestimated. Other things to note include: time of last anaesthetic and last oral intake; grade of intubation and size of endotracheal tube used and any analgesics administered.

**What would be your immediate management?**

Ensure good IV access is secured: the interosseous route may be required. Send blood for FBC, clotting and cross-match and a venous blood gas sample. Start fluid resuscitation. Give 20 ml/kg boluses of isotonic crystalloid. The volume required will be guided by frequent reassessment of clinical signs. Transfuse blood and blood products as required.

**What would you want to ensure prior to induction of anaesthesia?**

These can be very difficult cases to manage, so get senior help. Adequate preoperative fluid resuscitation is essential to prevent cardiovascular collapse at induction. Ensure you have the following equipment available:

- Two functioning suction devices with wide-bore tubing.
- An appropriate selection of endotracheal tubes; the size used previously and half a size smaller in case of oedema. Ensure two of each as they can become blocked with blood clots.
- A selection of laryngoscopes with appropriate sized blades.
- Wide-bore gastric tubes to empty the stomach of blood. This can be inserted once the airway is secured or under direct vision once haemostasis is achieved.

The surgical team should be scrubbed and ready in case an emergency tracheostomy becomes necessary.

**How would you induce anaesthesia?**

The two common techniques used are an inhalational induction in the head-down left lateral position or a modified rapid sequence induction (RSI) with cricoid pressure. There are pros and cons to both, so it is important that you use the technique you are most familiar and comfortable with.

**How would you extubate this patient?**

Once surgical haemostasis has been achieved the gastric tube can be suctioned to empty the stomach of blood and then be removed. After neuromuscular blockade reversal (if necessary), the patient should be extubated fully awake in the left lateral head-down position.

# Further reading

Allman K. G., Wilson I. H. (eds.) *Oxford Handbook of Anaesthesia*, 3rd edn. Oxford: Oxford University Press, 2011.

Ravi R., Howell T. Anaesthesia for paediatric ear, nose, and throat surgery. *Contin Educ Anaesth Crit Care Pain* 2007; 7(2): 33–7.

Sethi D., Smith J. Anaesthesia for bleeding tonsil. Available at http://www.frca.co.uk/documents/109 %20anaesthesia%20for%20the%20bleeding%20tonsil.pdf (accessed March 2015).

# ENT, maxillo-facial and dental: dental abscess

A 42-year-old man is listed for urgent surgery for incision and drainage of a dental abscess. His mouth opening is limited to 2 cm.

**Which of the following is the single best answer?**

a) This is not an urgent case
b) Any trismus should relax upon anaesthesia, allowing conventional laryngoscopy
c) An airway plan is needed
d) There is an indication for awake fibre-optic intubation

Answer: d)

It has been suggested that the term dental abscess should not be used, but rather a fascial or cervical space infection so as not to underestimate the condition. There are multiple interconnected potential spaces within the head and neck through which infection can easily and rapidly spread putting the airway at risk. Signs of advanced infection include trismus; dysphagia; altered speech; inability to protrude the tongue; intra-oral swelling; pharyngeal swelling; gross facial swelling; neck swelling; stridor and systemic signs of infection.

Trismus due to muscle spasm can improve on induction of anaesthesia; however, this may be minimal or not at all. Intra-oral and pharyngeal swelling may be present that was not elicited preoperatively owing to the poor view. A difficult airway should be anticipated. Of the cases reported to the 4th National Audit Project (NAP4) 39% were head and neck cases with nearly one-third of these involving poor airway management. Not planning for the worst case or not anticipating problems that may be encountered with each anaesthetic method may lead to problems. NAP4 concluded that with a potential difficult airway a single plan is insufficient, and a strategy or a coordinated logical sequence of plans, is required. Options include those shown in Table 20.1.

Owing to trismus an oral approach is often ruled out. This is an indication for awake nasal fibre-optic intubation and this should probably be the technique of choice. Potential difficulties which may arise during the process should be thought through in advance. Resources such as the Aintree Difficult Airway Management website can assist in highlighting problems with each technique and so contingency planning.

**Table 20.1** Options for securing the airway in a dental abscess case

| Asleep techniques | Awake techniques |
| --- | --- |
| Conventional laryngoscopy | Nasal fibre-optic intubation |
| Video laryngoscopy | Tracheostomy |
| Intubation via a supraglottic device | |
| The method of induction of anaesthesia (intravenous or inhalational) and the appropriate timing of muscle relaxation and the potential for a 'can't intubate can't ventilate' scenario must be considered | Consideration needs to be given to sedation techniques and the need to anaesthetize the airway |

## Further reading

Cook T., Woodall N., Frerk C. (eds.) 4th National Audit Project: Major Complications of Airway Management in the United Kingdom. London: RCoA, 2011.

Darshane S., Groom P., Charters P. Responsive Contingency Planning: a novel system for anticipated difficulty in airway management in dental abscess. *Br J Anaesth* 2007; 99(6): 898–905.

Morosan M., Parbhoo A., Curry N. Anaesthesia and common oral and maxillo-facial emergencies. *Contin Educ Anaesth Crit Care Pain* 2012; 12(5): 257–62.

Perry M. *Head, Neck and Dental Emergencies*. Oxford: Oxford University Press, 2005.

Schumann M., Biesler I., Borges A. et al. Tracheal intubation in patients with odentogenous abscesses and reduced mouth opening. *Br J Anaesth* 2014; 112(2): 348–54.

http://adam.liv.ac.uk/adam8/login.aspx (accessed 4 January 2016).

## Hepatobiliary anaesthesia and acute liver failure

A 24-year-old female with jaundice, encephalopathy and coagulopathy is transferred to a tertiary referral hospital. She has acute liver failure (ALF) following a significant paracetamol overdose 4 days ago.

**Which of the following statements are true or false?**

Regarding ALF:

a) In the UK, the commonest cause is paracetamol overdose
b) Sepsis is a common complication
c) This patient's ALF is hyperacute
d) The decision to offer transplantation depends on aetiology
e) Grade 1 encephalopathy is consistent with an alert, orientated patient

Answers: TTTFF

Worldwide, the commonest cause is viral hepatitis. Annually, 400 cases of ALF occur in the UK but high mortality is caused by cerebral oedema, multi-organ failure and sepsis. The time between onset of jaundice and onset of encephalopathy is used to classify ALF as hyperacute (less than 7 days), acute (8–28 days) or subacute (5–12 weeks). The severity of hepatic dysfunction affects prognosis. Prognostic scoring systems, e.g. the Model for End-stage Liver Disease (MELD), assist the decision to transplant. Hepatic encephalopathy is graded 0 to 4, with 0 being an alert, orientated patient.

Encephalopathy worsens and she is intubated. The multidisciplinary team decide to list her for transplantation.

**Preoperative considerations include which of the following?**

a) Coagulopathy is usually corrected prior to surgery
b) Intracranial pressure (ICP) monitoring may be required
c) Cardiac output is likely to be high, with reduced systemic vascular resistance
d) Renal failure affects 20% of patients after paracetamol overdose
e) Her family should be advised that there is a 70% mortality risk in the first year

Answers: FTTFF

Coagulopathy is not usually corrected unless there is active bleeding. INR is used in prognostication, e.g. in the MELD score. Risk of raised ICP may necessitate monitoring. Relative hypotension is common. Volume loading, guided by cardiac output monitoring may be required. Renal failure affects 70% of patients after paracetamol overdose. Renal replacement therapy with a lactate-free solution may be needed. There is a 70% 1-year patient survival.

**Intraoperative considerations include:**

a) Three distinct phases of a liver transplant are described
b) Desflurane is a suitable volatile agent
c) Nitrous oxide should be avoided
d) Post-operative epidural is commonly used
e) This patient should remain intubated for the next 48 hours

Answers: TTTFF

The phases are resection, anhepatic and post-reperfusion. Pharmacokinetics and dynamics are significantly altered in ALF. Desflurane undergoes little hepatic metabolism so allows quick recovery. Nitrous oxide is avoided as it can lead to bubble formation if veno-venous bypass is used to improve venous return. Coagulopathy often precludes an epidural; PCA is effective. Early extubation is often possible.

## Further reading

Fabbroni D., Bellamy M. Anaesthesia for hepatic transplantation. *Contin Educ Anaesth Crit Care Pain* 2006; 6: 171–5.
Fontana R. Acute liver failure including acetaminophen overdose. *Med Clin North Am* 2008; 92: 761–94.
Gimson A. Fulminant and late onset hepatic failure. *Br J Anaesth* 1996; 77: 90–8.
Vaja R., McNichol L., Sisley I. Anaesthesia for patients with liver disease. *Contin Educ Anaesth Crit Care Pain* 2010; 1: 15–19.

# Vascular: ruptured abdominal aortic aneurysm (AAA) management

Post-operative mortality rates following emergency open AAA repair are one of the highest for all surgical procedures, at approximately 38%, with only small improvements seen over the last few decades. Emergency repairs are generally carried out on elderly patients with significant co-morbidities and polypharmacy, with higher mortality rates seen in procedures undertaken out of hours. Endovascular repair under local anaesthesia confers lower mortality where feasible. All emergency repairs require two experienced anaesthetists, intravascular and cardiac output monitoring, rapid blood transfusion with cell salvage if available and post-operative recovery on an ICU.

**Which scoring systems can be used to predict hospital mortality?**

The two most commonly used scoring systems are the Hardman Index and the Glasgow Aneurysm Score. These, however, lack accuracy of predicting mortality at higher scores. The Vascular Study Group of New England (VSGNE) Ruptured AAA (RAAA) score more accurately predicts mortality, even in those at greatest risk. The VSGNE RAAA predictors are age >76, cardiac arrest, loss of consciousness and the requirement for suprarenal aortic clamp.

**What is the optimum target blood pressure during resuscitation of the patient with ruptured AAA?**

The IMPROVE trial showed that mortality rates significantly increased when the lowest systolic blood pressure (BP) was less than 70 mmHg, with a 13% increase in survival for each subsequent increase of 10 mmHg. There is no definitive optimal BP, but the chosen target should take into account cardiovascular and cerebrovascular co-morbidities.

**What are the potential causes of cardiovascular collapse during induction?**

The causes of cardiovascular collapse are:

a. Cardiovascular depression by inhalational and intravenous induction agents.
b. Reduction of venous return by IPPV.
c. Reduction in sympathetic tone.
d. Relaxation of abdominal muscles and loss of tamponade effect.

No specific induction agent is recommended but dose and effects must be considered carefully.

**How can the effects of application and removal of the aortic cross-clamp be ameliorated?**

Cross-clamping the aorta increases afterload, the effect of which depends on the patients' left ventricular function. Vasodilation, using specific agents such as GTN, or increasing the concentration of inhalational agent, can reduce afterload. Removal of the cross-clamp reverses this effect and, in combination with ischaemia-reperfusion release of lactic acid and potassium, causes profound cardiovascular depression. Expansion of intravascular volume should be undertaken prior to release, combined with readiness to rapidly administer vasopressor and inotropic agents.

## Further reading

IMPROVE trial investigators. Observations from the IMPROVE trial concerning the clinical care of patients with ruptured abdominal aortic aneurysm. *Br J Surg* 2014; 101(3): 216–24.

Leonard A., Thompson J. Anaesthesia for ruptured abdominal aortic aneurysm. *Contin Educ Anaesth CritCare Pain* 2008; 8(1): 11–15.

Robinson W. P., Schanzer A., Li Y. et al. Derivation and validation of a practical risk score for prediction of mortality after open repair of ruptured abdominal aortic aneurysms in a U.S. regional cohort and comparison to existing scoring systems. *J Vasc Surg* 2013; 57(2): 354–61.

Stoneham M., Murray D., Foss N. Emergency surgery: the big three – abdominal aortic aneurysm, laparotomy and hip fracture. *Anaesthesia* 2013; 69: 70–80.

The Vascular Study Group of New England Ruptured AAA score. www.vsgne.org (accessed 4 January 2016).

## Ophthalmics: penetrating eye injury

A 24-year-old presents with eye trauma following an accident at work. He has just eaten lunch. Airway examination is normal, vital signs are stable and Glasgow Coma Score (GCS) is 15. He is usually fit and well although a recent tendon repair under general anaesthesia caused severe nausea and vomiting. The ophthalmic surgeon suspects a penetrating eye injury; the patient requires examination under anaesthetic and repair.

**What are the key concerns?**

This patient has an open globe. Increased intraocular pressure (IOP) can therefore cause expulsion of the global contents and permanent loss of vision. Securing the airway to prevent aspiration should be balanced against the risk of raised IOP. This surgery often cannot wait until the patient is fasted and pain may cause gastric stasis, so the decision whether or not to use suxamethonium as part of the rapid sequence induction (RSI) needs to be made. Concerns about airway protection always take precedence. If surgery can wait, a laryngeal mask airway (LMA) may be used. This avoids the pressor response to laryngoscopy and reduces incidence of coughing on emergence. Although retrobulbar and peribulbar blocks produce akinetic anaesthesia, they are not usually considered possible because injecting around the globe increases IOP. The oculocardiac reflex may occur because of intraoperative pressure on the globe. Ophthalmic theatres may be remote from the main theatre complex.

**What is normal IOP? What affects it?**

Normal IOP is between 10 and 20 mmHg. An increase in either the volume of the globe or external pressure raises IOP. Many factors affect this; those relevant here include vomiting, coughing, laryngoscopy, hypercapnia, hypoxia and intra- or extra-global haemorrhage. By increasing extra-ocular muscle tone, suxamethonium transiently increases IOP but the clinical effects of this on the open globe are variable.

**Describe a possible approach to this anaesthetic**

Preoperative analgesia and antiemetics are given, avoiding opioids if possible to reduce the risk of vomiting. A prokinetic is given to reduce aspiration risk. A modified rapid sequence induction (RSI) is performed using rocuronium and sufficient time is given to avoid coughing. The pressor response to laryngoscopy is attenuated using alfentanil and a south-facing RAE endotracheal tube is inserted. IPPV is used to control $PaCO_2$ and its effects on IOP. A nerve stimulator reduces the risk of intraoperative coughing. Risk of coughing on emergence is reduced by maintaining depth of anaesthesia until surgery is finished and drapes removed. Propofol at 30–40 mg a few minutes before emergence also helps. Paracetamol, codeine and diclofenac are often adequate for post-operative analgesia. Further antiemetics may be required.

## Further reading

Allman K. G., Wilson I. H. (eds.) *Oxford Handbook of Anaesthesia*, 3rd edn. Oxford: Oxford University Press, 2011.

Gayer S. Rethinking anaesthesia strategies for patients with traumatic eye injuries: alternatives to general anaesthesia. *Trends Anaesth Crit Care* 2006; 17: 191–6.

Libonati M., Leahy J., Ellison N. The use of succinylcholine in open eye surgery. *Anaesthesiology* 1985; 62: 637–40.

Murgatroyd H., Bembridge J. Intraocular pressure. *Contin Educ Anaesth Crit Care Pain* 2008; 8: 100–3.

# Ophthalmics: regional eye blocks

An elderly gentleman has been scheduled for cataract surgery of his right eye. He has multiple co-morbidities which include; hypertension, ischemic heart disease (IHD) with angioplasty and stents insertion, chronic obstructive pulmonary disease with shortness of breath on lying flat and cerebrovascular disease (transient ischaemic attack in the past). His medication history includes ramipril, bisoprolol, clopidogrel, prednisolone and inhalers. He suffers from myopia with a globe axial length of 25 mm.

**Which of the following statements are true with regards to anaesthetic management?**

a) Clopidogrel should be stopped 7 days prior to surgery and peribulbar block should be performed

b) Clopidogrel should be continued for surgery and sub-Tenon (ST) block performed

c) If the patient was on warfarin, it could be continued in the perioperative period if the international normalized ratio (INR) < 2.5 and either peribulbar or ST block could be established
d) There is a higher risk of globe perforation with ST block
e) The risk of haemorrhagic complications is higher with the peribulbar block than the ST block

Answers: FTTFT

Options for regional anaesthesia for ophthalmic surgery are a sub-Tenon block, peribulbar block (an extra-conal block) and the retrobulbar block (an intra-conal block). Retrobulbar blocks have gone out of practice owing to higher risks of optic nerve injury and retrobulbar haemorrhage as compared to the other two.

General anaesthesia for cataract surgery should be reserved for the paediatric population or adults with learning difficulties, severe tremors or psychiatric illness. This patient is high risk for general anaesthesia. Even patients who suffer from shortness of breath on lying flat can usually be managed with regional techniques by adjusting the operating table and providing supplemental oxygen and reassurance.

Antiplatelet agents and anticoagulation drugs increase the incidence of bleeding and minor haemorrhage but serious complications such as sight-threatening bleeding are not seen with either a sharp needle or ST block. If the patient is on warfarin, anaesthesia and surgery may proceed with a therapeutic level of INR for the condition. The risks of thromboembolic events are higher when interrupting anticoagulation and hence, on balance, anticoagulation can be continued in the perioperative period.

The most commonly used technique currently is the ST block as it has a better safety profile. It is performed using a blunt, curved ST needle in the infero-nasal quadrant along the scleral curvature. If the curved needle is unavailable, a straight, blunt-tipped needle or a 22G cannula can be used to deposit local anaesthetic in the Tenon's capsule. This block is relatively contraindicated if the patients have had scleral bands for glaucoma or retinal detachment or pterygium surgery.

In extreme myopes, there is scleral thinning and increased risk of globe perforation with all types of blocks.

## Further reading
Benzimra J. D., Johnston R. L., Jaycock P. et al. The Cataract National Dataset electronic multi-centre audit of 55 567 operations: antiplatelet and anticoagulant medications. *Eye* 2009; 23: 10–16.
Parness G., Underhill S. Regional anaesthesia for intraocular surgery. *Contin Educ Anaesth Crit Care Pain* 2005; 5(3): 93–7.

## Bariatrics: adaptations in bariatrics
Twenty per cent of UK adults are obese and 1% are morbidly obese. Obesity is defined as a BMI $\geq 30$ kg/m$^2$. Morbid obesity refers to those with a BMI $\geq 40$ kg/m$^2$, or $\geq 35$ kg/m$^2$ in the presence of co-morbidity.

A 52-year-old male listed for an elective laparoscopic cholecystectomy weighs 154 kg with a BMI of 48 kg/m$^2$. He is hypertensive with stable angina. Regular medications include aspirin, ramipril and simvastatin. He reportedly snores and has apnoeic episodes overnight.

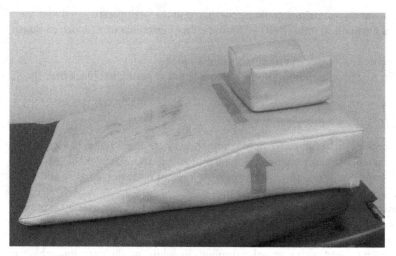

**Figure 20.1** Oxford Help pillow.

## What preparation in theatre is needed for this patient?

An experienced team is required. Induction of anaesthesia in theatre reduces the need for manual handling. Operating tables with an adequate maximum weight allowance must be used. An air hover mattress can assist patient transfers. Appropriately sized monitoring equipment must be available but invasive arterial pressure monitoring may be needed. Further equipment includes table extensions, arm boards and gel pads; nerve injuries and pressure sores are more common in obese patients. Ramping the patient prior to induction assists pre-oxygenation, reduces speed of desaturation and improves the position for intubation. The 'sniffing the morning air' position can be difficult to achieve because of body habitus; a wedge or blanket under the shoulders may help. Commercial solutions, e.g. the Oxford Help pillow are available (see Figure 20.1).

## What will be your anaesthetic technique?

Thorough preoperative assessment is required. A cardiorespiratory referral and investigations or continuous positive airway pressure (CPAP) for obstructive sleep apnoea (OSA) may be needed. Routine bloods and a preoperative ECG should be requested. Difficult intubation may be encountered although obesity alone is not a predictor for this; other signs, e.g. large neck circumference, and a Mallampati score $\geq 3$ are also required. A supine position may lead to airway obstruction and desaturation so awake intubation in a sitting position may be better tolerated in some patients. Minimize the time between induction and ventilation to avoid desaturation. Tracheal intubation is required and positive end-expiratory pressure (PEEP) should be used. A reverse Trendelenburg position is safe as long as patients are carefully secured to the table. This position may also improve respiratory compliance. Use calf compression devices for thromboprophylaxis. Antibiotic prophylaxis is important as postoperative wound infection is more common in obese patients. Consider using prokinetics and antacids. Short-acting anaesthetic agents, e.g. remifentanil, sevoflurane or desflurane,

THE SOCIETY FOR OBESITY AND BARIATRIC ANAESTHESIA SUMMARY

# ANAESTHESIA FOR THE OBESE PATIENT: BMI>35KG/M²

## Preoperative Evaluation

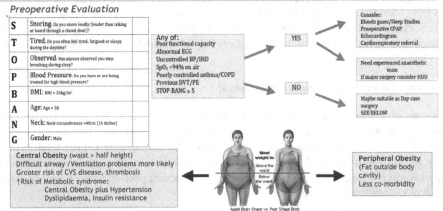

| S | Snoring. Do you snore loudly (louder than talking or heard through a closed door)? |
|---|---|
| T | Tired. Do you often feel tired, fatigued or sleepy during the daytime? |
| O | Observed: Has anyone observed you stop breathing during sleep? |
| P | Blood Pressure: Do you have or are being treated for high blood pressure? |
| B | BMI: BMI > 35kg/m² |
| A | Age: Age > 50 |
| N | Neck: Neck circumference >40cm (16 inches) |
| G | Gender: Male |

Any of:
Poor functional capacity
Abnormal ECG
Uncontrolled BP/IHD
SpO₂ <94% on air
Poorly controlled asthma/COPD
Previous DVT/PE
STOP-BANG ≥ 5

YES → Consider:
Bloods gases/Sleep Studies
Preoperative CPAP
Echocardiogram
Cardiorespiratory referral

Need experienced anaesthetic team
If major surgery consider HDU

NO → Maybe suitable as Day case surgery
SEE BELOW

Central Obesity (waist > half height)
Difficult airway /Ventilation problems more likely
Greater risk of CVS disease, thrombosis
↑Risk of Metabolic syndrome:
Central Obesity plus Hypertension
Dyslipidaemia, Insulin resistance

Peripheral Obesity
(Fat outside body cavity)
Less co-morbidity

Apple Body Shape vs. Pear Shape Body

## Intra Operative Management

### Suggested Equipment
Suitable bed/trolley & operating table
Gel padding, wide strapping, table extensions/arm boards
Forearm cuff or large BP cuff
Ramping device, step for anaesthetist, difficult airway equipment, ventilator capable of PEEP and pressure modes.
Hover mattress or equivalent.
Long spinal, regional and vascular needles.
Ultrasound machine.
Depth of anaesthesia and neuromuscular monitoring.
Enough staff to move patient.

### Ramping
Ear level with sternum. Reduces risk of difficult laryngoscopy, improves ventilation.

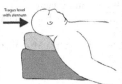

Tragus level with sternum

### Anaesthetic Technique
Consider premed antacid & analgesia, careful glucose control & DVT prophylaxis. Self-position on operating table.
Preoxygenate & intubate in ramped position +/- CPAP. Minimize induction to ventilation interval to avoid desaturation. Commence maintenance anaesthesia promptly.
Tracheal intubation is recommended.
Avoid spontaneous ventilation. Use PEEP.
Use short-acting agents e.g. desflurane or propofol infusion, short-acting opioids, multimodal analgesia. PONV prophylaxis.
Ensure full NMB reversal.
**Extubate and recover in head up position.**

### Drug dosing- what weight to use?
**Induction agents:** titrate to cardiac output- this equates to lean body weight in a fit patient.
**Competitive muscle relaxants:** use lean body weight.
**Suxamethonium** use total body weight
**Neostigmine:** Increase dose. Measure response
**Opioids:** Use Lean body weight. Care with obstructive apnoea!
**TCI propofol:** IBW plus 40% excess weight

*If in doubt, titrate and monitor effect!*

**Lean Body Weight** this exceeds Ideal body weight in the obese and plateaus ≈100kg for a man, ≈70kg for a woman.
**Ideal Body Weight in Kg** - Broca formula
Men: height in cm minus 100    Women: height in cm minus 105

### Suggested dosing regimes for anaesthetic drugs

| Lean Body Weight Males 100Kg Females 70Kg | Adjusted Body Weight Ideal plus 40% excess |
|---|---|
| Propofol induction | Propofol Infusion |
| Thiopentone | Alfentanil |
| Fentanyl | Lidocaine |
| Rocuronium | Neostigmine (max 5mg) |
| Atracurium | Sugammadex (see package insert) |
| Vecuronium | Antibiotics |
| Morphine | Low Molecular weight Heparin |
| Paracetamol | |
| Bupivacaine | |

## Post Operative Management
**PACU discharge:** Usual discharge criteria should be met. In addition, SpO₂ should be maintained at pre-op levels with minimal O₂ therapy, without evidence of hypoventilation.
**OSA or Obesity Hypoventilation Syndrome:** Sit up. Avoid sedatives and post-op opioids. Reinstate CPAP if using it pre-op. Additional time in recovery is recommended, only discharge to the ward if free of apnoeas without stimulation. Patients untreated or intolerant of CPAP who require postoperative opioids are at risk of hypoventilation and require continuous oxygen saturation monitoring. Level 2 care is recommended. Effective CPAP reduces this risk to near normal.
**Ward care:** Escalation to Level 1, 2 or 3 care may be required based on patient co-morbidity, the type of surgery undertaken and issues with hypoventilation discussed above. General ward care includes: multimodal analgesia, caution with long-acting opioids and sedatives, early mobilisation and extended thromboprophylaxis.

See www.SOBAuk.com for references          Updated November 2014

**Figure 20.2** SOBA Single Sheet Summary; Anaesthesia for the Obese Patient. Reproduced with kind permission from The Society for Obesity and Bariatric Anaesthesia.

help achieve rapid recovery and minimize post-operative hypoxaemia and hypoventilation. Reversal of neuromuscular block is essential; extubation and recovery should be in a head-up position. Pharmacokinetics are significantly affected by obesity. Drug dosing can be based on lean, ideal (height in cm minus 100 for men and 105 for women) or actual body weight. The Society for Obesity and Bariatric Anaesthesia (SOBA) have produced guidelines to assist drug dosage, which are part of their incredibly helpful single sheet guide, which can be found in Figure 20.2.

**What are the post-operative considerations?**

Patients with obesity-related co-morbidities have a greater risk of perioperative complications. Early mobilization reduces atelectasis and thromboembolism. Thromboprophylaxis should be started and continued post-operatively. This patient may require level 2 care in view of his co-morbidities. Adopt a multimodal approach to analgesia and avoid long-acting opioids where possible. If OSA is diagnosed he may require post-operative CPAP or continuous oxygen saturation monitoring.

## Further reading

Adams J. P., Murphy P. G. Obesity in anaesthesia and intensive care. *Br J Anaesth* 2000; 85: 91–108.
Association of Anaesthetists of Great Britain and Ireland. Peri-operative management of the obese surgical patient 2015. Available at http://www.aagbi.org/publications/publications-guidelines/M/R (accessed 4 January 2016).
Brodsky J. B., Lemmens H. J., Brock-Utne J. G., Vierra M., Saidman L. J. Morbid obesity and tracheal intubation. *Anesth Analg* 2002; 94: 732–6.

# Cardiothoracics: double lumen tube (DLT) management

You are anaesthetizing a patient for a right-sided upper lobectomy using a left-sided DLT. The patient is in the left lateral position. A few minutes after commencing surgery the patient's oxygen saturations fall to 88%.

**What are the indications for use of a DLT?**

**Table 20.2** Indications for use of a double lumen tube

| Absolute | Relative |
| --- | --- |
| Lung isolation to avoid contamination:<br>• Infection<br>• Massive haemorrhage | Non-thoracic surgical access:<br>• Spinal thoracic surgery |
| Control of distribution of ventilation:<br>• Bronchopleural fistula<br>• Tracheobronchial tree disruption<br>• Giant unilateral lung cyst/bulla<br>• Open surgery on main bronchi | Surgical access:<br>• Thoracic aortic aneurysm<br>• Pneumonectomy<br>• Mediastinal surgery<br>• Lobectomy<br>• Oesophagectomy |
| Unilateral bronchopulmonary lavage:<br>• Pulmonary alveolar proteinosis | Severe hypoxaemia due to unilateral lung disease |

## How would you verify correct placement of a DLT?

Most modern DLTs are based on Robertshaw's design (39–41 Fr or medium/large for men and 35–37 Fr or small/medium for women). A left-sided DLT is used more commonly because of the lower risk of obstructing the right upper lobe bronchus. The bronchial cuff of a right-sided DLT incorporates a side window for ventilating the right upper lobe.

The correct position of the DLT is confirmed by visual inspection, auscultation and fibre-optic bronchoscopy:

1. Inflate tracheal cuff and confirm ventilation of both lungs.
2. Usual insertion depth is 29 cm at teeth for patient of 170 cm height (+/−1 cm for every 10 cm change in height).
3. Confirm one-lung ventilation (OLV) via the bronchial lumen and inflate bronchial cuff. (If requires >4 ml air the DLT is malpositioned or too small.)
4. Confirm OLV via the tracheal lumen.
5. Confirm positioning of bronchial cuff (blue) just below level of carina with a bronchoscope.
6. If using a right-sided DLT confirm that side window of bronchial lumen is aligned with right upper lobe bronchus.
7. If moving patient to lateral position reconfirm adequacy of OLV and position of DLT bronchoscopically once positioned.

## How would you manage hypoxaemia during one-lung ventilation (OLV)?

Ventilate patient's lungs with 100% oxygen prior to OLV. Then ask yourself the following questions.

1. Is there a problem with oxygen delivery?
   - Check anaesthetic machine and breathing circuit.
   - Ventilate with 100% oxygen.

2. Is the airway pressure high or has it increased?
   - Check the position of the DLT with bronchoscope.
   - Suction to remove any sputum or blood.
   - Signs of bronchospasm? Give bronchodilators if needed.
   - Adequate paralysis?
   - Is there air trapping and hyperinflation? Decompress by disconnecting breathing circuit from DLT.
   - Is there a pneumothorax of the ventilated lung? Decompress with surgical assistance if required.

3. Is the hypoxaemia physiological?
   - Insufflate oxygen and apply CPAP to the non-ventilated lung to improve oxygenation of shunted blood.
   - Intermittent two-lung ventilation.
   - Consider early clamping of pulmonary artery to non-ventilated lung during planned lung resection.
   - Optimize haemoglobin, cardiac output and therefore oxygen delivery.

- Apply positive end-expiratory pressure (PEEP) to ventilated lung to improve functional residual capacity.
- Ensure adequate tidal volumes. The narrow lumen of the DLT may mean higher inspiratory pressures are required to achieve this.

## Further reading

Eastwood J., Mahajan R. One-lung anaesthesia. *Contin Educ Anaesth Crit Care Pain* 2002; 2(3): 83–7.

Sanders S. Isolation of the lungs. In: K. G. Allman, I. H. Wilson. *Oxford Handbook of Anaesthesia.* Oxford: Oxford University Press, 2001, pp. 368–73.

Ng A., Swanevelder S. Hypoxaemia during one-lung anaesthesia. *Contin Educ Anaesth Crit Care Pain* 2010; 10(4): 117–22.

# Cardiothoracics: emergency non-cardiac surgery in a high risk patient

You are asked to anaesthetize a 75-year-old man for an emergency laparotomy for large bowel obstruction secondary to a colonic carcinoma. The surgeon tells you that he has severe coronary artery disease (CAD) with an occluded left main stem, has type 2 diabetes, hypertension, and is currently awaiting coronary artery bypass grafting. He has deteriorated significantly, and they are keen to proceed as soon as possible.

**What further information would you want preoperatively?**

This gentleman is at high risk of suffering an adverse event in the perioperative period, and his coronary artery lesions mean that he has a significant risk of dying. Assessment of risk here is particularly important, and methods of risk stratification can be found in Chapter 23. In addition to a full medical and anaesthetic history, relevant investigations if available include:

- Coronary angiogram results
- Recent echocardiography: presence of valvular lesions, regional wall motion abnormalities, dilated chambers, overall function
- 12-lead ECG.

Some idea of cardiac function before you start is essential. It is important to continue beta blockade perioperatively as this has been shown to reduce the risk of myocardial events. As a general rule, most cardiac medication should be continued. Antiplatelet therapy may have been continued until presentation and this may preclude the use of regional anaesthesia for his post-operative analgesia. In cardiac patients, optimal pain control and the use of anxiolytics prior to surgery prevents sympathetic surges putting strain on a failing heart, avoiding tachycardia.

**What are the principles and priorities of anaesthesia in this patient?**

The haemodynamic goals for any patient with CAD are to balance supply and demand:

1. Preload – keep heart small, decrease wall tension, increase perfusion pressure
2. Afterload – maintain, hypertension better than hypotension
3. Contractility – depression is beneficial when left ventricular function adequate
4. Heart rate – slow, normal

5. Rhythm – usually sinus
6. $MVO_2$ – control of demand frequently not enough, monitor for and treat ischaemia.

Your choice of induction agent should bear the above in mind, and your main goal should be a smooth, balanced anaesthetic, avoiding swings in heart rate and blood pressure. Remember, by definition, he has areas of 'at-risk' myocardium which may become more ischaemic. Generally speaking, induction in this group of patients tends to be opiate-heavy (e.g. fentanyl 10–15 mcg/kg), minimizing the dose of hypnotic agent used. Although rapid sequence induction is required here, the traditional thio/sux approach is not recommended. Volatile agent choice may have some benefit: isoflurane theoretically enhances myocardial ischaemic preconditioning, although there is no evidence that it improves morbidity or mortality.

Invasive monitoring is essential to target haemodynamic goals. Here, arterial line, central venous catheter, urinary catheter and temperature monitoring should be used. Cardiac output monitoring will also guide fluid and inotrope therapy. This may be in the form of pulse contour analysis, trans-oesophageal echocardiography, or oesophageal Doppler. Intraoperative predictors of risk include:

- Choice of anaesthetic
- Site of surgery (thoracic/upper abdominal 2–3 × risk cf. extremity surgery)
- Anaesthetic duration (>3 hours increases morbidity and mortality)
- Emergency surgery (2–5 × risk cf. non-emergent).

Other options such as intra-aortic balloon pump may be considered should left ventricular failure ensue. If regional anaesthesia is contraindicated, analgesia will be opiate-based. Transversus abdominis plane (TAP) or rectus sheath blocks may be worth considering here. This patient will need managing on ICU post-operatively and this should be discussed before you begin.

## Further reading

Cardiac anaesthesia. Anaesthesia UK. Available at http://www.frca.co.uk/article.aspx?articleid=100660 (accessed 13 May 2015).
The Task Force for Preoperative Cardiac Risk Assessment and Perioperative Cardiac Management in Non-cardiac Surgery of the European Society of Cardiology (ESC) and endorsed by the European Society of Anaesthesiology (ESA). Guidelines for pre-operative cardiac risk assessment and perioperative cardiac management in non-cardiac surgery. *Eur Heart J* 2009; 30(22): 2769a. Available at http://eurheartj.oxfordjournals.org/content/ehj/30/22/2769.full.pdf (accessed 13 May 2015).

## Plastics and burns: free flap surgery

You are doing an elective plastic surgery list tomorrow. On your list is a 43-year-old patient for a free transverse rectus abdominis muscle (TRAM) myocutaneous flap breast reconstruction following mastectomy. She is otherwise fit and well.

**What is a free flap and what problems are associated with this type of tissue graft?**

Free flaps are often used to provide tissue cover following trauma or resection for malignancy. Microvascular surgical techniques allow the transfer of free vascularized tissue which may include skin, muscle, bone and bowel. Common flap donor sites include radial and ulnar forearm, latissimus dorsi and rectus abdominis.

The donor site neurovascular bundle is transplanted to the recipient site where it is microvascularly re-anastomosed. Once dissected out the flap is denervated; however, the feeding artery and vein still respond to physical, humeral and chemical stimuli such as cold, catecholamines and drugs.

Hypoperfusion and flap failure are major concerns. Blood flow to the flap often decreases to less than half during the immediate post-operative period and may take days or weeks to return to normal. Free flaps have no intact lymphatic drainage, making them very sensitive to extravasation of fluids and pressure effects.

**How can the conduct of your anaesthetic improve surgical outcome in free flap surgery?**

Anaesthesia can be an important factor in determining the success of this type of surgery. Regional anaesthesia, changes in blood volume and the use of vasoactive drugs may influence blood flow in the free flap. Requirements are a hyperdynamic circulation with a high cardiac output, peripheral vasodilatation and a large pulse pressure.

Monitoring:
- Invasive arterial monitoring allows blood pressure (BP) optimization and sampling.
- Central venous pressure monitoring/non-invasive cardiac output measurement to assess fluid balance and optimize cardiac output.
- Core and peripheral temperature: a difference of <2 °C indicates a warm, well-perfused patient.
- Urine output: aim 1 ml/kg/h.

Induction and maintenance:
- Vascular access: large bore.
- Active warming pre-induction. High ambient temperature in theatre.
- Positioning: prolonged cases so pressure area care important.
- Thromboprophylaxis: anti-embolism stockings/pneumatic compression boots.
- Maintenance with volatile/propofol infusion and remifentanil.
- IPPV to maintain normocapnia. Hypocapnia will cause vasoconstriction.
- Analgesia: regional blocks are useful for analgesia. The donor site should take priority for cover as sympathetic block will improve local blood flow and graft reperfusion.
- BP control: during the initial dissection phase of surgery blood loss may be reduced by controlled hypotension. Prior to harvesting the flap normotension should be achieved. There is little evidence that vasopressors adversely affect graft survival and raising the mean arterial pressure will usually improve graft perfusion.
- Fluid management: hypervolaemic haemodilution to a haematocrit of 0.3. Weigh swabs and aim for an Hb of >80 g/l.

Emergence and extubation:
- Coughing may increase BP and increase haematoma formation.
- Recovery: oxygen and warming should continue for 48 hours. Aims are normotension, normothermia, urine output >1 ml/kg/h. Avoid shivering.
- Flap monitoring: clinical observation (colour, capillary refill, surface temperature, turgor, bleeding) and Doppler flow.

## Further reading

Adams J., Charlton P. Anaesthesia for microvascular free tissue transfer. *Contin Educ Anaesth Crit Care Pain* 2003; 3(2): 33–7.

Prout J., Jones T., Martin D. *Advanced Training in Anaesthesia: The Essential Curriculum*. Oxford: Oxford University Press, 2014, pp. 540–1.

## Plastics and burns: anaesthesia for burns dressings

A 25-year-old is admitted to the burns ward with 30% burns over her arms and abdomen. She requires regular change of dressings every 2 days on the burns ward. She is very anxious and IV cannulation is difficult with very few sites available.

**What would your anaesthetic plan be for her next dressing change?**

a) Premedication with oral midazolam and Entonox during the dressing change

b) Premedication with oral ketamine and intermittent boluses of IV alfentanil once intravenous access is secured

c) Entonox to facilitate IV cannulation and then intermittent boluses of intravenous ketamine and midazolam

d) Oral morphine premedication and continue with titrated doses of morphine and midazolam once intravenous access is established

e) Oral midazolam premedication and Entonox to assist IV cannulation and then intermittent boluses of intravenous ketamine and alfentanil

Answer: c)

Burns wound dressing removal has been perceived as the greatest procedural pain with the pain continuing in the post-procedure period. Inadequately controlled procedural pain is detrimental; it leads to heightened anxiety and may add to the post-traumatic stress disorder. Repeated dressing changes are essential to promote healing.

The key principles of providing analgesia for these procedures are aimed at controlling severe acute pain with short-acting, potent analgesics titrated to effect and prevent excessive sedation, which can compromise airway reflexes. Prolonged starvation should be avoided as it can affect nutritional goals. Entonox is a good analgesic and can be used for small dressing changes but is not usually sufficient for bigger procedures. It is a good agent to assist with cannulation.

Intravenous opioids are effective analgesics but drugs such as morphine have a delayed onset when compared with alfentanil and fentanyl. Additionally, morphine also has a long-lasting effect, which can cause respiratory depression and sedation in the post-procedure period.

Titrated doses of IV ketamine are the mainstay of treatment in these cases. It is a potent analgesic and maintains airway reflexes. The main limiting factor of ketamine is its side effect of hallucinations. Midazolam given along with ketamine decreases the risk of side effects. The anaesthetic induction dose of ketamine is 1–2 mg/kg when used intravenously but sub-anaesthetic doses of 0.5 mg/kg can be used as boluses for analgesia. With repeated dressing change, the dose requirement of these patients can increase significantly.

Small amounts of titrated alfentanil (boluses of 10 mcg) can work synergistically to provide optimal analgesia if needed. Midazolam can be used as an anxiolytic premedication in this patient but it may be difficult to titrate oral doses and hence it is often avoided. Other drugs which can be used are low dose infusions of propofol and/or remifentanil.

## Further reading

Latarjet J. The management of pain associated with dressing changes in patients with burns. *EWMA Journal* 2002; 2(2): 5–9.

Norman A. T., Judkins K. C. Pain in the patient with burns. *Contin Educ Anaesth Crit Care Pain* 2004; 4(2): 57–61.

Chapter

# Patient safety

*This chapter focusses on topics that are often the subject of statutory and mandatory training sessions: infection control, safeguarding, blood transfusion. Whilst not perhaps as interesting as clinical dilemmas, they are important in terms of patient safety. The chapter ends with some MCQs to help you to refresh your memory of the newer agents used to prevent venous thromboembolism.*

## Theatre list management: infection control

You are anaesthetizing for a vascular list and there has been a below knee amputation added at the beginning of the list. On assessing the patient you establish they have cellulitis and are MRSA positive. They are isolated on the ward and barrier nursed. There are also two fem-pop bypasses on the list.

**The most appropriate plan to be made at the morning team briefing is?**

a) Postpone the amputation until the patient has completed MRSA eradication and has had two sets of negative swabs

b) Run to the order of the list but inform theatre staff of the positive MRSA status of the first patient and recommend everyone uses gloves and aprons

c) Run to the order of the list but have the theatre deep cleaned and left empty for 60 minutes following the infected case

d) Suggest to the surgeons that the order of the list should be changed to put the infected case at the end of the day

e) Suggest that the infected case be postponed to a list with other 'dirty' procedures in order that the two 'clean' cases can proceed without additional risk of cross-infection

Answer: d)

Anaesthetists will be involved in the care of patients who may be actively infected with, or carriers of, pathogenic organisms. This may or may not be known to them. Therefore, infection control precautions should be routine practice. Trusts should have Infection Control committees and teams that are responsible for making policies and monitoring compliance. A member of the anaesthetic department should be identified as lead for infection control. It is their responsibility to liaise with the Trust's infection control teams and occupational

*Returning to Work in Anaesthesia*, ed. Emma Plunkett, Emily Johnson and Anna Pierson.
Published by Cambridge University Press. © Cambridge University Press 2016.

health to ensure relevant standards are established and monitored in all areas of anaesthetic practice.

There should be a Trust policy that covers management of known infected cases coming to theatres. This would likely govern the local management of this example. The Association of Anaesthetists of Great Britain and Ireland (AAGBI) recommendation is that there is a policy requiring accurate printed theatre lists to be available before the date of surgery. 'Dirty' cases should be identified before surgery and staff notified. These cases should be scheduled last on a list to minimize risk. Where this is not possible the Hospital Infection Society (HIS) advises that a plenum-ventilated operating theatre should require a minimum of 15 minutes before proceeding to the next case following a 'dirty' operation. Other recommendations include:

- Standard precautions for every case, including single-use gloves. Additional precautions for specific procedures and patients including fluid-resistant masks with face shields and gowns.
- Appropriate cleaning of the operating theatre between all patients, which includes surfaces of anaesthetic machines and monitoring equipment, particularly when visibly soiled.
- Local policies to govern the cleaning with detergent of equipment not in contact with patients on a daily basis.
- Movement into and out of the theatre complex to be kept to a minimum and doors shut to aid ventilation systems.
- Bed linen to be handled with care and bagged by the bed or trolley to reduce the release of small fomite particles into the air.

## Further reading

Association of Anaesthetists of Great Britain and Ireland. Guidelines: Infection control in anaesthesia. *Anaesthesia* 2008; 63: 1027–36. Available at http://www.aagbi.org/sites/default/files/infection_control_08.pdf (accessed 29 April 2015).

Woodhead K., Taylor E. W., Bannister G. et al. Behaviours and rituals in the operating theatre. A report from the Hospital Infection Society Working Group on Infection Control in Operating Theatres. *J Hosp Infect* 2002; 51(4): 241–55.

## Safeguarding: child protection

A 7-year-old girl presents to the paediatric day case unit for dental extractions. While examining her airway you notice a torn and bruised upper labial frenulum, sub-aponeurotic haematoma and also some bruising on her right arm. Her mother says the girl fell off her bike 2 days ago causing these injuries.

**Your actions should include which of the following?**

a) Take a history and examine the child fully, documenting your findings carefully
b) Inform your consultant or manager and the local child protection team that you are concerned the girl is being abused
c) The injuries are consistent with the history given by the mother: therefore take no further action and proceed with the anaesthetic

d) Contact the police, as these injuries are indicative of physical abuse and the child may be in immediate danger

e) Check with social services whether the child's name appears on the child at risk register

Answer: b)

It is not uncommon for children presenting for multiple dental extractions to be experiencing some form of neglect. Their parents or guardians are responsible for ensuring the child has an appropriate diet and adequate dental hygiene. In this case, however, it is physical abuse that is suspected.

The mother's history does not fit with the injuries. A torn labial frenulum is a sign of potential child abuse if there is no history that is consistent with the injury. A sub-aponeurotic haematoma is a sign suggesting that the girl's hair has been pulled with considerable force.

As a result of the Laming enquiry into the death of Victoria Climbié it was deemed that everyone involved in the care of children in the UK has a responsibility to act if child abuse is suspected. All NHS Trusts must have a named lead for child protection, and often this named lead will be part of a child protection team. The child protection team is able to coordinate a response to a child protection enquiry and appoint experienced personnel to undertake a full examination of the child.

To avoid unnecessary distress for the child and to ensure that physical signs are not missed, it is advisable that the child is fully examined once and by an experienced trained member of the child protection team. It could be argued that to check whether the child's name appears on the child at risk register would be helpful and worthwhile, but in practice this is often a time-consuming task.

Prior to specialist child protection teams being established, the distribution of information between the hospital, general practitioner and various agencies could be a challenging process. Child protection teams are able to coordinate this much more efficiently.

## Further reading

General Medical Council. Consultation on new child protection guidance. Available at www.gmc-uk .org/guidance/news_consultation/8411.asp (accessed 28 November 2011).

National Institute for Health and Clinical Excellence. When to Suspect Child Maltreatment. NICE Clinical Guideline 89. 2009. Available at http://guidance.nice.org.uk/CG89 (accessed 20 January 2015).

Royal College of Paediatrics and Child Health. Looked after children: knowledge, skills and competences of Health Care Staff. 2015. Available at rcpch.adlibhosting.com/Details/resources/ 700000184 (accessed 9 January 2016).

The Victoria Climbié Inquiry: Report of an Inquiry by Lord Laming. 2003. Available online at www .dh.gov.uk/dr_consum_dh/groups/dh_digitalassets/documents/digitalasset/dh_110711.pdf (accessed 20 January 2015).

## Safeguarding vulnerable adults

You are on call for intensive care and have been referred a 78-year-old lady who is a residential home resident. She has presented with septic shock secondary to a urinary tract infection. You are in the emergency department seeing the patient and notice that the patient's clothes are dirty and there are some unusual bruises on her limbs. On further inspection you find a sacral pressure sore.

**What are your concerns and how should you proceed?**

This patient is a vulnerable adult and there are signs here that are suggestive of abuse. There are a number of risk factors that result in people being vulnerable which include being elderly and frail; living alone at home or in a care home (especially with little family support); having mental health needs, physical disabilities or learning difficulties. Everyone is entitled to live a life free from harm or abuse. We have a duty as healthcare professionals to protect all patients, but there are certain groups who are less able to look after themselves and who therefore need particular care: children, young people and vulnerable adults.

Vulnerable adults are at risk of many different types of abuse; physical, emotional (bullying), neglect and sexual abuse, but also include financial abuse, discriminatory abuse, institutional abuse and forced marriage. As is the case in paediatrics, the perpetrator of the abuse is often someone well known to the person abused. There are many signs of abuse but general ones include changes in personality or behaviour of the person being abused or frequent arguments between the person and their carer.

We have a duty of care to report any concerns if we have reason to believe that someone is a victim of abuse. Concerns should be reported to the appropriate person within your organization as soon as possible (within one working day) and any immediate protection needs for the person in question should be addressed. This is a 'Safeguarding Alert' and should be to your supervising consultant (line manager) or the Safeguarding Adults lead. A decision then needs to be made as to whether to refer the case on to the local authority with a 'Safeguarding Adults referral'. You should also keep the patient in question informed, although in this situation she may be too unwell. You do not need to question the patient regarding the possibility of abuse, but if any information is given, it should be recorded verbatim in the notes. In a different situation, if there were to be any 'evidence', you should leave this where it is, unless it is necessary to provide essential care or treatment.

Not relevant in this case, but something else that you should be aware of when caring for vulnerable adults is The Deprivation of Liberty Safeguards 2009. This is an extra safeguard for vulnerable adult and forms part of the Mental Capacity Act. It is relevant in situations where it is necessary to restrain patients, for example when patients are acutely confused and at risk of injuring themselves or others. Restraint is lawful if it is necessary to prevent harm but it must be the last option, for as little time as possible and with minimal force.

## Further reading

Safeguarding Adults. e-LfH open access sessions. Part A and Part B. http://www.e-lfh.org.uk/ programmes/safeguarding-adults/open-access-sessions/ (accessed 1 April 2015).

Safeguarding Adults. Patient.co.uk leaflet. http://www.patient.co.uk/health/safeguarding-adults-leaflet (accessed 1 April 2015).

## Safe blood transfusion

Anaesthetists are frequently involved in the transfusion of blood products and it is vital you have good up-to-date knowledge of both the national guidance and your local Trust guidance on the administration of blood products. This section aims to give a refresher on blood groups and compatibility, followed by an overview of the practicalities of transfusion and the associated risks.

**Consider the following true/false questions:**

a) Group AB RhD +ve patients can receive any group of blood cells
b) Group O RhD −ve females of childbearing age should only receive group O RhD −ve blood
c) The majority of wrong blood transfusion incidents are due to clerical errors in the transfusion laboratory
d) Red blood cells can be returned to the lab unused within 4 hours
e) In the event of a suspected transfusion reaction the blood should be immediately discontinued and discarded

Answers: TTFTF

Serious Hazards of Transfusion (SHOT) is the UK's haemovigilance scheme that collects data on serious adverse events and reactions and makes recommendations to improve safety. SHOT identified the biggest risk from the transfusion of blood products is receiving the incorrect blood component. *All errors identified could have been prevented with a final bedside check prior to administration.*

## Blood group serology

The ABO group is the most important: patients should receive blood of their own ABO group. In a life-threatening situation group O can be given as it has no antibodies on the red blood cells. Table 21.1 shows the antigen and antibody status of the ABO blood groups.

The Rhesus D (RhD) system is the second most important as the RhD antigen is highly immunogenic. Red cells carrying this antigen are known as RhD positive. RhD +ve individuals (85% of the population) can be transfused any type of RhD blood (+ve or −ve). The 15% who are RhD −ve can ONLY be given RhD −ve blood. Exposure to RhD +ve cells via transfusion or pregnancy can lead to development of anti-D antibodies. In women of childbearing age this can threaten future pregnancies as maternal antibodies can attack RhD +ve fetal cells, causing haemolytic disease of the newborn, which can be fatal.

**Table 21.1** ABO blood group serology

| Blood group | Patient blood cell antigens | Patient plasma antibodies | % UK population |
|---|---|---|---|
| A | A antigen | Anti-B | 42 |
| B | B antigen | Anti-A | 8 |
| AB | AB antigen | None | 3 |
| O | No antigens | Anti-A + Anti-B | 47 |

## Practicalities of transfusion

### 1. Decision to transfuse

Signed consent is not a legal requirement in the UK; however, the patient needs to be informed in a timely manner of the reason for transfusion, risks and alternatives. The discussion should be documented. Usually this is part of the surgical consent process but should also be discussed at your preoperative assessment.

## 2. Requesting procedure

The minimum patient identification data set is: first name; last name; date of birth; hospital number or other unique identifier; gender (optional – check your local transfusion policy).

Other information such as the test/components required is also necessary. In short – complete the whole request form accurately and make sure you sign it.

## 3. Sample testing pre-transfusion

Group and Screen/Save. ABO and RhD group can be identified within 5–10 minutes. The antibody screen is then used to detect the 1% of the population who will have an atypical red cell antibody. The components will then be selected on the basis of being the correct ABO and RhD group. The sample can then be saved for up to 7 days.

Cross-match. After a Group and Screen, a cross-match can usually be performed within 20–30 minutes. Request for cross-match for surgical patients should be guided by the Maximum Surgical Blood Ordering Schedule (MSBOS); a locally agreed tariff indicating the number of units that should be ordered for specific procedures to avoid wastage.

## 4. Sample collection

Proper procedure must be followed by portering staff for collection of blood products.

Different products are stored at different temperatures, with varying shelf lives. However, the consistent advice is that all products should be transfused within 4 hours of either removal from fridge (red blood cells), agitation rack (platelets) or after thawing (FFP and cryoprecipitate).

## 5. Sample administration

There are several checks that must be made prior to transfusion. These include:

1. Baseline observations, including temperature. These will already be being done in theatre.
2. Inspection of the unit, including expiry date and time.
3. Confirm with patient (or second person) the name and DOB of the patient.
4. Check details on the laboratory-produced label attached to the blood component against the patient's ID wristband. You MUST check all the details of the minimum patient identification data set.
5. Check the laboratory-produced label attached to the blood component against the blood component. You must check the donor component numbers are the same, the blood groups are the same, the RhD types are the same, whether there are any special requirements, e.g. CMV negative.

A number of hospitals have introduced a one registered health professional check, others still require a two-man check. Once checks are completed sign the transfusion documentation, record the donor component number and fully complete traceability documentation and return to the lab as per local policy.

### 6. Monitoring for transfusion reaction

The minimum observations recommended are: temperature, pulse, blood pressure, respiratory rate. These should be checked pre-transfusion (no more than 60 minutes before starting); during transfusion (15 minutes after start of each unit) and on completion of each unit. Signs of a reaction include:

- MILD – pyrexia (2 above baseline), urticaria, rash
- SEVERE – pyrexia, rigors, hypotension, back/loin pain, anxiety, pain at infusion site, respiratory distress, dark urine, tachycardia, disseminated intravascular coagulopathy.

Management of a severe transfusion reaction includes:

- STOP the transfusion and assess the patient – ABCDE
- Check compatibility of unit with patient identification band
- Replace the administration set and preserve IV access with IV fluid to maintain systolic blood pressure
- Inform the lab and return the remaining product in its packaging to the lab accompanied by the paperwork
- Check urine for signs of haemoglobinuria
- Reassess the patient and treat appropriately, seeking expert advice if they deteriorate.

Acute transfusion reactions (ATRs) are defined as 'a reaction occurring during or up to 24 hours after transfusion of blood or blood components'. Often an ATR is evident within 30 minutes of starting a transfusion. The ATR definition excludes complications that may arise as a result of transfusion and have similar signs, for example: acute haemolysis (including ABO incompatibility); bacterial contamination; transfusion-related lung injury (TRALI); transfusion-associated circulatory overload (TACO) or worsening of the pre-existing condition of course.

## Further reading

http://www.shotuk.org (accessed 4 January 2016).
www.transfusionguidelines.org.uk (accessed 4 January 2016).
British Committee for Standards in Hematology. Guidelines on the administration of blood components. 2009. Available at www.bcshguidelines.com (accessed 4 January 2016).

## Patient safety: venous thromboembolism (VTE) prophylaxis

There are several new anticoagulant drugs that have been introduced in recent years. Learning about their different pharmacological profiles and indications can be a bit dry.

**Here are a series of MCQs with key facts about each one to give you an overview.**

1. Rivaroxiban
   a) Is a factor Xa agonist
   b) Requires regular monitoring of international normalized ratio (INR)
   c) Should be considered for patients with AF and poor INR control on warfarin
   d) Should be considered for patients with AF and no other risk factors for stroke or other VTE
   e) Should be omitted for 24 hours before insertion of neuraxial block

Answers: FFTFT

Rivaroxiban directly inhibits activated factor X (factor Xa). It is administered as a fixed daily dose of 20 mg PO. Its effects can be monitored with PT, APTT and Heptest. The National Institute for Health and Care Excellence (NICE) suggests that rivaroxiban is indicated for patients with AF and at least one additional risk factor for VTE, such as congestive heart failure, hypertension, age 75 years or older, diabetes mellitus, prior stroke or transient ischaemic attack (CHADS$_2$ score of 1 and above). Twenty-two to twenty-six hours must elapse between administration of rivaroxiban and neuraxial block.

2. Fondaparinux
   a) Is a low molecular weight heparin
   b) Is administered as a subcutaneous, daily dose
   c) Can be monitored using factor Xa assays
   d) Is not a contraindication for use of an indwelling neuraxial catheter
   e) Can be administered 2 hours after surgery

Answers: FTTFF

Fondaparinux is a factor Xa inhibitor. The use of neuraxial catheters in patients receiving fondaparinux is not recommended. Neuraxial blocks should be performed with extreme caution, using an atraumatic, single-shot technique. The first dose should be administered 6 hours after surgery.

3. Lepirudin
   a) Is a direct thrombin inhibitor
   b) Is indicated for patients who have heparin-induced thrombocytopenia (HIT)
   c) Is administered as a twice daily, intravenous dose
   d) Is predominantly eliminated via the kidneys
   e) Has no specific antidote

Answers: TTFTT

Lepuridin is a recombinant hirudin. It is administered as a continuous infusion, with activity measured by APTT, usually aiming for a target ratio of 2.0–3.0. Dosing depends on presence of thrombosis and renal function/use of haemofiltration. Approximately 90% is renally excreted.

1. Abciximab
   a) Is a heparinoid mixture
   b) Is administered orally
   c) Is indicated for patients with acute myocardial infarction undergoing percutaneous coronary intervention
   d) Is required to be discontinued for 48 hours before platelet function can be considered to be normal
   e) Has a peak effect within minutes of administration

Answers: FFTTT

Abciximab is a platelet glycoprotein IIb/IIIa receptor antagonist. It is administered as an intravenous infusion or directly into coronary vessels. It should be discontinued 48 hours prior to insertion of a neuraxial block.

The management of patients for regional anaesthesia with abnormalities of coagulation is the subject of an AAGBI guideline and is discussed in Chapter 25.

## Further reading

Barker R. C., Marval P. Venous thromboembolism: risks and prevention. *Contin Educ Anaesth Crit Care Pain* 2011; 11(1): 18–23.

Horlocker T. T. Regional anaesthesia in the patient receiving antithrombotic and antiplatelet therapy. *Br J Anaesth* 2011; 107(Suppl 1): i96–106.

National Institute for Health and Clinical Excellence. Venous thromboembolism: reducing the risk for patients in hospital. 2010. Available at http://www.nice.org.uk/guidance/CG92 (accessed 4 January 2016).

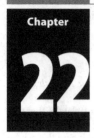

**Chapter**

# 22

# Ethical and legal issues

*Ethical principles underpin the duties of doctors. The main focus of this chapter is information governance and consent – two important topics for anaesthetists. The chapter covers consent in three different situations: children, elderly patients and obstetrics. The starting points are similar in all of the scenarios: establishment of whether the patient has capacity. Chapter 24 also has more information about consent and documentation.*

## Can a patient see their notes?

You have gone to the ward to perform a preoperative assessment on a patient whom you previously looked after whilst they were on ITU. They recognize you and have some questions regarding their care. They also ask to look in their ITU notes as they wish to clarify something.

**What legislation covers the rights of access to health records?**

The Data Protection Act (DPA) 1998 applies to living individuals and permits access to both electronic and manual health records, including those held by the NHS, private health companies, GPs, dentists and opticians. Applications can be made by an individual or their authorized representative. The Access to Health Records Act 1990 applies for accessing deceased individuals' health records.

**Would it be legal for you to informally show the patient their ITU notes?**

Yes, there is nothing within the law that prevents a healthcare professional from informally showing a patient their own notes, although copies can only be provided following a formal application.

**How can a patient make a formal application to see their notes?**

Formal requests are made under The Data Protection Act 1998. Individuals are not required to provide a reason for the request, unless it is with a view to commencing legal proceedings (pursuant to the Clinical Negligence Pre-action Protocol). Requests can be made in writing or via email; this is known as the Subject Access Request (SAR). These should be sent directly to the GP/practice manager, or for hospital records to the Health Records Manager at the Trust in question. All requests should be met within 40 days. Fees do apply; these are between £10 and £50 depending on whether copies are requested. There is no charge to view records added within the last 40 days.

---

*Returning to Work in Anaesthesia*, ed. Emma Plunkett, Emily Johnson and Anna Pierson.
Published by Cambridge University Press. © Cambridge University Press 2016.

An appointment will be made in order for the individual to view their notes. A member of staff should be present to offer support, explain medical terms and ensure the notes are not altered.

If copies have been requested they must be written in language understandable by a layperson, therefore medical terminology/abbreviations must be explained.

### When might access be denied?

- If it is felt that information held within the notes is likely to cause serious harm to the individual or another party.
- If applying on behalf of someone else, when the patient gave information on the understanding that it would remain confidential.
- If the records contain details about a third party who has not given their consent for disclosure.
- If it is restricted by an order of the courts or if the records are subject to legal professional privilege.

### How long are healthcare records held?

Hospital records are normally held for 8 years after completion of treatment; exceptions include maternity, children and mental health records. GP records are held for 10 years following treatment completion, death or leaving the UK; again exceptions apply.

## Further reading

British Medical Association. Access to health records – Guidance for health professionals in the United Kingdom. 2014. www.bma.org.uk (accessed March 2015).

Department of Health. Guidance for Access to Health Records Requests. 2010. http://systems.hscic .gov.uk/infogov/links/dhaccessrecs.pdf (accessed March 2015).

NHS. How do I access my medical records (health records)? 2014. www.nhs.uk (accessed March 2015).

## Consent and the child: Gillick competence

In which one of the following circumstances has the process of obtaining consent been most appropriate:

a) A 19-year-old patient with autism has his consent provided by his mother.
b) A 14-year-old girl presents with her partner for surgical termination – she provides consent, but insists her parents are not told.
c) A 17-year-old boy with osteosarcoma of his tibia declines potentially life-saving lower limb amputation – despite his parents' pleas, surgery does not take place.
d) A 15-year-old Jehovah's Witness girl declines the use of blood products ahead of scoliosis surgery, but her mother requests that she receives blood in the case of life-threatening haemorrhage.
e) A 1-year-old boy presents with his parents for a religious circumcision – although the father provides consent, the mother does not appear happy.

Answer: d)

Parental responsibility encompasses a large range of roles, amongst which is the legal requirement to provide consent for the child, following due consideration of the benefits and risks involved. For the provider obtaining the consent, this process is much easier whilst the child and parents are in accord, but can become a legal minefield when disagreement arises.

Once a child reaches 18, parents no longer have the legal ability to provide consent, whatever that child's capacity of understanding may be. Should anyone over the age of 18 not be judged to have sufficient capacity to produce consent, then it remains for the doctor to prove this, and potentially have this corroborated with a second opinion.

Following the case of Gillick vs. Norwich and Wisbech AHA (1986) the House of Lords held that a child under 16 could provide consent for treatment if they showed '... sufficient maturity and intelligence to understand the nature and implications of the proposed treatment'. Although this case was specifically about contraception, further cases have expanded the argument to other areas of medical practice. However, the declaration also expounded that efforts should be made to persuade the child to tell her parents, or to allow the doctor to tell them.

When there is disagreement between an older child and the parents, particularly when the child could be deemed Gillick competent, the scenario becomes particularly difficult. Although the age of consent is 16, young people under the age of 18 cannot give a binding refusal for treatment. Parental responsibility overrides the child's wishes in this life-saving scenario. It would be justified to delay surgery in order to explore the patient's fears; however, if a consensus to treat could not be reached, a legal review should be sought.

Consent from only one parent with parental responsibility is required in law. However, if there is disagreement, particularly in the elective setting, it would be unwise to proceed with surgery. The onus lies with the clinician to obtain a consensus. If this should prove impossible and the treatment is deemed urgent, then the Doctrine of Best Interest may be applied. Obtaining and documenting the independent opinion of a colleague would be prudent.

## Further reading

General Medical Council. Consent: patients and doctors making decisions together. 2008. Available at http://www.gmc-uk.org/static/documents/content/Consent_-_English_0911.pdf (accessed 25 January 2015).

Wheeler R. Consent for non-therapeutic male circumcision: an exception to the rule? *Arch Dis Child* 2008; 93: 825–6.

Williams C., Perkins R. Consent issues for children: a law unto themselves. *Contin Educ Anaesth Crit Care Pain* 2011; 11(3): 99–103.

## Definition of capacity

A 75-year-old lady is admitted to hospital with a history of vomiting and abdominal pain. General surgeons have identified an obstructing sigmoid tumour. They have booked her for an urgent laparotomy. During your anaesthetic assessment, she tells you that she does not wish to proceed with surgery, as she does not believe that she will survive. You assess her as slightly confused with an abbreviated mental test score of 9/10, although she assures you that she has understood the implications of her decision. Her daughter tells you that she has a power of attorney document to make the decision to proceed on her behalf, and that she feels that her mother is not herself.

**How would you assess the lady's capacity to make a decision about refusing surgery?**

It is the responsibility of the decision maker to assess capacity. The Mental Capacity Act 2005 makes clear that a person must be assumed to have capacity unless it can be established that they do not. The Act makes clear that all practicable steps must be taken to assist someone to have capacity and a person does not lack capacity just because they make an unwise choice. Importantly, capacity is time and decision specific so mild confusion on its own does not necessarily preclude a person having capacity. Practical steps to enhance this lady's capacity may include: facilitating a further discussion with the surgeons; ensuring she has hearing aids/glasses if needed or providing her with written information about the procedure.

A person lacks capacity if, at the time they need to make the decision, they have 'an impairment of or disturbance in the functioning of the mind or brain'. It does not matter whether the impairment is temporary or permanent. A person will lack capacity to make a decision if the impairment or disturbance of mind or brain means they are unable to 'understand the information relevant to the decision, retain the information, use or weigh that information as part of the decision-making process or communicate a decision'. If she is felt to have capacity to decide and her refusal is likely to have a life-threatening consequence it would be wise to get a second opinion from a senior colleague if possible.

If it is felt she does not have capacity, the Mental Capacity Act dictates that actions must be in the person's best interests. You should check whether she has a valid and applicable advanced directive, a valid lasting power of attorney (LPOA) or a court appointed deputy. If none of these exist you must identify the person's best interests by considering the individual's past and present wishes, values, beliefs and feelings, consult relatives or those involved in the individual's care as to their views of what the person would have wanted and consider whether the decision can be postponed until the person regains capacity. If there is disagreement regarding an individual's capacity to make a decision or what is in their best interests, legal advice can be sought from the hospital solicitors and if necessary they can seek advice from the Court of Protection.

**What is the document that she is referring to, and what are its implications?**

A lasting power of attorney (LPOA) is a legal document that allows another person (an attorney) to make decisions on behalf of a person who lacks capacity that are as valid and binding as if the person was consenting/refusing themselves. LPOAs can be created for personal welfare decisions (including consent to medical treatment) or for property and financial affairs. Prior to the Mental Capacity Act 2005, individuals could create an enduring power of attorney but these only relate to property and financial affairs.

In this case the first step would still be to clarify whether the patient has capacity to consent to treatment. If she has capacity then it is not relevant what document the daughter has as the patient must be allowed to make her own decision. If the patient lacks capacity then it would be important to see the document to establish whether it was a valid LPOA appointing the daughter as an attorney for personal welfare decisions. If the LPOA for personal welfare decisions is to be relevant in this situation it must be registered with the Office of the Public Guardian and must expressly authorize the attorney to make decisions regarding life-sustaining treatment. If the daughter's LPOA is valid and applicable then her consent to treatment is legally binding.

# Further reading

http://www.legislation.gov.uk/ukpga/2005/9/section/9 (accessed 4 January 2016).
https://www.gov.uk/government/uploads/system/uploads/attachment_data/file/224660/Mental_
    Capacity_Act_code_of_practice.pdf (accessed 4 January 2016).

We would like to acknowledge the contribution of Dr Sara Ormerod, Consultant Liaison Psychiatrist for her work on the question above. Thank you.

# Consent in obstetrics

A 30-year-old primip is requesting an epidural for labour analgesia. She had planned to deliver in the midwife-led birth centre attached to your unit and her birth plan states that she wishes to have minimal interventions and did not want to have an epidural. She has no medical or obstetric history of note. Her cervix is 5 cm dilated and she is distressed with pain and using Entonox.

**Regarding this patient giving consent for an epidural, which of the following statements are true?**

a) The patient cannot give consent: she lacks capacity as she is so distressed
b) Her partner can refuse consent on her behalf
c) The midwife can consent for the patient as she will be acting in her best interests
d) It is not necessary to obtain consent as this can be considered an emergency
e) Her birth plan should be considered an advance directive and must be followed
f) Consent must be taken in writing

Answers: all are false.

In order to give their consent a person must be able to make a decision for themselves, i.e. have capacity. (Please refer to the previous question for a definition of capacity.) In the case of women in labour, although their level of distress and the intermittent use of Entonox may lead to questioning of whether they have capacity, all current evidence and guidance would support the view that unless circumstances are exceptional, they do. It is correct that consent may be via an appropriately made advanced decision; however, a patient with capacity is able to change their mind at any point. The key point in this situation is that she is most likely to have capacity and therefore is able to change her mind from her previously written birth plan and give consent to insertion of an epidural. Remember that consent is a process and it may be necessary to reaffirm this at intervals throughout the procedure. If you are concerned that she does not have capacity, then further advice should be sought and her birth plan may be considered an advanced directive in the meantime.

Unless someone has been given lasting powers of attorney or has been appointed by the courts, no one can give or withhold consent to treatment on behalf of an another adult. The consent process must be voluntary and the patient must be free from coercion, including by a partner or relative, when making her decision. It is occasionally seen in obstetrics that the strong opinions of a birth partner are influencing a patient's decision regarding options for analgesia. In the situation described above, if a partner is present it might be worth explaining to them the reasoning and rationale for you proceeding despite the documented birth plan.

Good medical practice states that the doctor providing the treatment or performing the procedure has a responsibility to discuss it with the patient. This may be delegated to a suitable person and for anaesthesia it is not uncommon for one anaesthetist to take consent on behalf of another.

Previously, the courts considered that the amount of information about the risks of a procedure that was required to be given was judged according to the Bolam principle: that which would have been given by a responsible body of clinical opinion. The case of Montgomery vs. Lanarkshire Health Board has changed this and made it clear that the patient should be informed of all the risks that a reasonable person in their position might consider significant. It is argued in the editorial listed below that this is not new, but merely brings the law in line with good medical practice, putting the patient and their wishes at the centre of the process of consent.

If patients insist they do not wish to know about the risks, then they do not need to have the information forced on them, although the consequences of not informing them about the risk should be conveyed. Ideally information would have been provided in the antenatal setting to reduce the need for extensive information to be provided to the labouring woman.

At present a written consent form is not a requirement for anaesthesia (general or regional) as verbal consent is considered acceptable. However, the General Medical Council (GMC) advises that you must record your meeting with the patient including information discussed, any specific requests, any written visual or audio information given and the decisions made. Many hospitals have included details of consent on obstetric anaesthesia records to facilitate this. In this case it may be prudent to ask the patient to co-sign your documentation of the conversation, in case of any confusion in the future.

Consent forms used within the NHS are:

Form 1 for adults or competent children
Form 2 for parental consent for a child or young person
Form 3 for when a patient will remain alert and no anaesthetist is involved
Form 4 for adults unable to consent for themselves.

A consent form does not provide proof of consent but is evidence that consent has been given.

## Further reading

Association of Anaesthetists Great Britain and Ireland. Consent for Anaesthesia. 2006. (Due to be updated in 2016.)

Department of Health. Reference guide to consent for examination or treatment, 2nd edn. London: HMSO, 2009.

General Medical Council. Good medical practice (2013). Available at http://www.gmc-uk.org/guidance/good_medical_practice.asp (accessed 2 January 2016).

McCombe K., Bogod D. G. Paternalism and consent: has the law finally caught up with the patient? *Anaesthesia* 2015; 70(9): 1016–19.

# Guidelines, Updates and Checklists

## Introduction

Welcome to Section 3. This section contains summaries of important guidelines that you may wish to refresh your knowledge of just before you return to work or in the first few days or weeks back at work. And perhaps after that too. We doubt that you will be reading this section from beginning to end, but rather that you will dip in and out of the section as required.

We have included national and international guidelines such as those from the Royal College of Anaesthetists, Association of Anaesthetists, European Society of Anaesthesiology, Resuscitation Council, Difficult Airway Society and National Institute of Health and Care Excellence. Where relevant we have reproduced (with kind permission – thank you) copies of the guideline summaries and also given a short commentary on them to highlight salient points. We have included a number of checklists too. Some, such as the World Health Organization (WHO) checklist, are embedded into everyday practice. Others, such as our preoperative assessment checklist, are more of a practical summary of the subject. We hope that collating all this information together will be useful for you. It has been good revision for us too!

We realize that guidelines are updated periodically. We have included the latest versions available to us at the time of going to print. We intend to update the text at regular intervals but in between print runs we will update the accompanying website to point you towards the latest versions. Please let us know if you find anything that has subsequently been updated.

Chapter

# 23

# Preoperative assessment and anaesthetic planning

Katy Miller, Anna Costello and Emma Plunkett

*The purposes of preoperative assessment are to minimize the risks of anaesthesia, plan the anaesthetic and gain consent for the anaesthetic and associated procedures. This section will summarize key issues in this area as well as relevant guidance. Included in the section is a checklist which you may find useful when performing preoperative assessments in your first few days back at work. Other pertinent information may be found in the Consent, Drug calculator and Difficult Airway Society guidelines sections that follow.*

The following subjects are covered in this chapter:

- Airway assessment
- National Institute for Health and Care Excellence (NICE) guidelines for preoperative investigations
- Preoperative assessment checklist
- Operative risk scoring systems
- Paediatric issues
  - Heart murmurs
  - Recent upper respiratory tract infections
  - Immunizations
  - Child protection
- ECG interpretation
- Pacemakers and implantable cardioverter defibrillators
- Basic echocardiography
- Pulmonary function tests
- ESA preoperative starvation guidelines
- Remote site anaesthesia

## Airway assessment

The aim of airway assessment is to predict or anticipate a difficult airway, either for face mask ventilation or intubation, and therefore avoid the anaesthetic nightmare of a 'can't intubate, can't ventilate' situation. There are many different tests for assessing the airway and each of us is likely to have a select few we feel provide us with the 'optimum assessment'. Remember that it is all very well doing the tests but you need to know the significance of the results. Unfortunately, none of the tests are perfect and, in general, have both a low specificity and

*Returning to Work in Anaesthesia*, ed. Emma Plunkett, Emily Johnson and Anna Pierson.
Published by Cambridge University Press. © Cambridge University Press 2016.

positive predictive value (patients with concerning test results do not turn out to be difficult to manage) and a low sensitivity (many cases of difficult intubation are not detected).

## Difficult ventilation

The following factors, remembered using the mnemonic OBESE, are associated with difficult mask ventilation, so consider them in your history and examination.

- Overweight (BMI > 26)
- Bearded
- Elderly (age > 55)
- Snoring
- Edentulous.

The presence of two of these has a sensitivity and specificity >70%. The patient's BMI alone is a poor predictor of difficult ventilation and the distribution of the patient's fat deposition should be taken into consideration. Other concerning factors include facial or jaw abnormalities and a history of obstructive sleep apnoea. The single most important factor predicting impossible mask ventilation is neck irradiation[1].

## Difficult intubation

The following factors can all contribute to and help to predict a difficult intubation. (The list is not exhaustive.)

- Limited mouth opening (the standard Macintosh blade requires 3 cm between incisors)[1]
- Narrow or high arching palate
- Limited neck extension
- Retrognathia
- Thyromental distance < 6.5 cm or a sternomental distance < 12.5 cm
- Mallampati grade 3 and 4
- Barrel chest or large breasts (the effect of this can be limited by using the ramp position)
- Increased fat deposition in the neck
- Stridor
- Pre-existing oral/glottic pathology (including vocal cord palsy, tumours, trauma).

Table 23.1 summarizes airway assessment and a reminder of factors which should be a cause for concern[2].

## Preoperative investigations (NICE guidelines)

In 2016 NICE updated their 2003 guidance regarding the use of routine preoperative investigations[3]. The guidance is based on the best available evidence, which in this case is all level IV (expert opinion from the consensus development process and clinical experience). This makes the recommendations grade D. The guidance tailors the recommended investigations according to:

- Patient's ASA grade
- Co-morbidity

**Table 23.1** Assessment of the airway

| Test | Details | Result predicting difficult intubation | Statistics* |
|---|---|---|---|
| Mallampati | Oropharyngeal view with mouth maximally open, tongue out and without phonation | 3 (only soft palate visible) and 4 (only hard palate visible) | Sensitivity 50% 90% false-positive rate |
| Thyromental distance | Extend neck. Measure from tip of thyroid cartilage to tip of mandible Normal > 7 cm | <6 cm | Positive predictive value 75% When combined with Mallampati: sensitivity 81%, specificity 97% |
| Sternomental distance | Extend neck. Close mouth. Upper border of manubrium to tip of mandible | <12.5 cm | Positive predictive value 82% |
| Mouth opening (inter-incisor gap) | Distance between incisors (or gums) with mouth maximally open | <3 cm (<2.5 cm LMA insertion difficult and <2 cm impossible) | |
| Jaw protrusion | Class A: lower incisors anterior to upper Class B: lower incisors level with upper Class C: lower incisors cannot meet upper | Class B and C | |
| Dentition | Buck teeth, poor dentition with loose teeth and anterior gaps | | |
| Neck movements | Finger on chin and occipital protuberance. Extend head maximally. Normal if finger on chin higher | Level fingers, moderate restriction Occipital finger higher = severe limitation | |
| Wilson's Score (Complicated therefore less practical) | Weight Head and neck movement Jaw movement Receding mandible Buck teeth | ≥ 2 (each factor scored 0, 1 or 2) | Positive predictive value 75% Sensitivity 88% |

\* Sensitivity = probability of identification of true positives, i.e. detects a difficult case that is difficult. When low, lots of false negatives occur meaning you fail to predict difficult cases.

Specificity = probability of identification of true negatives, i.e. detects a normal case that is normal. When low, lots of false positives occur.

Positive predictive value = the probability of a positive result being a true positive, i.e. it is the % of patients found to be difficult out of all those predicted to be difficult.

- Cardiovascular (including diabetes)
- Respiratory
- Renal
- Obesity
- The grade of complexity of the surgery (see Table 23.2 below).

The tests are summerised in the form of colour-coded table using a traffic light system: red = not recommended; yellow = consider; green = recommended.

**Table 23.2** Surgical complexity

| Surgical complexity | Examples |
|---|---|
| Minor (grade 1) | I&D abscess |
| Intermediate (grade 2) | Inguinal hernia, tonsillectomy, arthroscopy |
| Major (grade 3 or 4) | TAH, TURP, Joint replacement, bowel resection |

**Table 23.3** Routine preoperative investigations (**bold = recommended;** italics = consider)

| | Complexity of surgery | | |
|---|---|---|---|
| ASA | Minor | Intermediate | Major |
| 1 | | | **FBC**, *ECG if > 65 & not within 12 months, U&E if at risk of AKI** |
| 2 | | *ECG, U&E if at risk* | **FBC, U&E, ECG** |
| 3 or 4 | *U&E if at risk of AKI, ECG if no result within 12 months* | *FBC,* **U&E, ECG**, *consider haemostasis tests if chronic liver disease, consider lung function tests.* | **FBC, U&E, ECG,** *haemostasis tests if chronic liver disease, consider lung function tests.* |

\* AKI = acute kidney injury
Patients with diabetes should also have an HbA1c result within 3 months.

Table 23.3 above summarizes the green and yellow recommendations which are further condensed onto the preoperative assessment checklist. These guidelines cover elective surgery only and urgent or emergency cases are likely to require additional investigations

## Sickle cell test

By adulthood sickle cell disease will be evident. Testing patients may reveal carrier status but this will not affect management and so it is not routinely recommended. Patients should be asked about their own and their family's sickle cell status to guide management.[3]

## Pregnancy test

All women of childbearing age should be asked whether or not there is a chance they may be pregnant. Women should be made aware of the risks to the fetus that surgery and anaesthesia entails and a pregnancy test should be performed with consent if there is any doubt as to the result.

## Preoperative assessment checklist

Figure 23.1 is a preoperative assessment checklist which summarises the key points in the anaesthetic history and examination and the NICE recommendations for preoperative investigations.

Pre-operative assessment checklist

| History | Medications | Direct questions |
|---|---|---|
| □ Of surgical problem<br>□ Anaesthesia & problems including PONV<br>□ Or family history GA problems<br>□ Past Medical History (PMH) | □ Regular + prn - omit or give usual meds?<br>□ Anticoagulation<br>□ Allergies<br>□ Ok with NSAIDs?<br>□ Check drug chart for recently given medication<br>□ Pre-med? | □ Exercise tolerance<br>□ Reflux<br>□ Snoring<br>□ Motion sickness<br>□ Smoking / EtOH / Drugs<br>□ Recent URTI / illness<br>□ Dentition<br>□ Starvation |
| **Observations** | **Examination** | **Airway** |
| □ Weight + Height (BMI)<br>□ Pulse<br>□ Blood pressure<br>□ Temperature<br>□ Oxygen saturations<br>□ BM if diabetic | □ Cardiovascular<br>□ Respiratory<br>□ Other? | □ Mallampati (MP)<br>□ Jaw protrusion<br>□ Thyromental distance (TM)<br>□ Neck movement |

≥ 2 "OBESE" factors (overweight, beard, elderly, snoring, edentulous): Think difficult ventilation
MP 3 or 4, Jaw protrusion Class B or C, TM < 6 cm, limited neck movement: Think difficult intubation

| Routine preoperative investigations (from NICE guidance 2016) | | |
|---|---|---|
| **ECG** | **FBC** | **U&E** |
| • Major surgery (consider if ASA 1 & ≥ 65 & not done within 12 months)<br>• ASA 3 or 4 (consider if minor surgery & not done within 12 months)<br>• Consider if ASA 2 & intermediate surgery | • All major surgery<br>• Consider for ASA 2 patients and intermediate surgery | • Major surgery<br>• ASA 3 or 4<br>• If at risk of acute kidney injury (AKI) |

- HbA1c within 3 months if patient has diabetes
- Consider haemostasis tests in liver disease; use point of care testing if possible
- Pregnancy test (with consent) if any chance may be pregnant
- Sickle test not routine; ask about PMH or family history
- CXR not routinely required

| Consent | | | |
|---|---|---|---|
| □ GA | □ Additional procedures for e.g. invasive monitoring | □ Regional anaesthesia | □ Peripheral nerve blockade |

| Surgical issues to consider and discuss during WHO checklist |
|---|
| • Position + access to patient, IV access sites<br>• Blood loss / Risk of major bleeding / Tourniquet – check G&S / X-match<br>• Antibiotic prophylaxis<br>• Thromboembolism prophylaxis<br>• Temperature management<br>• Length of surgery / who is operating |

**Figure 23.1** Preoperative assessment checklist.

# Operative risk scoring systems

A patient should be considered high risk if their predicted mortality is greater than 5%. The Royal College of Surgeons suggests that the following patients should always be considered high risk.

Patients undergoing major gastrointestinal or vascular surgery who are either:

1) Aged > 50 years;
    And undergoing urgent, emergency or redo surgery,
    Or have acute or chronic renal impairment (serum creatinine > 130 μmol/l),
    Or have diabetes mellitus (even if only diet controlled),
    Or have or are strongly suspected clinically to have any significant risk factor for cardiac or respiratory disease.
2) Aged > 65 years.
3) Have shock of any cause, any age group[4].

In 2010 the Association of Anaesthetists of Great Britain and Ireland (AAGBI) published guidelines covering the preoperative management of patients. These guidelines list the following factors for survival prediction: age (risk increases after the age of 10); sex (males 1.7 × > females); socioeconomic class (low social class increases risk); aerobic fitness (increased fitness decreases risk and vice versa) and medical history (1.5 × increased risk with a diagnosis of myocardial infarction, heart failure, cerebrovascular accident, peripheral arterial disease and renal failure)[5].

Multiple scoring systems exist to try and predict the patient's morbidity and mortality with surgery. None are perfect and they range from the simple (e.g. ASA grade) to the multifaceted (e.g. P-POSSUM).

# ASA

Grade 1:  Normal healthy patient (without clinically important co-morbidity)
Grade 2:  Patient with mild systemic disease
Grade 3:  Patient with severe systemic disease
Grade 4:  Patient with severe systemic disease, constant threat to life
Grade 5:  Moribund patient who is not expected to survive 24 hours with or without surgery
Grade 6:  Brain dead patient, organ donation

# Revised Cardiac Risk Index

The Revised Cardiac Risk Index was devised in 1999 to predict the risk of a cardiac event in patients undergoing non-cardiac surgery. Each factor is assigned one point.

- High-risk surgical procedures
    - Intraperitoneal
    - Intrathoracic
    - Supra-inguinal vascular
- History of ischaemic heart disease
    - History of myocardial infarction
    - History of a positive exercise test
    - Current history of ischaemic chest pain

- Use of nitrate therapy
- ECG with pathological Q waves
- History of congestive heart failure
  - History of congestive heart failure
  - Pulmonary oedema
  - Paroxysmal nocturnal dyspnoea
  - Bilateral rales or S3 gallop
  - Chest x-ray showing pulmonary vascular redistribution
- History of cerebrovascular disease
  - History of transient ischaemic attack or stroke
- Preoperative treatment with insulin
- Preoperative serum creatinine > 2.0 mg/dl.

The risk of a major cardiac event (which includes myocardial infarction, pulmonary oedema, ventricular fibrillation, cardiac arrest and complete heart block) is calculated as follows[6]:

- 0 points risk 0.4%
- 1 point risk 0.9%
- 2 points risk 6.6%
- 3 or more points risk 11%.

# P-POSSUM

The Physiological and Operative Severity Score for the enUmeration of Mortality and Morbidity (POSSUM) was originally developed as a retrospective tool. It was found to overestimate mortality and morbidity in the lower-risk population and hence the Portsmouth modification (P-POSSUM) was developed. The parameters used (listed in Table 23.4) should be readily available from the patient's charts and following discussion with the surgeons.

**Table 23.4** Variables included in the P-POSSUM score

| Physiological variables | Operative variables |
| --- | --- |
| Age | Operative severity |
| Cardiac signs | Multiple procedures |
| Dyspnoea | Total blood loss |
| Blood pressure | Peritoneal soiling |
| Pulse | Malignancy |
| Glasgow Coma Scale | Mode of surgery |
| Haemoglobin | |
| White cell count | |
| Urea | |
| Sodium | |
| Potassium | |
| ECG | |

The Vascular Anaesthesia Society of Great Britain and Ireland have a useful calculator on their website that predicts POSSUM morbidity and mortality and P-POSSUM mortality[7].

## METs

Metabolic equivalents are an important way to assess the physical ability of a patient prior to surgery. This can be tested formally or by asking the patient about their level of exercise and physical ability without restriction or limitations.

One MET is the basal metabolic rate of a 40-year-old 70 kg man, which is an oxygen consumption of approximately 3.5 ml/kg/min[8]. Climbing two flights of stairs is equivalent to 4 METs and inability to do this is associated with increased incidence of post-operative cardiac events[9]. In fact, the number of METs achieved is inversely proportional to anaesthetic risk.

# Paediatric anaesthesia

The paediatric population presents a unique set of problems for the anaesthetist preoperatively. The age and the development of the child will affect their level of understanding and dictate the interaction with them and their parents. Cancelling children's operations is disruptive for the child and other family members. Additionally, a number of factors need to be considered when anaesthetizing the child.

## Heart murmurs

It is important to distinguish between the innocent and the pathological murmur as the latter may require cancellation of the proposed operation. Upon discovering a murmur, the chances are that it will be innocent; however, some features may be of greater concern (see Table 23.5).

If the child is under the age of one, then the finding of a murmur should prompt referral and investigation prior to anaesthesia, even if asymptomatic. In the older child, any additional symptoms require a referral to cardiology.

**Table 23.5** Assessing paediatric heart murmurs[10]

| Features | Innocent | Pathological |
| --- | --- | --- |
| Cardiac symptoms | Asymptomatic | Symptomatic |
| Timing of murmur | Early systolic Continuous | Diastolic; pansystolic; late systolic |
| Quality of murmur | Blowing; musical; vibratory | Variable; harsh |
| Precordial thrill | Never | Sometimes |
| Variation with posture | Often | Rarely |

## Upper respiratory tract infections

Upper respiratory tract infections (URTI) are very common in children and will affect the administration of anaesthesia. The main risks of proceeding in a child with a concurrent URTI are laryngospasm and bronchospasm. Postponing surgery may be prudent if the child shows signs of any systemic symptoms (e.g. malaise, fever), purulent nasal discharge, a productive cough, and signs on chest auscultation and in children < 1 year old[10]. Confirmation from the parents that the child has been unwell may also lead to cancellation. Depending on the severity of the URTI, then rescheduling should take place from 2 weeks (mild) to 4–6 weeks (severe) to limit the risk of laryngospasm.

## Immunization

The timing of surgery with vaccination has been summarized by the Association of Paediatric Anaesthetists of Great Britain and Ireland.

- Inactivated vaccine
  - Delay surgery by 48 hours to avoid confusion of perioperative and post-vaccination symptoms.
  - Vaccination can be administrated post-operatively providing child has recovered.
- Live attenuated vaccine
  - No need to delay surgery as long as child is well[11].

## Child protection

Every anaesthetist who has contact with children has a responsibility to that child. Within the hospital there will be designated child protection professionals with whom the concerns can be raised and discussed. There will be a person who can be contacted irrespective of the time of day; check who this is within your Trust.

## ECG interpretation

This section provides a quick refresher on salient points to remember about ECGs. Firstly, we provide a reminder of basic 12-lead ECG interpretation, information on accompanying symptoms or arrhythmias which require further investigation and, finally, some ECG patterns not to be missed.

- Rate:                 300 divided by the number of large squares in between R waves
- PR interval:      0.12–0.24 ms (3–6 small squares)
- QRS complex:    0.8–0.12 ms (2–3 small squares)
- Electrical axis:    Lead I and aVF positive – normal axis
  Lead I positive and II and aVF negative – left axis deviation
  Lead I negative and aVF positive – right axis deviation
- Bundle branch block: Prolonged QRS with RSR pattern, looks like an M in V1, W in V6 – right bundle branch block (MoRRow)
  Prolonged QRS, looks like a W in V1, M in V6 – left bundle branch block (WiLLiam).

When presented with an ECG it is important to identify those that will warrant further investigation and, potentially, cancellation. Certain adverse signs in the presence of arrhythmia should prompt immediate treatment. According to the Resuscitation guidelines 2015, these adverse signs are:

- Shock – hypotension (systolic blood pressure < 90 mmHg), pallor, sweating, cold and clammy extremities, confusion or impaired consciousness
- Syncope

- Myocardial ischaemia – typical ischaemic chest pain and/or ECG evidence of a myocardial event
- Heart failure – pulmonary oedema and/or raised jugular venous pressure[12].

Bradyarrhythmias with an inherent risk of asystole are: complete heart block with widened QRS complexes; second-degree heart block type 2 and ventricular pauses greater than 3 seconds.

## Wolff–Parkinson–White

Additional aberrant muscular tissue in the form of the bundle of Kent conducts more quickly than the AV node and hence, one side of the ventricle is excited early. This results in the following:

- Short PR interval
- Prolonged QRS deflection on the upslope
- Normal length interval between start of P wave and end of QRS[13].

Atrial premature beats have the potential to cause paroxysmal supraventricular tachycardias. There is an increased risk of atrial fibrillation and deterioration to ventricular fibrillation. Perioperatively there needs to be avoidance of drugs and events that may precipitate antero-grade conduction via the accessory pathway.

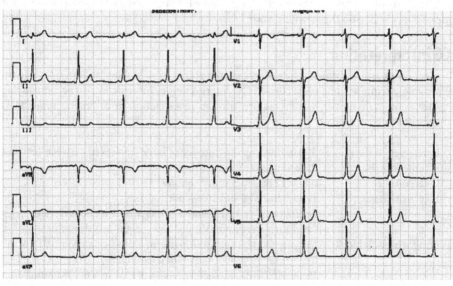

**Figure 23.2** ECG of Wolff-Parkinson-White. Reproduced with kind permission from ECGlibrary.com, the accompanying website to the book, ECGs by Example, D. Jenkins and S. Gerred.

## Prolonged QT syndrome

The acquired or congenital electrical abnormality predisposes to syncope and polymorphic ventricular tachycardia. An ECG should be performed on patients with a family history of sudden cardiac death. The abnormality is:

- Prolonged QTc > 460–480 ms.

Stop precipitant drugs (including isoflurane and sevoflurane) wherever possible. Electrolyte abnormalities, particularly hypomagnesaemia, should be corrected should deterioration occur. Esmolol is the anti-arrhythmic drug of choice intraoperatively. Phenytoin should be considered post-operatively[14].

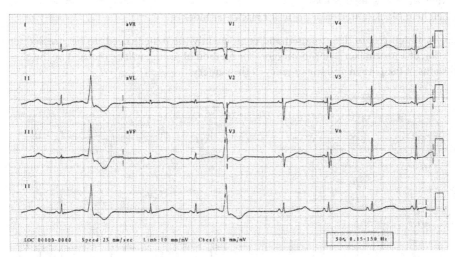

**Figure 23.3** ECG of prolonged QT syndrome. Reproduced with kind permission from ECGlibrary.com, the accompanying website to the book, ECGs by Example, D. Jenkins and S. Gerred.

## Complete heart block

A complete dissociation between the atria and ventricles. On inspection of the ECG there is no relationship between the P wave and QRS complexes. The broader the QRS complex and the slower the rate, the further down the bundle the ventricular response is being initiated.

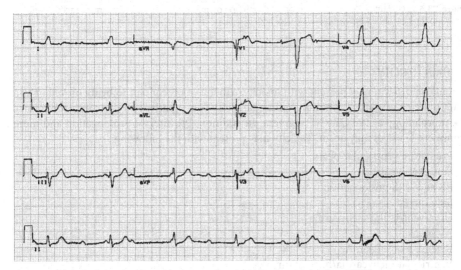

**Figure 23.4** ECG of complete heart block. Reproduced with kind permission from ECGlibrary.com, the accompanying website to the book, ECGs by Example, D. Jenkins and S. Gerred.

## Trifascicular block

This is the combination of the following:

- Prolonged PR interval
- Right bundle branch block
- Left hemiblock (anterior or posterior fascicular block).

There is a high risk of deterioration and consequently the patient needs to be assessed for insertion of a pacemaker prior to surgery. The method of pacing will be dictated by the clinical status of the patient and the urgency of the surgery.

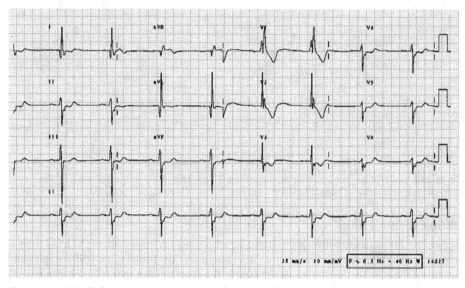

**Figure 23.5** ECG of trifascicular block. Reproduced with kind permission from ECGlibrary.com, the accompanying website to the book, ECGs by Example, D. Jenkins and S. Gerred.

## Digoxin toxicity

Patients on digoxin may present with toxicity, either as a precipitant to being unwell or as a result of being unwell. A common finding on an ECG of a patient on digoxin is the reverse tick morphology of the QRS/ST segment. In addition, PR interval prolongation and more prominent U waves may occur. Toxicity may present with the following:

- Premature ventricular beats
- Sinus bradycardia
- PR and QRS prolongation
- Sinus arrest
- Supraventricular tachycardia
- AV block
- Bigeminy or trigeminy
- Ventricular tachycardia/fibrillation[15].

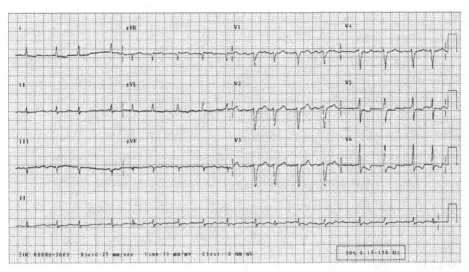

**Figure 23.6** ECG of digoxin toxicity. Reproduced with kind permission from ECGlibrary.com, the accompanying website to the book, ECGs by Example, D. Jenkins and S. Gerred.

Blood tests may not be readily available, therefore treatment may be considered prior to any laboratory results.

## Brugada syndrome

Associated with sudden cardiac death and often difficult to diagnose as there may be periods where the ECG returns to normal. It is characterized by:

- Right bundle branch block
- ST elevation in leads V1–V3 (often with an upward convexity to an inverted T wave)
  - Type 1: elevated ST segment (≥2 mm) descends with an upward convexity to an inverted T wave – coved type pattern
  - Type 2: elevated ST segment (≥2 mm) with a saddleback ST-T wave configuration where the ST segment remains above the baseline and rises again to the T wave[16].

The ECG changes may be brought on by the use of sodium channel blockers and in fact this is used in the HRS/EHRA/APHRS expert consensus statement on the diagnosis and management of patients with inherited primary arrhythmia syndromes[17]. Ultimately these patients will need to be fitted with an implantable cardioverter defibrillator (ICD) and a discussion with a cardiologist as to whether this is required preoperatively is needed.

## Pacemakers and implantable cardioverter defibrillators

### Pacemakers

In 2002 the North American Society of Pacing and Electrophysiology and the British Pacing and Electrophysiology Group (NASPE/BPEG) revised the pacemaker code[18].

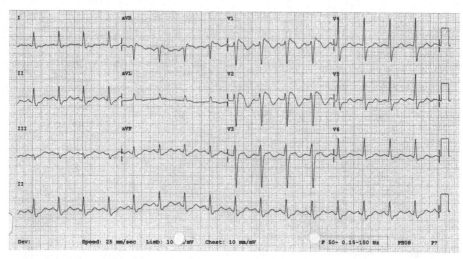

**Figure 23.7** ECG of Brugada syndrome. Reproduced with kind permission from Life in the Fast Lane lifeinthefastlane.com.

Whilst this may not cover every single device on the market it is useful in identifying the type of pacemaker present and likely perioperative management.

Prior to anaesthesia, it is important to clarify the type of pacemaker and indication for its insertion. Interrogation of the device is helpful, as is an ECG and a review of the patient's notes. Irrespective of the type of pacemaker it is no longer recommended that a magnet is used owing to variable and undesired results. Within theatre, ensure that there is a back-up mode of pacing which may include precordial or transcutaneous pacing.

The main source of interference is monopolar diathermy and this should be avoided if possible. Lithotripsy is thought to be safe. Should defibrillation be required, the pads need to be placed away from the pacemaker box. Positioning of the patient is important to avoid lead displacement.

**Table 23.6** Revised NASPE/BPEG generic code for antibradycardia pacing

| Letter position | I | II | III | IV | V |
|---|---|---|---|---|---|
| Category | Chamber paced | Chamber sensed | Response to sensing | Rate modulation | Multisite pacing |
| Letters | O – None | O – None | O – None | O – None | O – None |
| | A – Atrium | A – Atrium | T – Triggered | R – Rate modulation | A – Atrium |
| | V – Ventricle | V – Ventricle | I – Inhibited | | V – Ventricle |
| | D – Dual (A & V) | D – Dual (A & V) | D – Dual (T & I) | | D – Dual (A & V) |

# Implantable cardioverter defibrillators (ICD)

Once again, the indication for the device is of importance. The electrophysiology department are able to interrogate the device and assist with identification, should the patient be unable to inform you. These multifunctional devices are often able to deliver a shock and pace a patient. Prior to surgery it is important that the defibrillator element is turned off so that there is no risk of inadvertent shocks due to interference. An alternative mode of defibrillation should ideally be available, i.e. ensure transcutaneous pads in situ. If the device has an anti-tachycardia mode then this should also be deactivated.

Use of magnets is not recommended owing to unpredictable consequences. Once surgery is complete it is important that any device (pacemaker or ICD) should be reverted back to the patient's pre-existing mode unless there is a clinical reason not to.

## Basic echocardiography

In the adult population it would be ideal if all murmurs heard could be investigated by transthoracic echo to provide a complete perioperative assessment. Table 23.7 should assist in the classification of valvular disease determined from the echocardiogram.

Severity of cardiac disease correlates well with an increased probability of problems during induction and maintenance of anaesthesia. Criteria for defining the severity of the lesion are listed in Table 23.7.

**Table 23.7** Valve lesion and disease severity

| Valve lesion | Mild | Moderate | Severe |
|---|---|---|---|
| Mitral stenosis | Valve area: $> 1.5\,cm^2$ Mean gradient $< 5\,mmHg$ | Valve area: $1.0–1.5\,cm^2$ Mean gradient $5–10\,mmHg$ | Valve area: $< 1.0\,cm^2$ Mean gradient $> 10\,mmHg$ |
| Mitral regurgitation | Regurgitant fraction $< 20\%$ | Regurgitant fraction $20–40\%$ | Regurgitant fraction $> 60\%$ ($40–60\% =$ moderate to severe) |
| Aortic stenosis* | Valve area: $1.6–2.5\,cm^2$ Mean gradient $< 25\,mmHg$ | Valve area: $1.0–1.5\,cm^2$ Mean gradient $25–40\,mmHg$ | Valve area: $< 1.0\,cm^2$ Mean gradient $> 40\,mmHg$ |
| Aortic regurgitation | Regurgitant fraction $< 30\%$. Central jet width $< 25\%$ of LVOT | | Regurgitant fraction $> 50\%$ or regurgitant orifice area $> 0.3\,cm^2$ |
| Pulmonary stenosis | Valve area: $> 1.0\,cm^2$ Peak gradient $< 36\,mmHg$ | Valve area: $0.5–1.0\,cm^2$ Peak gradient $36–64\,mmHg$ | Valve area: $< 0.5\,cm^2$ Peak gradient $> 64\,mmHg$ |
| Pulmonary hypertension | Mean PAP $25–35\,mmHg$ | Mean PAP $35–44\,mmHg$ | Mean PAP $> 45\,mmHg$ |
| LV impairment | EF $40–50\%$ | EF $30–40\%$ | EF $< 30\%$ |

* Critical aortic stenosis is categorized by a valve area: $< 0.6\,cm^2$ and mean gradient $> 70\,mmHg$.
EF, ejection fraction; LVOT, left ventricular outflow tract; PAP, pulmonary artery pressure.

## Aortic stenosis

Ideally, all patients require an echocardiogram (time permitting) irrespective of presenting symptoms. Should this not be possible, then you should treat the patient as if they have a significant valvular lesion with a possible reduction in cardiac output. This requires maintenance of systemic vascular resistance and avoidance of hypotension. Consideration should be given to regional but not neuraxial techniques and any procedure should be discussed with the patient, as there will be significant morbidity and mortality. Invasive blood pressure monitoring should be considered before induction. A central venous catheter provides additional monitoring and a means of delivering inotropes.

## Mitral regurgitation

This lesion should be quantified wherever possible prior to surgery. Should you need to proceed emergently, worst case scenario should be assumed, i.e. a significant lesion. It is therefore imperative to avoid increasing the systemic vascular resistance and decreasing the heart rate as both of these have the potential to increase the regurgitation.

## Aortic regurgitation

The principles of anaesthesia are to maintain forward flow within the heart and into the aorta. Preventing or rapidly treating any reduction in heart rate and preventing a rise in systemic vascular resistance can maintain this.

# Pulmonary function testing

Pulmonary function tests are useful in patients with chronic lung disease to assess disease severity, reversibility and progression, as well as being part of the assessment process for lobectomy/pneumonectomy. The most commonly used facets of this are spirometry, lung volumes and flow-volume loops. Here is a quick recap of the differences.

## Normal lungs

Spirometry

- FEV1/FVC ratio approximately 75%

Flow-volume loops

- Rapid initial increase in flow rate
- Subsequent steady decrease in flow rate
- Relatively straight curve during expiration
- Squarer inspiratory curve.

## Obstructive disease

Spirometry

- FEV1/FVC ratio decreased

Flow-volume loops

- Reduced peak expiratory flow rate
- Larger residual volume (shift to left on x-axis)
- Increased concavity to expiratory curve
- Relatively preserved inspiratory curve, may have decreased flow rates.

## Restrictive disease

Spirometry

- FEV1/FVC ratio maintained or raised

Flow-volume loops

- Reduced total lung capacity (shift to right on x-axis)
- Reduced peak expiratory flow rate
- Similar shaped expiratory and inspiratory curves to normal.

# Guidance for perioperative starvation

The European Society of Anaesthesiology published guidelines for perioperative fasting in 2011[19]. Their work reviewed 87 studies between 1950 and 2009 regarding preoperative fasting, effects of carbohydrate-based drinks on gastric emptying and post-operative recovery and how early post-operative feeding impacts the recovery from anaesthesia. Below is a summary of the main finding from this guideline.

## Preoperative

There is significant evidence suggesting clear fluid up to 2 hours before surgery is safe[20-23]. In fact, more recent work has identified that prolonged fasting can be detrimental. Many now believe that small quantities of milk, in hot drinks, will act like clear fluids and are therefore safe. However, there is little evidence to support this and any advice you offer should reflect your professional opinion. Solid food should be stopped 6 hours before surgery.

Patients with potential for delayed gastric emptying (e.g. pregnancy, obesity, diabetes) should be advised in the same way; 6 hours for solid food and clear fluids until 2 hours preoperatively.

Smoking and chewing gum can reduce gastric pH and increase gastric fluid volume respectively but there is no evidence to suggest a change in gastric emptying. Recommendation is that patients are not cancelled for smoking or chewing gum in the preoperative period[24]. (NB There is slight variation in the guidance on this, the Royal College of Nursing Guidance[25] suggests that chewing gum should not be permitted on the day of surgery and the AAGBI recommend that it may be allowed only 2 hours before induction[5].)

Prophylactic use of $H_2$ antagonists and proton pump inhibitors is common. They increase gastric pH and reduce gastric fluid volume. However, there is no evidence that they reduce aspiration risk in the non-obstetric population[26-28].

## Obstetrics and paediatrics

The risk of aspiration in children is less significant than previously thought[29]. Clear fluids should be encouraged until 2 hours preoperatively. Breast milk and formula milk should be stopped 4 and 6 hours before surgery respectively. Cows' milk behaves as a solid and should be stopped 6 hours preoperatively. In trauma, best practice is to assume a full stomach. Current guidance for post-operative feeding is to allow the child to eat and drink as they wish with no need to enforce a meal before discharge for day case procedures.

Labouring women are at risk of needing operative intervention and are preferably kept fasted. However, the risk of ketosis and dehydration is high. Isotonic sports drinks are helpful and can reduce ketosis but do not increase intra-gastric volumes. Solid food should be discouraged as it confers no medical benefit. However, the risks of aspiration are low owing to high rates of regional anaesthesia. During labour, women should be allowed to consume clear fluids, including sports drinks, as they feel necessary.

For elective surgery, clear fluids should be allowed, and encouraged, until 2 hours before surgery. Post operative oral fluids are encouraged but more caution is needed with commencing solid foods. Ranitidine should be prescribed for the night before and the morning of surgery.

In an emergency, intravenous ranitidine is recommended with 30 ml of citrate if general anaesthesia is planned.

# Carbohydrate loading

Evidence in favour of carbohydrate-rich drinks until 2 hours preoperatively is strong. The body has an impaired stress response after a period of prolonged fasting[30]. Carbohydrate loading also reduces post-operative insulin resistance. Oral carbohydrate is more effective than intravenous in terms of subjective well-being and insulin resistance[31-36].

---

**Summary points**

- Stop solid food 6 hours before surgery
- Encourage clear fluids up to 2 hours before elective surgery
- $H_2$ antagonists and proton pump inhibitors have minimal effect on gastric emptying in the non obstetric population
- For babies, breast milk can be offered until 4 hours before surgery, with clear fluids until 2 hours
- Formula milk needs to be stopped 6 hours before surgery, with clear fluids until 2 hours preoperatively
- Labouring women should be encouraged to have clear fluids and isotonic sports drinks to reduce the risks of ketosis and dehydration.

---

# Remote site anaesthesia

Looking after patients in remote areas can be challenging, even for experienced anaesthetists. It is an added stress during the return to work phase. You should not be expected to be a solo anaesthetist in a remote area in your first few weeks when returning to work and, as always, if you feel you need help you must ask for it.

In this section we will look at what is a remote site, the potential problems posed and recommendations for how to make things run more smoothly when anaesthetizing in a remote area.

## What is remote site anaesthesia?

The Royal College of Anaesthetists describes a remote site as any site where anaesthesia or sedation is provided away from the main theatre area and when the help of another anaesthetist cannot be guaranteed[37]. Normally, anaesthesia in remote sites should be performed by a consultant with appropriate experience. However, there will be occasions when competent specialty doctors/trainees are asked to anaesthetize in remote sites, particularly during out-of-hours work. In these situations, a consultant must be directly responsible for them at all times[38].

## What are the potential problems with anaesthetizing in remote sites?

Unless you regularly perform anaesthesia remotely, one of the biggest problems is unfamiliarity with the environment. The equipment may be different, especially in the magnetic resonance imaging department, and the staff may be less well known to you. Some of the equipment you prefer may not be available or possible to use in the area you are working. There may be unfamiliarity with the patient's procedure and finally, and perhaps most importantly, the ability to get instant help or communicate with other anaesthetists may be limited.

## How to make working in a remote site more manageable

- Familiarize yourself with the location. This should be part of departmental induction but if it does not happen, try to find time to go for a look around.
- Equipment should be standardized but this is not always the case. Check which equipment is used in your Trust and attend any equipment training sessions.
- Check that senior backup is available and that they know where you are going and with whom. If you are unsure about any aspect, ask for help.
- Ensure full patient monitoring is available.
- A phone must be available so you can call for back-up if required.
- A fully trained anaesthetic assistant should be available at all times[39,40].
- Check all equipment as you would in a standard operating theatre, including the machine check and emergency drug availability.
- Prioritize patient safety and complete safety checks; the World Health Organization (WHO) checklist is mandatory.
- Ensure a provision for recovery. This may be in the remote area or involve a transfer to theatre recovery[41,42]. If a transfer is involved, prepare accordingly (see Chapter 10 in Section 2).
- If post-procedure intensive care may be required, confirm availability prior to commencing the case.
- Document all events and clinical observations fully.

Remote site anaesthesia can be challenging even before an extended period away from work. This guidance aims to help you to anticipate and deal with potential problems. Above all, if you are unsure ask someone to help.

## References

1. S. M. Crawley, A. J. Dalton. Predicting the difficult airway. *Contin Educ Anaesth Crit Care Pain* [Online] November 11, 2014. Available at: bjaed.oxfordjournals.org/content/15/5/253 (accessed 9 January 2016).
2. R. Vaughan. Predicting difficult airways. *BJA CEPD Rev* 2001; 1(2), 44–7.
3. NICE. Preoperative tests: Routine preoperative tests for elective surgery. 2016. [Online] Available at www.nice.org.uk/guidance/ng45/resources/routine-preoperative-tests-for-elective-surgery-1837454508997 (accessed 19 July 2016).
4. The Royal College of Surgeons of England / Department of Health. The Higher Risk General Surgical Patient: towards improved care for a forgotten group. 2011. [Online] Available from: https://www.rcseng.ac.uk/publications/docs/higher-risk-surgical-patient/ (accessed 29 March 2015).
5. Association of Anaesthetists of Great Britain and Ireland (AAGBI). AAGBI Safety Guideline: Pre-operative Assessment and Patient Preparation. The Role of the Anaesthetist. London: AAGBI, 2010. Available at http://www.aagbi.org/sites/default/files/preop2010.pdf (accessed 4 January 2016).
6. T. H. Lee, E. R. Marcantonio, C. M. Mangione et al. Derivation and prospective validation of a simple index for prediction of cardiac risk of major noncardiac surgery. *Circulation* 1999; 100: 1043–9.
7. VASGBI The Vascular Anaesthesia Society of Great Britain and Ireland. POSSUM calculator. 2013. [Online] Available at https://www.vasgbi.com/riskscores.php (accessed: 29 March 2015).
8. N. Shah, M. Hamilton. Clinical review: can we predict which patients are at risk of complications following surgery. *Crit Care* 2013; 17(3): 226.

9. The Task Force for Preoperative Cardiac Risk Assessment and Perioperative Cardiac Management in Non-cardiac Surgery of the European Society of Cardiology (ESC) and endorsed by the European Society of Anaesthesiology (ESA). Guidelines for pre-operative cardiac risk assessment and perioperative cardiac management in non-cardiac surgery. *Eur Heart Journal* 2009; 30(22): 2769a. Available at http://eurheartj.oxfordjournals.org/content/ehj/30/22/2769.full .pdf (accessed 13 May 2015).

10. N. Bhatia, N. Barber. Dilemmas in the preoperative assessment of children. *Contin Educ Anaesth Crit Care Pain* 2011; 11(6): 214–18.

11. APA. The timing of vaccination with respect to anaesthesia and surgery. [Online] Available at http://www.apagbi.org.uk/sites/default/files/images/Final%20Immunisation%20apa.pdf (accessed 29 March 2015).

12. J. Nolan, J. Soar, A. Lockey et al. (ed.). *Advanced Life Support*, 6th edn. London: Resuscitation Council (UK), 2011.

13. W. F. Ganong. *Review of Medical Physiology*, 19th edn. Connecticut: Appleton and Lange, 1999.

14. R. L. Hines, K. E. Marschall (ed.). *Handbook for Atoelting's Anesthesia and Co-Existing Disease*, 3rd edn. Philadelphia: Saunders Elsevier, 2002.

15. S. G. Myerson, R. P. Choudhury, A. R. J. Mitchell (eds.). *Emergencies in Cardiology*. Oxford: Oxford University Press, 2006.

16. A. S. Sheikh, K. Ranjan. Brugada syndrome: a review of the literature. *Clin Med* 2014; 14(5): 482–9.

17. S. G. Priori, A. A. Wilde, M. Horie et al. Executive summary: HRS/EHRA/APHRS expert consensus statement on the diagnosis and management of patients with inherited primary arrhythmia syndromes. *Europace* 2013; 15(10): 1389–406.

18. A. D. Bernstein J. C. Daubert, R. D. Fletcher et al. The revised NASPE/BPEG generic code for antibradycardia, adaptive-rate, and multisite pacing. *Pacing Clin Electrophysiol* 2002; 25(2): 260–4.

19. I. Smith, P. Kranke, I. Murat et al. European Society of Anaesthesiology. Perioperative fasting in adults and children: guidelines from the European Society of Anaesthesiology. *Eur J Anaesthesiol* 2011; 28(8): 556–69.

20. J. R. Maltby, A. D. Sutherland, J. P. Sale, E. A. Shaffer. Preoperative oral fluids: is a five-hour fast justified prior to elective surgery? *Anesth Analg* 1986; 65: 1112–16.

21. S. Phillips, S. Hutchinson, T. Davidson. Preoperative drinking does not affect gastric contents. *Br J Anaesth* 1993; 70: 6–9.

22. E. Søreide, K. E. Stromskag, P. A. Steen. Statistical aspects in studies of preoperative fluid intake and gastric content. *Acta Anaesthesiol Scand* 1995; 39: 738–43.

23. E. Søreide, L. I. Eriksson, G. Hirlekar et al. Preoperative fasting guidelines: an update [review]. *Acta Anaesthesiol Scand* 2005; 49: 1041–7.

24. E. Søreide, H. Holst-Larsen, T. Veel, P. A. Steen. The effects of chewing gum on gastric content prior to induction of general anesthesia. *Anesth Analg* 1995; 80: 985–9.

25. Perioperative fasting in adults and children: An RCN guidance for the multidisciplinary team. London: Royal College of Nursing, 2005.

26. M. S. Iqbal, M. Ashfaque, M. Akram. Gastric fluid volume and pH: a comparison of effects of ranitidine alone with combination of ranitidine and metoclopramide in patients undergoing elective caesarean section. *Ann King Edward Medical College* 2000; 6: 189–91.

27. J. Y. Hong. Effects of metoclopramide and ranitidine on preoperative gastric contents in day-case surgery. *Yonsei Med J* 2006; 47: 315–18.

28. I. Bala, K. Prasad, I. Bhukal et al. Effect of preoperative oral erythromycin, erythromycin-ranitidine, and ranitidine-metoclopramide on gastric fluid pH and volume. *J Clin Anesth* 2008; 20: 30–4.

29. R. P. Flick, G. J. Schears, M. A. Warner. Aspiration in pediatric anesthesia: is there a higher incidence compared with adults? *Curr Opin Anaesthesiol* 2002; 15: 323–7.

30. O. Ljungqvist, J. Nygren, A. Thorell. Insulin resistance and elective surgery [review]. *Surgery* 2000; 128: 757–60.

31. J. Hausel, J. Nygren, M. Lagerkranser et al. A carbohydrate-rich drink reduces preoperative discomfort in elective surgery patients. *Anesth Analg* 2001; 93: 1344–50.
32. M. Soop, J. Nygren, P. Myrenfors et al. Preoperative oral carbohydrate treatment attenuates immediate postoperative insulin resistance. *Am J Physiol Endocrinol Metab* 2001; 280: E576–83.
33. M. Soop, J. Nygren, A. Thorell et al. Preoperative oral carbohydrate treatment attenuates endogenous glucose release 3 days after surgery. *Clin Nutr* 2004; 23: 733–41.
34. J. Nygren, M. Soop, A. Thorell et al. Preoperative oral carbohydrate administration reduces postoperative insulin resistance. *Clin Nutr* 1998; 17: 65–71.
35. Z. G. Wang, Q. Wang, W. J. Wang, H. L. Qin. Randomized clinical trial to compare the effects of preoperative oral carbohydrate versus placebo on insulin resistance after colorectal surgery. *Br J Surg* 2010; 97: 317–27.
36. H. Helminen, H. Viitanen, J. Sajanti. Effect of preoperative intravenous carbohydrate loading on preoperative discomfort in elective surgery patients. *Eur J Anaesthesiol* 2009; 26: 123–7.
37. The Royal College of Anaesthetists. Anaesthetic services in remote sites. London: The Royal College of Anaesthetists, 2014. Available at http://www.rcoa.ac.uk/system/files/REMOTE-SITES-2014_3.pdf (accessed 4 January 2016).
38. The Royal College of Anaesthetists. Clinical supervision: the obligation to patients (6.1). Curriculum for a CCT in Anaesthetics. London: The Royal College of Anaesthetists, 2010. Available at http://www.rcoa.ac.uk/system/files/TRG-CU-CCT-ANAES2010_1.pdf (accessed 4 January 2016).
39. The Royal College of Anaesthetists. Guidance for the provision of anaesthetic services for intra-operative care. London: The Royal College of Anaesthetists, 2014. Available at http://www.rcoa.ac.uk/document-store/guidance-the-provision-of-anaesthesia-services-intra-operative-care-2014 (accessed 4 January 2016).
40. The Association of Anaesthetists for Great Britain and Ireland. The anaesthesia team 3. London: The Association of Anaesthetists for Great Britain and Ireland, 2010. Available at http://www.aagbi.org/sites/default/files/anaesthesia_team_2010_0.pdf (accessed 4 January 2016).
41. The Royal College of Anaesthetists. Guidance for the provision of anaesthetic services for post-operative care. London: The Royal College of Anaesthetists, 2014. Available at http://www.rcoa.ac.uk/document-store/guidance-the-provision-of-anaesthesia-services-post-operative-care-2014 (accessed 4 January 2016).
42. The Association of Anaesthetists of Great Britain and Ireland. Immediate post-anaesthesia recovery. London: The Association of Anaesthetists of Great Britain and Ireland, 2013. Available at http://www.aagbi.org/publications/guidelines/immediate-post-anaesthesia-recovery-2013 (accessed 4 January 2016).

# Chapter 24

# Consent and documentation

Anna Costello

*Taking consent and documenting an anaesthetic record are routine parts of daily practice and are important to get right. This chapter provides a recap of the role of the anaesthetist in taking consent and how to ensure record keeping and documentation meet the required standard. In the first section, consent is defined and the impact of the anaesthetic consent process is explored. Formal written consent is not required at present but some record of the consent process is needed. There are situations when formal written consent for anaesthetic procedures is necessary and these are highlighted in this chapter. Quoting risks for anaesthetic procedures can be difficult. You will find tables with risks to quote to your patients for some of the most common types of anaesthetic listed in this chapter. The final part of the chapter emphasizes the importance of good record keeping. The main discussions, observations and events to document are examined and the chapter ends with a summary of the key things that need to be recorded. There are also relevant sections in Chapter 22 (Ethical and legal issues) and Chapter 34 (National Audit Project (NAP) summaries).*

## Consent

Good medical practice tells us to take valid consent before we perform any examination, test or investigation on a patient, before we start any treatment and before we ask a patient to be involved in teaching or research[1]. When a patient consents to treatment, they are giving their permission for a test, examination or procedure to go ahead. Consent forms part of medical ethical principles and human rights law. It can be given in writing, verbally or be implied and should be voluntary, informed and the patient must have capacity for the consent to be valid. Capacity is the ability for a patient to understand the information given to them, retain the information, be able to weigh up the details to make a decision and communicate their decision to the medical practitioner.

Consent should ideally be taken by the doctor or clinician who will be performing the procedure for which consent is required. However, this is not always possible or practical and in those circumstances, the task can be delegated. However, the person taking consent must be suitably trained and have good knowledge of the proposed procedure, fully understanding the risks involved[2].

### How does consent affect anaesthetists?

At present written consent for an anaesthetic is not required if it is being performed as part of another procedure. The surgical consent form includes a section about the anaesthetic.

*Returning to Work in Anaesthesia*, ed. Emma Plunkett, Emily Johnson and Anna Pierson.
Published by Cambridge University Press. © Cambridge University Press 2016.

By signing the surgical consent, the patient agrees to the anaesthetic as well. However, it is important that pre-assessment details are recorded including the risks quoted to the patient for the anaesthetic technique planned, documenting the risks, benefits and any alternatives discussed[3]. If a procedure is being performed independently of a surgical operation then a consent form should be completed. For example, a tracheostomy on intensive care, a chest drain or an epidural blood patch. If a central line is being sited for a ward patient then formal consent should be taken and documented. It is not common practice to complete consent forms for central vascular access provided for intensive care patients.

## What should we tell our patients?

After completing a thorough pre-assessment (see Chapter 23) it is our responsibility to explain the anaesthetic technique planned. As part of this we need to quote any relevant risks of the various stages of the anaesthetic. Some patients prefer potential risks quoted in numbers, e.g. 1 in 100 risk; others prefer a broader description, such as 'common' or 'rare'. Figure 24.1 links these two descriptions.

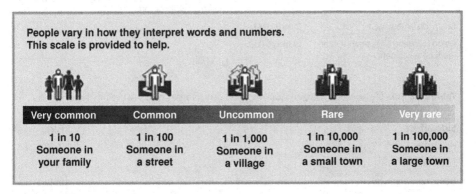

**Figure 24.1** Scale to help describe the frequency of risks. Reproduced with permission from the Royal College of Anaesthetists.

Quoting risks can be difficult as the exact numbers will vary from case to case depending on patient factors, the type of surgery being performed, the types of drugs likely to be administered and of course, the grade and skill of the anaesthetist. However, it is good practice to have a grasp of the risks for an average patient having an average operation and these are listed in Table 24.1[4]. The same risks for a child in good health having minor surgery are quoted in Table 24.2[5].

Taking consent can be particularly challenging in the labouring woman. One may argue that when someone is in significant pain that they no longer have capacity to give consent. In the case of an emergency caesarean section, it is rare, but not unheard of, for a mother to refuse the treatment to save her unborn child. This would involve a multidisciplinary team approach so you would never be alone in this situation, and is beyond the scope of this book. A more likely situation to find oneself in is a labouring mother asking for an epidural when she had previously stated she would not want to have an epidural. In these situations we have to rely on the opinions of relatives, midwives, a birthing plan if available and our own expert judgement. Trying to explain the risks of an epidural to a woman in labour can be difficult. In some trusts ladies are given written information about pain relief in labour when at antenatal

**Table 24.1** Risks of side effects and complications from a general anaesthetic in adults

| Side effect | Risk | Other information |
| --- | --- | --- |
| Nausea | 1 in 3 | Dependent on operation type, drugs used, gender etc |
| Sore throat (ETT) | 2 in 5 | |
| Sore throat (LMA) | 1 in 5 | |
| Shivering | 1 in 4 | |
| Damage to tongue/lips | 1 in 20 | |
| Damage to teeth | 1 in 4500 | |
| Damage to eyes | 1 in 2800 | |
| Post-operative chest infection | 1 in 5 | For major abdominal surgery |
| Accidental awareness | 1 in 20 000 | From NAP5 data. Smaller interview studies have suggested the risk to be as high as 1 in 1000 |
| Anaphylaxis | 1 in 10 000–20 000 | |
| Nerve damage | 1 in 1000 | E.g. ulnar or common peroneal nerve injury from compression |
| Death/brain damage | 1 in 100 000 | |
| Death following Caesarean section (general anaesthetic) | 17 in 100 000 | |

**Table 24.2** Risks of side effects and complications from a general anaesthetic in a healthy child having a minor procedure

| Side effect | Risk |
| --- | --- |
| Headache | 1 in 10 |
| Sore throat | 1 in 10 |
| Nausea and vomiting | 1 in 10 |
| Dizziness | 1 in 10 |
| Agitated on waking | 1 in 5 |
| Severe allergic reaction | 1 in 10 000 |
| Death | 1 in 100 000 |

clinic. However, it remains prudent to offer some information to the labouring women at the time of request for help. It is important to at least ask them if they would like to hear the risks and encourage them to read the information card, if your Trust supplies one. It is preferable to quote the main risks as listed in Table 24.3[6]. Since the publication of the NAP3 report many people use its results to inform the consent process. Please see Chapter 34 for more information.

Consent for regional anaesthesia can prove more challenging as many of the potential problems are less easy to understand for the lay person than potentially having a sore throat or feeling sick. It is therefore important to emphasize the degree of risk in a way the patient will understand. Table 24.4 will help with this[7].

When taking consent for a peripheral nerve block the risks will vary according to the block being performed, e.g. a 1 in 100 risk of a Horner's syndrome when having an

**Table 24.3** Risks associated with regional anaesthesia

| Side effect | Risk |
| --- | --- |
| Epidural not working perfectly | 1 in 8 |
| Hypotension | 1 in 50 |
| Headache | 1 in 100 |
| Nerve damage (temporary) | 1 in 1000 |
| Nerve damage (longer than 6 months) | 1 in 13 000 |
| Epidural abscess | 1 in 50 000 |
| Meningitis | 1 in 100 000 |
| Epidural haematoma | 1 in 170 000 |
| Reduced Glasgow Coma Score (GCS) | 1 in 100 000 |
| Severe injury/paralysis | 1 in 250 000 |

**Table 24.4** Risks of regional anaesthesia according to frequency of occurrence

| Side effect | Very common–common (1 in 10 to 1 in 100) | Common–uncommon (1 in 100 to 1 in 1000) | Rare–very rare (1 in 10 000 to 1 in 100 000) |
| --- | --- | --- | --- |
| Hypotension | X | | |
| Itching | X | | |
| Urinary retention | X | | |
| Pain during injection | X | | |
| Headache (benign) | X | | |
| Headache (PDPH) | | X | |
| Nerve injury | | | X |

PDPH, post-dural puncture headache.

interscalene block. In more broad terms, the risk of nerve injury following any peripheral nerve block is 1 in 10 for short-term (<48 hours) nerve injury and 1 in 2000–5000 for more permanent nerve injury[8].

# Record keeping and documentation

We have been taught that we must write legibly in black ink and record all discussions, observations and interventions in a timely manner. However, that is not always possible during an operating list with lots of short cases or in the more challenging scenario when a patient becomes very sick and our attention is a long way away from writing down the most recent blood pressure and heart rate. There are ways to try to accommodate for these situations such as electing a scribe during times when normalizing the patient's physiology is the primary focus; major haemorrhage for example or profound hypotension.

The Royal College of Anaesthetists have published a document called Good Practice which dictates what is deemed appropriate for record keeping. The General Medical Council (GMC) also discuss record keeping in their document, Good medical practice. They state that 'Clinical records should include relevant clinical findings, the decisions made and actions agreed, and who is making the decisions and agreeing the actions, the information given to patients, any drugs prescribed or other investigation or treatment and who is making the record and when'[1]. Our role, as anaesthetists, is to provide written evidence of preoperative assessment, document relevant perioperative observations, describe intraoperative events such as significant changes in physiology and how these were managed and why management decisions were made. We also have a major role in the post-operative period and, as such, should document a clear plan for this phase of the patient pathway. In some situations, such as day case surgery, we also have a duty to make recommendations for discharge planning and again, this should all be recorded[9,10].

Any documentation we make should provide enough information for another anaesthetist to be able to replicate the anaesthetic you planned and delivered. It should provide instructions for ongoing care in recovery, on the ward or at home and should be clear and easy to follow by nursing and ward staff. It is important to document the ranges of physiological parameters that are acceptable and who to call if the observations stray from the ranges set.

Having good record keeping does not ablate the need for a good handover for ongoing care but it can make the handover an easier one and can help reduce the need for a phone call to clarify things in the hours that follow.

A full and clear record of events is of great benefit in the event of legal proceedings which can happen many months or years after the date of the anaesthetic or the time you were involved in the patient care. In fact, 'an untidy, illegible, scantily completed chart may be taken as indirect evidence of shoddy or inattentive care'[10,11]. Specific things that are important to document include the following[9,10,12]:

- Patient identification
- Date of procedure
- Name and grade of anaesthetist and surgeon (named consultant anaesthetist if trainee)
- Anaesthetic pre-assessment, consent and risks explained
- Procedure planned and procedure performed
- Anaesthetic equipment and machine check completion
- WHO checklist completion
- Pre-induction observations
- Anaesthetic technique and agents used, including IV site
- Drugs given (including fluids); doses and timing
- Monitoring
- Record of observations during case (5-minute interval) and significant changes in physiology
- Post-operative instructions.

For those working in critical care, the Royal College of Anaesthetists suggests a full review of each patient should be performed at least once in any 24-hour period. This should record any abnormal test results and an agreed management plan and the reasons for this plan.

# References

1. General Medical Council. Good medical practice (2013). Available at http://www.gmc-uk.org/guidance/good_medical_practice.asp (accessed 2 January 2016).
2. General Medical Council. Consent: patients and doctors making decisions together. 2008. Available at http://www.gmc-uk.org/static/documents/content/Consent_-_English_0911.pdf (accessed 25 January 2015).

3. Association of Anaesthetists of Great Britain and Ireland. Consent for Anaesthesia. 2006. (Due to be updated in 2016.)
4. The Royal College of Anaesthetists. Information for patients; risks associated with your anaesthetic. London: The Royal College of Anaesthetists, 2013. Available at http://www.rcoa.ac.uk/system/files/PI-RISK-SERIES-2013_2.pdf (accessed 4 January 2016).
5. The Royal College of Anaesthetists (RCoA), Association of Anaesthetists of Great Britain and Ireland (AAGBI) and Association of Paediatric Anaesthetists of Great Britain and Ireland (APAGBI). Your child's general anaesthetic, Information for parents and guardians of children. London: RCoA, AAGBI and APAGBI, 2014. Available at http://www.rcoa.ac.uk/document-store/your-childs-general-anaesthetic (accessed 4 January 2016).
6. Epidural Information Card. A summary card from The Obstetric Anaesthetic Association. Available at http://www.labourpains.com/assets/_managed/editor/File/Info%20for%20Mothers/EIC/2008_eic_english.pdf (accessed 4 January 2016).
7. The Royal College of Anaesthetists (RCoA) and Association of Anaesthetists of Great Britain and Ireland (AAGBI). Your spinal anaesthetic, Information for patients. London: RCoA and AAGBI, 2014. Available at http://www.rcoa.ac.uk/document-store/your-spinal-anaesthetic (accessed 4 January 2016)
8. Regional Anaesthesia United Kingdom. Patient consent for peripheral nerve blocks. 2015. Available at http://www.ra-uk.org/index.php/guidelines-standards/5-guidelines/detail/255-patient-consent-for-peripheral-nerve-blocks (accessed 4 January 2016).
9. Royal College of Anaesthetists. Raising the Standards: a compendium of audit recipes, 3rd edn. 2012. Available at http://www.rcoa.ac.uk/ARB2012 (accessed 4 January 2016).
10. Royal College of Anaesthetist and the Association of Anaesthetists for Great Britain and Ireland. Good Practice: A guide for departments of anaesthesia, critical care and pain management, 3rd edn. 2006. Available at http://www.aagbi.org/sites/default/files/goodpractice%20_guidefordepartments06.pdf (accessed 4 January 2016).
11. J. E. Utting. Pitfalls in anaesthetic practice. *Br J Anaesth* 1987; 59: 888–90.
12. The Association of Anaesthetists of Great Britain and Ireland, Recommendations for Standards of Monitoring during anaesthesia and recovery, 4th edn. 2007. Available at https://www.aagbi.org/sites/default/files/standardsofmonitoring07.pdf (accessed 9 January 2016).

# AAGBI guidelines

Maria Garside

**25**

*In this chapter a selection of six of the safety guidelines from the Association of Anaesthetists of Great Britain and Ireland (AAGBI) are reviewed in the context of returning to work in anaesthesia. Each guideline is summarized, and key points are highlighted. The AAGBI's A4 summary sheets are included where appropriate. The aim is to help you refresh your memory of the guidelines on safe anaesthetic practice (checking anaesthetic equipment, monitoring standards and regional blockade and coagulopathy), and management of emergencies (anaphylaxis, severe local anaesthetic toxicity and malignant hyperthermia). The AAGBI has published many other guidelines and you will find examples of these summarized or referenced in almost every chapter of the book. The guidelines included here are particularly widely applicable and were felt to be worthy of additional revision.*

## AAGBI guidelines

The Association of Anaesthetists of Great Britain and Ireland (AAGBI) have been producing guidelines on various aspects of anaesthetic practice since 1989. These are consensus documents formed by working parties of experts set up for each topic, and sometimes in conjunction with other professional bodies. Previously provided as A5 booklets (glossies), they are now best accessed online. They are available through the AAGBI Guideline App for mobile devices, and at www.aagbi.org > Publications > Guidelines. Many of the guidelines, such as the machine check and management of emergencies, are summarized on A4 sheets which can be laminated and kept in relevant clinical areas. Through a number of routes, the information is readily available and informs our daily practice in many areas. The AAGBI is developing a Quick Reference Handbook, which is a collection of guidelines to help manage emergencies in anaesthesia. This is expected to be published in the middle of 2016 and will be available to download from the AAGBI website.

## Checking Anaesthetic Equipment 2012[1]

Incidents reported to the Medicines and Healthcare Products Regulatory Agency (MHRA), National Patient Safety Agency (NPSA) and the AAGBI have contributed to identifying

*Returning to Work in Anaesthesia*, ed. Emma Plunkett, Emily Johnson and Anna Pierson.
Published by Cambridge University Press. © Cambridge University Press 2016.

priority checks included in this guidance. The guidance is too detailed for all the points to be covered here. We recommend that you read the full document.

The bottom line is that a machine check by an anaesthetist trained and competent in the equipment's use is essential to patient safety. On returning to work, it is imperative that you receive training for any new equipment, and refresh your knowledge of the details of equipment you may not have used for a while. Quickly running through how a machine works just before having to use it is not acceptable.

'It must be emphasized that failure to check the anaesthetic machine $+/-$ breathing system features as a major contributory factor in many anaesthetic misadventures, including some that result in hypoxic brain damage or death.'[1]. Hence, the machine check is now also part of the World Health Organization (WHO) Surgical Safety Checklist[2], and also features in the FRCA examination. A record of the checks should be made on the anaesthetic record, as well as in a document kept with the anaesthetic machine (the latter can be done by an anaesthetic assistant). A full check is required at the start of each operating session, with a limited check repeated before each case. (See Figure 25.1.)

In the 2012 guidance, the 'two-bag check' was added to the full pre-list check. Firstly, the breathing system, ventilator and vaporizers must be checked individually. Then, a second bag, or 'test lung', is added to the patient end of the breathing system. Through this test, the patency and absence of leaks in the whole system is checked. The 'test lung' should then be left attached, as this prevents intrusion of foreign bodies into the circuit between the end of the check and attaching the machine to a patient.

Before each case, the two-bag-test, checking of vaporizers, breathing circuits and gas outlet should be repeated. Patient harm has resulted from failure of the latter. This is particularly important when there are small children and larger patients on the same list. Ensure you check the gas outlet selected before every anaesthetic you give.

The 'manual leak test', whereby vaporizers are manually put under pressure, is no longer routinely recommended. This test can cause damage to some modern anaesthetic machines, and so you must consult the manufacturer's guidance before performing this test.

Do not forget:

- Self-inflating bag
- Trolley/table tilt
- Difficult airway equipment
- Resuscitation equipment and drugs (availability of dantrolene, sugammadex, lipid emulsion)
- Pumps, and infusion equipment
- Electrical back-up.

Beware of changes to circuit, or anaesthetist, part way through an operating session. Failure to check for leaks if a vaporizer is changed during use is a common cause of critical incidents. Include confirmation of the machine check in any handover.

Make all of the above part of your routine as you return to work. Just as when we are learning things for the first time, by not cutting corners, we establish foundations of good practice which then continue throughout our careers. This is a great opportunity to ensure you include each important detail of the most recent guidance on equipment checks in your daily practice. Start as you mean to go on, and you will embed this crucial part of safe patient care into your daily practice for good.

# Checklist for Anaesthetic Equipment 2012
## AAGBI Safety Guideline

### Checks at the start of every operating session
### Do not use this equipment unless you have been trained

**Check self-inflating bag available**

**Perform manufacturer's (automatic) machine check**

| | |
|---|---|
| **Power supply** | • Plugged in<br>• Switched on<br>• Back-up battery charged |
| **Gas supplies and suction** | • Gas and vacuum pipelines – 'tug test'<br>• Cylinders filled and turned off<br>• Flowmeters working (if applicable)<br>• Hypoxic guard working<br>• Oxygen flush working<br>• Suction clean and working |
| **Breathing system** | • Whole system patent and leak free using 'two-bag' test<br>• Vaporisers – fitted correctly, filled, leak free, plugged in (if necessary)<br>• Soda lime - colour checked<br>• Alternative systems (Bain, T-piece) – checked<br>• Correct gas outlet selected |
| **Ventilator** | • Working and configured correctly |
| **Scavenging** | • Working and configured correctly |
| **Monitors** | • Working and configured correctly<br>• Alarms limits and volumes set |
| **Airway equipment** | • Full range required, working, with spares |

**RECORD THIS CHECK IN THE PATIENT RECORD**

| | |
|---|---|
| **Don't Forget!** | • Self-inflating bag<br>• Common gas outlet<br>• Difficult airway equipment<br>• Resuscitation equipment<br>• TIVA and/or other infusion equipment |

This guideline is not a standard of medical care. The ultimate judgement with regard to a particular clinical procedure or treatment plan must be made by the clinician in the light of the clinical data presented and the diagnostic and treatment options available.

© The Association of Anaesthetists of Great Britain & Ireland 2012

**Figure 25.1** Checklist for Anaesthetic Equipment 2012. Reproduced with the kind permission of the Association of Anaesthetists of Great Britain and Ireland.

## CHECKS BEFORE EACH CASE

| | |
|---|---|
| **Breathing system** | Whole system patent and leak free using 'two-bag' test<br>Vaporisers – fitted correctly, filled, leak free, plugged in (if necessary)<br>Alternative systems (Bain, T-piece) – checked<br>Correct gas outlet selected |
| **Ventilator** | Working and configured correctly |
| **Airway equipment** | Full range required, working, with spares |
| **Suction** | Clean and working |

## THE TWO-BAG TEST

**A two-bag test should be performed after the breathing system, vaporisers and ventilator have been checked individually**

i.  Attach the patient end of the breathing system (including angle piece and filter) to a test lung or bag.

ii. Set the fresh gas flow to 5 l.min$^{-1}$ and ventilate manually. Check the whole breathing system is patent and the unidirectional valves are moving. Check the function of the APL valve by squeezing both bags.

iii. Turn on the ventilator to ventilate the test lung. Turn off the fresh gas flow, or reduce to a minimum. Open and close each vaporiser in turn. There should be no loss of volume in the system.

This checklist is an abbreviated version of the publication by the Association of Anaesthetists of Great Britain and Ireland 'Checking Anaesthesia Equipment 2012'. It was originally published in *Anaesthesia*.
(Endorsed by the Chief Medical Officers)

If you wish to refer to this guideline, please use the following reference: Checklist for anaesthetic equipment 2012. *Anaesthesia* 2012; **66:** pages 662–63. http://onlinelibrary.wiley.com/doi/10.1111/j.1365-2044.2012.07163.x/abstract

**Figure 25.1** (*cont.*)

# Recommendations for standards of monitoring during anaesthesia and recovery[3]

The presence of an anaesthetist, along with minimum monitoring standards, is considered essential from before induction of anaesthesia until after recovery from anaesthetic. This applies regardless of length, type or location of procedure, including patient transfer both within and outside of the hospital. The same standards apply whether for general, regional or local anaesthetic, and for sedation for surgery.

The presence of an anaesthetist is the main determinant of patient safety. A stethoscope must always be available for clinical assessment. Monitoring devices supplement clinical observation, and their correct use reduces the risk of incidents and accidents occurring.

Audible alarm limits should be set appropriately before each case. This includes patient monitoring and equipment alarms (e.g. ventilator and infusion pump alarms). When this is done, alarms give early warning of problems, whether or not they are due to fault or error.

## Essential during anaesthesia

Pulse oximetry, blood pressure monitering, ECG, airway gases (oxygen, carbon dioxide and vapours) and airway pressures where relevant are essential, though more complex cases may require additional monitoring. Temperature measurement for cases >30 minute duration, and a nerve stimulator for anyone who has received a muscle relaxant, must also be immediately available.

## Essential during recovery

Pulse oximetry and blood pressure measurement are essential, with ECG, temperature measurement and a nerve stimulator immediately available.

Supplemental advice (2011) on continuous capnography recommends its use in **all** patients who are:

– anaesthetized
– intubated (excluding tracheostomy without ventilatory support)
– receiving deep sedation
– receiving cardiopulmonary resuscitation, for continuous monitoring of tracheal tube position, and early signalling of return of spontaneous circulation[4].

Depth of anaesthesia monitoring should be chosen on a case-by-case basis, and should be considered in all patients with a high risk of awareness, such as when using a total intravenous anaesthesia (TIVA) technique with neuromuscular blockade[3,5].

Observations from essential monitoring should be recorded every 5 minutes, or more frequently. The AAGBI advocates the use of electronic record keeping systems where available.

# Suspected anaphylactic reactions[6]

This 2009 update from the AAGBI is much more than just a guideline for the management of suspected anaphylactic reactions. It forms a good resource for information on many aspects of anaesthetic allergy.

Appendix 1 of the guideline is 'Frequently Asked Questions', and is worth reading. Amongst others, it provides a detailed answer to the question 'What should I do if a patient with a convincing history of cardiovascular collapse during a previous anaesthetic presents for emergency surgery without having been investigated for anaphylaxis?' It is very useful to know where to access such advice. There is also a discussion of how to manage a case of suspected anaphylaxis in Chapter 8.

### THE ASSOCIATION OF ANAESTHETISTS
*of Great Britain & Ireland*

## Management of a Patient with Suspected Anaesthesia During Anaesthesia
## SAFETY DRILL

(Revised 2009)

## Immediate management

- Use the ABC approach (Airway, Breathing, and Circulation). Team-working enables several tasks to be accomplished simultaneously.

- Remove all potential causative agents and maintain anaesthesia, if necessary, with an inhalational agent.

- CALL FOR HELP and note the time.

- Maintain the airway and administer oxygen 100%. Intubate the trachea if necessary and ventilate the lungs with oxygen.

- Elevate the patient's legs if there is hypotension.

- If appropriate, start cardiopulmonary resuscitation immediately according to Advanced Life Support Guidelines.

- Give adrenaline i.v.

  ○ Adult dose: 50 µg (0.5 ml of 1:10 000 solution).
  ○ Child dose: 1.0 µg.kg⁻¹ (0.1 ml.kg⁻¹ 1:100 000 solution).

- Several doses may be required if there is severe hypotension or bronchospasm. If several doses of adrenaline are required, consider starting an intravenous infusion of adrenaline.

- Give saline 0.9% or lactated Ringer's solution at a high rate via an intravenous cannula of an appropriate gauge (large volumes may be required).

  ○ Adult: 500 - 1 000 ml
  ○ Child: 20 ml.kg⁻¹

- Plan transfer of the patient to an appropriate Critical Care area.

### CONTINUED OVERLEAF

© The Association of Anaesthetists of Great Britain & Ireland 2009

**Figure 25.2** A4 sheet Management of a Patient with Suspected Anaphylaxis During Anaesthesia. Reproduced with the kind permission of the Association of Anaesthetists of Great Britain and Ireland.

## Secondary management

- Give chlorphenamine i.v.

  | | |
  |---|---|
  | Adult: | 10 mg |
  | Child 6 - 12 years: | 5 mg |
  | Child 6 months - 6 years: | 2.5 mg |
  | Child <6 months: | 250 µg.kg$^{-1}$ |

- Give hydrocortisone i.v.

  | | |
  |---|---|
  | Adult: | 200 mg |
  | Child 6 - 12 years: | 100 mg |
  | Child 6 months - 6 years: | 50 mg |
  | Child <6 months: | 25 mg |

- If the blood pressure does not recover despite an adrenaline infusion, consider the administration of an alternative i.v. vasopressor according to the training and experience of the anaesthetist, e.g. metaraminol.

- Treat persistent bronchospasm with an i.v. infusion of salbutamol. If a suitable breathing system connector is available, a metered-dose inhaler may be appropriate. Consider giving i.v. aminophylline or magnesium sulphate.

## Investigation

- Take blood samples (5 - 10 ml clotted blood) for **mast cell tryptase:**

  - Initial sample as soon as feasible after resuscitation has started – do not delay resuscitation to take the sample.

  - Second sample at 1 - 2 h after the start of symptoms.

  - Third sample either at 24 h or in convalescence (for example in a follow-up allergy clinic). This is a measure of baseline tryptase levels as some individuals have a higher baseline level.

- Ensure that the samples are labelled with the time and date.

- Liaise with the hospital laboratory about analysis of samples.

## Later investigations to identify the causative agent

The anaesthetist who gave the anaesthetic or the supervising consultant anaesthetist is responsible for ensuring that the reaction is investigated. The patient should be referred to a specialist Allergy or Immunology Centre (see www.aagbi.org for details). The patient, surgeon and general practitioner should be informed. Reactions should be notified to the AAGBI National Anaesthetic Anaphylaxis Database (see www.aagbi.org).

**Figure 25.2** (cont.)

## Malignant hyperthermia (MH)

This guideline contains three parts. The first outlines the recognition, management and follow-up of MH. The second recommends a team structure for dealing with MH. This list of task allocations is useful because there are many tasks which need to be carried out simultaneously. The third gives the recommended contents of a Malignant Hyperthermia Management kit, so that all necessary equipment is to hand in a crisis[7].

Copies of these should be readily available in areas wherever anaesthetics are given. This also goes for the guidelines on management of suspected anaphylaxis and local anaesthetic toxicity.

You should check where these guidelines are kept as you are introduced to new clinical areas at the start of your return to work. If they are not readily accessible, maybe standardizing the availability of the AAGBI guideline summaries in relevant clinical areas can be your next project!

## Management of severe local anaesthetic toxicity

Bear in mind the possible presenting signs and symptoms of local anaesthetic toxicity whenever using large doses of local anaesthetic. These may be delayed, and may or may not include seizures. Any arrhythmia, including bradycardia, tachyarrhythmia or asystole, can be a feature. Remember that arrhythmias in this context may be resistant to normal treatments. The use of 20% lipid emulsion is required in cases of cardiovascular collapse unresponsive to conventional management.

Lipid emulsion (such as Intralipid[R]) is used to treat toxicity from local anaesthetics, and other lipophilic drugs. Although propofol may sometimes be used in small doses to control convulsions, it is not sufficient management for lipophilic drug toxicity owing to the amount of cardiovascular depression which would ensue.

The AAGBI guidelines give example doses for a 70 kg man. Remember to adjust the dose accordingly. You should use lean body weight in the obese. Always give 5 minutes for a response before giving another bolus or changing the dose.

A blood sample for later analysis from the time of the event is useful. However, this should not delay emergency management. Pancreatitis is a recognized complication of treatment with lipid emulsion. Therefore, it is necessary to check amylase 24 hours following its use.

## Regional anaesthesia and abnormalities of coagulation[8]

This is a consensus document in conjunction with Obstetric Anaesthetists' Association (OAA) and Regional Anaesthesia UK (RA-UK). Their aim was to give concise guidance that would be helpful in the clinical setting, regardless of the cause of the coagulation abnormality. The guidelines are set out in the form of four tables.

'Risk is a continuum running from normal risk to very high risk.'[9]. This guidance is to be used in conjunction with assessment of each clinical situation.

The first table in the guidelines (see Table 25.1) is an extremely useful reference in deciding plans for the anaesthetic management of patients with altered coagulation, whether the clotting abnormality is due to drug therapy or patient pathology. We are often faced with the choice of giving a regional anaesthetic, and must balance its benefits with its risks in the presence of abnormal clotting. Also, patients should be given all the information necessary for them to make a fully informed choice[9]. Different regional blocks carry different bleeding risks. The second table, with accompanying notes, summarizes this information.

# Malignant Hyperthermia Crisis

## AAGBI Safety Guideline

Successful management of malignant hyperthermia depends upon early diagnosis and treatment; onset can be within minutes of induction or may be insidious. The standard operating procedure below is intended to ease the burden of managing this rare but life threatening emergency.

### 1 Recognition

- Unexplained increase in ETCO2 **AND**
- Unexplained tachycardia **AND**
- Unexplained increase in oxygen requirement
  (Previous uneventful anaesthesia does **not** rule out MH)
- Temperature changes are a late sign

### 2 Immediate management

- **STOP** all trigger agents
- **CALL FOR HELP.** Allocate specific tasks (action plan in MH kit)
- Install clean breathing system and **HYPERVENTILATE** with **100% O2 high flow**
- Maintain anaesthesia with intravenous agent
- **ABANDON/FINISH** surgery as soon as possible
- Muscle relaxation with non-depolarising neuromuscular blocking drug

### 3 Monitoring & treatment

- Give **dantrolene**

- Initiate active **cooling** avoiding vasoconstriction

- **TREAT:**

  - **Hyperkalaemia:** calcium chloride, glucose/insulin, NaHCO3⁻

  - **Arrhythmias:** magnesium/amiodarone/metoprolol **AVOID** calcium channel blockers - interaction with dantrolene

  - **Metabolic acidosis:** hyperventilate, NaHCO3⁻

  - **Myoglobinaemia:** forced alkaline diuresis (mannitol/furosemide + NaHCO3⁻); may require renal replacement therapy later

  - **DIC:** FFP, cryoprecipitate, platelets

- Check plasma CK as soon as able

**DANTROLENE**
2.5mg/kg immediate iv bolus.
Repeat 1mg/kg boluses as required to max 10mg/kg

**For a 70kg adult**

- **Initial bolus: 9 vials dantrolene** 20mg (each vial mixed with 60ml sterile water)

- Further boluses of 4 vials dantrolene 20mg repeated up to 7 times.

**Continuous monitoring**
Core & peripheral temperature
ETCO2
SpO2
ECG
Invasive blood pressure
CVP

**Repeated bloods**
ABG
U&Es (potassium)
FBC (haematocrit/platelets)
Coagulation

### 4 Follow-up

- Continue monitoring on ICU, repeat dantrolene as necessary
- Monitor for acute kidney injury and compartment syndrome
- Repeat CK
- Consider alternative diagnoses (sepsis, phaeochromocytoma, thyroid storm, myopathy)
- Counsel patient & family members
- Refer to MH unit (see contact details below)

The UK MH Investigation Unit, Academic Unit of Anaesthesia, Clinical Sciences Building, Leeds Teaching Hospitals NHS Trust, Leeds LS9 7TF. Direct line: 0113 206 5270. Fax: 0113 206 4140. Emergency Hotline: 07947 609601 (usually available outside office hours). Alternatively, contact Prof P Hopkins, Dr E Watkins or Dr P Gupta through hospital switchboard: 0113 243 3144.

**Your nearest MH kit is stored** ............................................................

This guideline is not a standard of medical care. The ultimate judgement with regard to a particular clinical procedure or treatment plan must be made by the clinician in the light of the clinical data presented and the diagnostic and treatment options available.

© The Association of Anaesthetists of Great Britain & Ireland 2011

**Figure 25.3** Malignant Hyperthermia Crisis. AAGBI Safety Guidelines. Reproduced with the kind permission of the Association of Anaesthetists of Great Britain and Ireland.

# Malignant Hyperthermia Crisis Task Allocations
## AAGBI Safety Guideline

The successful management of a malignant hyperthermia crisis requires multiple simultaneous treatment actions. This is made far easier through effective teamwork and specific task allocation.

### 1st anaesthetist - commence immediate management (on guideline sheet)
The anaesthetist diagnosing MH or the most senior anaesthetist responding should assume the role of clinical leader once immediate management actions have been undertaken and avoid becoming focused on a single task.

### 2nd anaesthetist - resuscitation
- Ensure dantrolene is given in correct dose (2.5mg/kg initially then 1mg/kg every 10-15min)
- Commence TIVA
- Management of hyperkalaemia
- Management of arrhythmias
- Management of acidosis
- Renal protection (forced alkaline diuresis)

### 1st anaesthetic nurse/ODP
- Collect MH kit
- Collect cold saline & insulin
- Set up lines (arterial/CVC)
- Runner for resuscitation drugs/equipment

### 2nd anaesthetic nurse/ODP (ideally two people)
- Draw up dantrolene as requested by anaesthetist in charge of resuscitation

### 3rd anaesthetist - lines/investigations
- Site arterial line
- Send bloods for
  - ABG – repeated (approx every 30 min initially)
  - U&Es
  - CK
  - FBC
  - Coagulation screen
  - Cross match
- Central venous access
- Urinary myoglobin
- Monitor core and peripheral temperatures

### Surgical team
- Catheterise
- Complete/abandon surgery as soon as feasible
- Undertake cooling manoeuvres

Adapted from the Malignant Hyperthermia Australia and New Zealand (MHANZ) MH Resource Kit with permission

**Figure 25.4** Malignant Hyperthermia Crisis Task Allocations. Reproduced with the kind permission of the Association of Anaesthetists of Great Britain and Ireland.

# AAGBI Safety Guideline

## Management of Severe Local Anaesthetic Toxicity

### 1 Recognition

**Signs of severe toxicity:**
- Sudden alteration in mental status, severe agitation or loss of consciousness, with or without tonic-clonic convulsions
- Cardiovascular collapse: sinus bradycardia, conduction blocks, asystole and ventricular tachyarrhythmias may all occur
- Local anaesthetic (LA) toxicity may occur some time after an initial injection

### 2 Immediate management

- Stop injecting the LA
- Call for help
- Maintain the airway and, if necessary, secure it with a tracheal tube
- Give 100% oxygen and ensure adequate lung ventilation (hyperventilation may help by increasing plasma pH in the presence of metabolic acidosis)
- Confirm or establish intravenous access
- Control seizures: give a benzodiazepine, thiopental or propofol in small incremental doses
- Assess cardiovascular status throughout
- Consider drawing blood for analysis, but do not delay definitive treatment to do this

### 3 Treatment

| IN CIRCULATORY ARREST | WITHOUT CIRCULATORY ARREST |
|---|---|
| • Start cardiopulmonary resuscitation (CPR) using standard protocols<br>• Manage arrhythmias using the same protocols, recognising that arrhythmias may be very refractory to treatment<br>• Consider the use of cardiopulmonary bypass if available | Use conventional therapies to treat:<br>• hypotension,<br>• bradycardia,<br>• tachyarrhythmia |
| **GIVE INTRAVENOUS LIPID EMULSION**<br>(following the regimen overleaf)<br><br>• Continue CPR throughout treatment with lipid emulsion<br>• Recovery from LA-induced cardiac arrest may take >1 h<br>• Propofol is not a suitable substitute for lipid emulsion<br>• Lidocaine should not be used as an anti-arrhythmic therapy | **CONSIDER INTRAVENOUS LIPID EMULSION**<br>(following the regimen overleaf)<br><br>• Propofol is not a suitable substitute for lipid emulsion<br>• Lidocaine should not be used as an anti-arrhythmic therapy |

### 4 Follow-up

- Arrange safe transfer to a clinical area with appropriate equipment and suitable staff until sustained recovery is achieved
- Exclude pancreatitis by regular clinical review, including daily amylase or lipase assays for two days
- Report cases as follows:
  in the United Kingdom to the National Patient Safety Agency (via www.npsa.nhs.uk)
  in the Republic of Ireland to the Irish Medicines Board (via www.imb.ie)
  If Lipid has been given, please also report its use to the international registry at www.lipidregistry.org. Details may also be posted at www.lipidrescue.org

**Your nearest bag of Lipid Emulsion is kept** ...............................................................................................

This guideline is not a standard of medical care. The ultimate judgement with regard to a particular clinical procedure or treatment plan must be made by the clinician in the light of the clinical data presented and the diagnostic and treatment options available.
© The Association of Anaesthetists of Great Britain & Ireland 2010

**Figure 25.5** Management of Severe Local Anaesthetic Toxicity. Reproduced with the kind permission of the Association of Anaesthetists of Great Britain and Ireland.

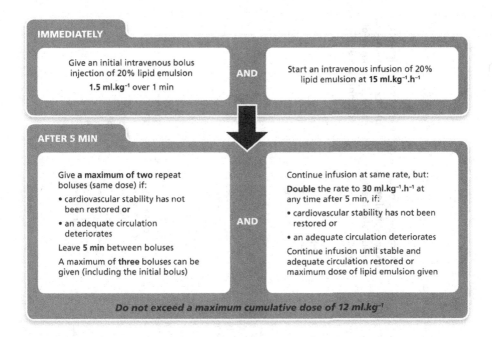

An approximate dose regimen for a 70-kg patient would be as follows:

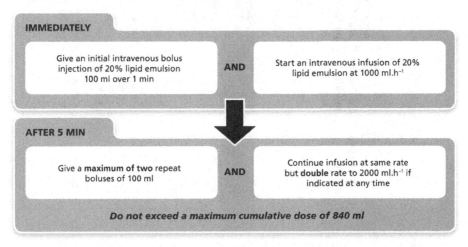

 This AAGBI Safety Guideline was produced by a Working Party that comprised:
Grant Cave, Will Harrop-Griffiths (Chair), Martyn Harvey, Tim Meek, John Picard, Tim Short and Guy Weinberg.

**This Safety Guideline is endorsed by the Australian and New Zealand College of Anaesthetists (ANZCA).**

© The Association of Anaesthetists of Great Britain & Ireland 2010

**Figure 25.5** (cont.)

**Table 25.1** Recommendations regarding regional anaesthesia in the presence of drugs used to modify coagulation. Reproduced with the kind permission of the Association of Anaesthetists of Great Britain and Ireland

| Drug | Time to peak effect | Elimination half-life | Acceptable time after drug for block performance | Administration of drug while spinal or epidural catheter in place[1] | Acceptable time after block performance or catheter removal for next drug dose |
|---|---|---|---|---|---|
| **Heparins** | | | | | |
| UFH sc prophylaxis | <30 min | 1–2 h | 4 h or normal APTTR | Caution | 1 h |
| UFH iv treatment | <5 min | 1–2 h | 4 h or normal APTTR | Caution[2] | 4 h |
| LMWH sc prophylaxis | 3–4 h | 3–7 h | 12 h | Caution[3] | 4 h[3] |
| LMWH sc treatment | 3–4 h | 3–7 h | 24 h | Not recommended | 4 h[4] |
| **Heparin alternatives** | | | | | |
| Danaparoid prophylaxis | 4–5 h | 24 h | Avoid (consider anti-Xa levels) | Not recommended | 6 h |
| Danaparoid treatment | 4–5 h | 24 h | Avoid (consider anti-Xa levels) | Not recommended | 6 h |
| Bivalirudin | 5 min | 25 min | 10 h or normal APTTR | Not recommended | 6 h |
| Argatroban | <30 min | 30–35 min | 4 h or normal APTTR | Not recommended | 6 h |
| Fondaparinux prophylaxis[5] | 1–2 h | 17–20 h | 36–42 h (consider anti-Xa levels) | Not recommended | 6–12 h |
| Fondaparinux treatment[5] | 1–2 h | 17–20 h | Avoid (consider anti-Xa levels) | Not recommended | 12 h |
| **Antiplatelet drugs** | | | | | |
| NSAIDs | 1–12 h | 1–12 h | No additional precautions | No additional precautions | No additional precautions |
| Aspirin | 12–24 h | Not relevant; irreversible effect | No additional precautions | No additional precautions | No additional precautions |
| Clopidogrel | 12–24 h | | 7 days | Not recommended | 6 h |
| Prasugrel | 15–30 min | | 7 days | Not recommended | 6 h |
| Ticagrelor | 2 h | 8–12 h | 5 days | Not recommended | 6 h |
| Tirofiban | <5 min | 4–8 h[6] | 8 h | Not recommended | 6 h |
| Eptifibatide | <5 min | 4–8 h[6] | 8 h | Not recommended | 6 h |
| Abciximab | <5 min | 24–48 h[6] | 48 h | Not recommended | 6 h |
| Dipyridamole | 75 min | 10 h | No additional precautions | No additional precautions | 6 h |

| Oral anticoagulants | | | | | After catheter removal |
|---|---|---|---|---|---|
| Warfarin | 3–5 days | 4–5 days | INR <1.4 | Not recommended | 6 h |
| Rivaroxaban prophylaxis[5] (CrCl > 30 ml.min⁻¹) | 3 h | 7–9 h | 18 h | Not recommended | 6 h |
| Rivaroxaban treatment[5] (CrCl > 30 ml.min⁻¹) | 3 h | 7–11 h | 48 h | Not recommended | 6 h |
| **Dabigatran prophylaxis or treatment**[7] | | | | | |
| (CrCl > 80 ml.min⁻¹) | 0.5–2.0 h | 12–17 h | 48 h | Not recommended | 6 h |
| (CrCl 50–80 ml.min⁻¹) | 0.5–2.0 h | 15 h | 72 h | Not recommended | 6 h |
| (CrCl 30–50 ml.min⁻¹) | 0.5–2.0 h | 18 h | 96 h | Not recommended | 6 h |
| Apixaban prophylaxis | 3–4 h | 12 h | 24–18 h | Not recommended | 6 h |
| **Thrombolytic drugs** | | | | | |
| Alteplase, anistreplase, reteplase, streptokinase | <5 min | 4–24 min | 10 days | Not recommended | 10 days |

UFH, unfractionated heparin; sc, subcutaneous; APTTR, activated partial thromboplastin time ratio; iv, intravenous; LMWH, low molecular weight heparin; NSAIDs, non-steroidal anti-inflammatory drugs; INR, international normalized ratio; CrCl, creatinine clearance.

### Notes to accompany Table 1

1  The dangers associated with the administration of any drug that affects coagulation while a spinal or epidural catheter is in place should be considered carefully. There are limited data on the safety of the use of the newer drugs in this Table, and they are therefore not recommended until further data become available. The administration of those drugs whose entry in this column is marked as 'caution' may be acceptable, but the decision must be based on an evaluation of the risks and benefits of administration. If these drugs are given, the times identified in the column to the left ('Acceptable time after drug for block performance') should be used as a guide to the minimum time that should be allowed between drug administration and catheter removal.

2  It is common for intravenous unfractionated heparin to be given a short time after spinal blockade or insertion of an epidural catheter during vascular and cardiac surgery. Local clinical governance guidelines should be followed and a high index of suspicion should be maintained if any signs attributable to vertebral canal haematoma develop.

3  Low molecular weight heparins are commonly given in prophylactic doses twice daily after surgery, but many clinicians recommend that only one dose be given in the first 24 h after neuraxial blockade has been performed.

4  Consider increasing to 24 h if block performance is traumatic.

5  Manufacturer recommends caution with use of neuraxial catheters.

6  Time to normal platelet function rather than elimination half-life.

7  Manufacturer recommends that neuraxial catheters are not used.

There is guidance regarding neuraxial blockade in obstetric patients in the third table. The fourth table refers to the special situations of trauma, liver failure, sepsis, uraemia, massive transfusion and disseminated intravascular coagulopathy.

The view that an experienced anaesthetist should perform the block in a patient who is at higher risk of bleeding complications is supported by the AAGBI. The more experienced anaesthetist may have fewer attempts, with greater chance of achieving a successful block.

Rare haematological conditions are not covered and decisions should be made in conjunction with a haematologist, who will often advise on clotting factor replacement which can reduce the risk of bleeding complications during regional anaesthesia.

# References

1. Association of Anaesthetists of Great Britain and Ireland. Checking Anaesthetic Equipment 2012. *Anaesthesia* 2012; 67: 660–8.
2. National Patient Safety Agency. WHO Surgical Safety Checklist NPSA/2009/PSA002/ u1, January 2009, London: NPSA, 2009. Available at www.safesurg.org/uploads/1/0/9/0/1090835/ npsa_checklist.pdf (accessed 4 January 2016).
3. Association of Anaesthetists of Great Britain and Ireland. Recommendations for Standards of Monitoring during Anaesthesia and Recovery, 4th edn. 2007.
4. Association of Anaesthetists of Great Britain and Ireland. AAGBI Safety Statement. The use of capnography outside the operating theatre. 2011. Available at http://www.aagbi.org/sites/default/ files/Capnographyaagbi090711AJH%5B1%5D_1.pdf (accessed 4 January 2016).
5. J. J. Pandit, T. M. Cook, The NAP5 Steering Panel. NAP5. Accidental Awareness During General Anaesthesia. London: The Royal College of Anaesthetists and Association of Anaesthetists of Great Britain and Ireland, 2014 ISBN 978–11–900936–11–8.
6. Association of Anaesthetists of Great Britain and Ireland. Suspected anaphylactic reactions associated with anaesthesia. *Anaesthesia* 2009; 64: 199–211.
7. http://www.aagbi.org/sites/default/files/MH%20recommended%20contents%20for%20web.pdf (accessed 2 January 2016).
8. Association of Anaesthetists of Great Britain and Ireland, Obstetric Anaesthetists' Association and Regional Anaesthesia UK. Regional anaesthesia and patients with abnormalities of coagulation. *Anaesthesia* 2013; 68: 966–72.
9. D. Sokol. Update on the UK law on consent. *BMJ* 2015; 350: h1481 doi:10.1136.

Chapter

# 26

# WHO Safer Surgery Checklist

Emma Plunkett

*This chapter is a reminder of the process behind the introduction of the ubiquitous World Health Organization (WHO) Surgical Safety Checklist and also briefly considers how to ensure it is used effectively.*

## The World Health Organization (WHO) Surgical Safety Checklist

This checklist is now firmly embedded in anaesthetic culture in most hospitals in the UK, although not everyone is convinced of its utility. After all, wrong site surgery (a Never Event) still happens, and antibiotics and venous thromboembolism prophylaxis occasionally get missed. The problem is that the checklist is done so often that we rattle off the answers automatically. That is not its point. When done properly it should stop us from using our automatic, reflex, fast thinking (sometimes known as System 1 thinking) and force us into deliberate, reasoned, slower thinking (System 2 thinking), which is less prone to biases and mistakes[1].

In his book describing the inception of the WHO checklist, Atul Gawande describes how checklists are used for complex tasks in many different industries[2]. Patients, systems and procedures are incredibly complicated, and increasingly so, and we cannot expect ourselves to remember everything, every time. Because we are human and because of the complexity of the work we do, we need help from checklists to make sure we get things right.

The WHO checklist was revealed in 2008 as part of the WHO Second Global Patient Safety Challenge: Safe Surgery Saves Lives. The paper describing the success of the pilot project was published in *The New England Journal of Medicine* in January 2009[3], following which an NPSA Alert was released, requiring all trusts to implement the checklist by the 1 February 2010. The WHO checklist forms the middle section of the '5 steps to safer surgery' approach designed and promoted by Patient Safety First.

Briefing → Sign in → Time out → Sign out → Debriefing

The key to safe surgical care is effective team work and communication in combination with the use of evidence-based interventions. The WHO checklist combines all of these.

The implementation of the WHO checklist has been reviewed by Patient Safety First with a survey to all trusts[4]. All those who responded were implementing the checklist and about 60% reported positive change as a result. Factors which were identified as leading to successful introduction were all related to engagement with staff; having a clinical champion, early adopter and clinician and nurse enthusiasm. Challenges included it being seen as a tick box

*Returning to Work in Anaesthesia*, ed. Emma Plunkett, Emily Johnson and Anna Pierson.
Published by Cambridge University Press. © Cambridge University Press 2016.

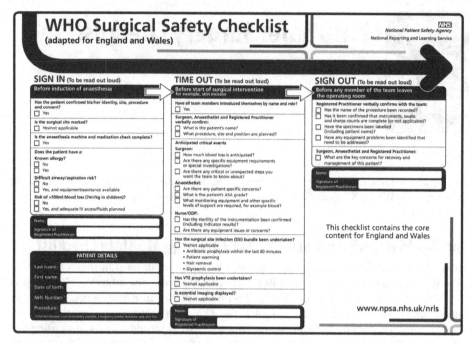

**Figure 26.1** The NPSA WHO Surgical Safety Checklist. Available at: http://www.nrls.npsa.nhs.uk/resources/ ?entryid45=59860. Contains public sector information licensed under the Open Government Licence v3.0.

exercise, and difficulties getting staff engagement when it is not seen as a priority or under time pressures.

Trusts can adopt the checklist and a version has also been created for maternity cases. We have included a standard copy of the checklist (Figure 26.1), to remind you of what it includes.

The WHO checklist is incorporated into the National Safety Standards for Invasive Procedures (NatSSIPs) published in September 2015[5]. These are recommended minimum standards developed in response to the Surgical Never Events Taskforce Report. Based on the NatSSIPs, local standards (LocSSIPS) will be developed for all invasive procedures (within and outside theatre) with the aim of systematically eliminating never events.

# References

1. D. Kahneman. *Thinking Fast and Slow*. London: Penguin, 2012.
2. A. Gawande. *The Checklist Manifesto: How to Get Things Right*. London: Profile Books, 2011.
3. A. B. Haynes, T. G. Weiser, W. R. Berry et al. Safe Surgery Saves Lives Group. A surgical safety checklist to reduce morbidity and mortality in a global population. *N Engl J Med* 2009; 360: 491–9.
4. Patient Safety First. Implementing the Surgical Safety Checklist: the journey so far … 2010. www.scribd.com/doc/284954207/Implementing-the-Surgical-Safety-Checklist-the-Journey-So-Far-2010-06-21-FINAL#scribd (accessed 9 January 2016).
5. NHS England Patient safety alert. Supporting the introduction of National Safety Standards for Invasive Procedures. 14 September 2015. Available online at https://www.england.nhs.uk/wp-content/uploads/2015/09/psa-natssips.pdf (accessed 11 July 2016).

Chapter

# Drug doses

Anna Pierson and Emma Plunkett

**27**

*Administering pharmacological and fluid therapies is a significant part of any anaesthetist's daily practice. However, after a break from clinical practice, it is inevitable that knowledge of drug choices and doses is not as intuitive as before. For those times when we need a helping hand to recall such information, this chapter provides the reader with a reference guide to commonly used drugs, their dosing regimen and some additional tips/information. The tables are divided into relevant sections for ease of use, with the inclusion of a 'key tips' fluids box at the end.*

## Drug dosing: handy hints and reference guide

Taking a significant break from work and focussing on another area of your life undoubtedly means that, often, skills or knowledge once taken as read seem rather less sharp and may take some time to return. As anaesthetists we administer a vast variety of drugs and fluid therapies on a daily basis. When we are in full flow in our jobs, familiarity with drug dosing is expected of us. However, we have all found ourselves in an anaesthetic room after time away, struggling to recall how to dilute adrenaline to make a 10 mcg/mL solution, or what the paediatric dose of a drug is.

This chapter is here to help you during those moments. We have included tables of commonly used anaesthetic drugs with doses and concentrations, along with a few other handy hints. If this is something you think you may find useful, you may want to make a copy and keep it in your pocket to refer to on your return to work.

Each table gives you a quick guide to drug dose, the concentration either in the ampoule or once diluted, the average adult dose given and, finally, any particular points to note. This is by no means an exhaustive list, but should suffice in the short term following your return to clinical practice.

*Returning to Work in Anaesthesia*, ed. Emma Plunkett, Emily Johnson and Anna Pierson.
Published by Cambridge University Press. © Cambridge University Press 2016.

# Induction agents

**Table 27.1** Induction agents

| Drug | Dose | Concentration | Average dose for 70 kg patient | Notes |
|------|------|---------------|-------------------------------|-------|
| Propofol | 2–4 mg/kg | 10 mg/ml (1%) 20 mg/ml (2%) | 200 mg = 20 ml (1%) | TCI induction Ce4–8 mcg/ml, then 3–6 mcg/ml |
| Thiopentone | 5–6 mg/kg | 25 mg/ml | 350 mg = 14 ml | NAP5 recommended min. 5 mg/kg |
| Etomidate | 0.1–0.4 mg/kg | 2 mg/mL | 14 mg = 7 ml | More cardiostable. Adrenal suppression |
| Ketamine | 1–2 mg/kg slowly. After 10–15 min 0.5 mg/kg top-up or 5–10 mg/kg IM. Maintenance 3–5 mg/kg after 20–30 min | | | |

# Inhalational agents

**Table 27.2** Inhalational agents

| Agent | MAC in $O_2$ | MAC in 66% $N_2O$ | Notes |
|-------|-------------|-------------------|-------|
| Desflurane | 6.0 | 4.5 | 8% induction, 4–5% maintenance. Airway irritant, unsuitable for gas induction |
| Isoflurane | 1.15 | 0.5 | 5% induction, 1–1.5% maintenance |
| Sevoflurane | 2.2 | 0.66 | Better in asthmatics |
| Nitrous oxide | 104 (alone) | - | Analgesic |

MAC, minimum alveolar concentration.

# Muscle relaxants and reversal

**Table 27.3** Muscle relaxants and reversal

| Drug | Dose | Concentration | Average dose for 70 kg patient | Notes |
|------|------|---------------|-------------------------------|-------|
| Suxamethonium | 1–1.5 mg/kg | 50 mg/ml | 100 mg = 2 ml | $K^+$/burns/neuro |
| Rocuronium | 0.6–1.2 mg/kg | 10 mg/ml | 70 mg = 7 ml (for RSI) | Works in 60 s, repeat after 30–40 min |
| Atracurium | 0.5 mg/kg | 10 mg/ml | 35 mg = 3.5 ml | Works in 90 s, repeat after 20–30 min Avoid in asthma. Safe in renal failure |
| Mivacurium | 0.15 mg/kg | | | Works in 2 min, repeat after 10–20 min Avoid in asthma |
| Vecuronium | 0.1 mg/kg | 2 mg/ml | 7 mg = 3.5 ml | Avoid in renal failure Action in 90 s, repeat after 20–30 min |
| Pancuronium | 0.04–0.1 mg/mg | | | Vagolytic and sympathomimetic. Duration 45–60 min |
| Neostigmine | 50 mcg/kg | 2.5 mg/ml | 2.5 mg = 50 kg patient | Give with glycopyrrolate to avoid bradycardia |
| Glycopyrrolate | 10 mcg/kg | 200 mcg/ml | 500 mcg = 50 kg patient | |
| Sugammadex | 2–16 mg/kg | | | Moderate block: 2 mg/kg; profound block: 4 mg/kg Immediate reversal after RSI: 16 mg/kg |

RSI, rapid sequence induction.

# Analgesics

**Table 27.4** Analgesics

| Drug | Dose | Concentration | Average dose 70 kg | Paediatrics | Notes |
|---|---|---|---|---|---|
| Fentanyl | 1–5 mcg/kg | 50 mcg/mL | | 1 mcg/kg | Epidural 50–100 mcg; spinal 5–25 mcg; PCA dose 10–20 mcg |
| Alfentanil | 5–10 mcg/kg | | 250–750 mcg | | Fast acting, bolus lasts 10 mins |
| Diamorphine | 0.05 mg/kg | | 2.5–5 mgs | 50 mcg/kg | Epidural: 2–3 mgs, Spinal: 0.25 – 0.5 mg |
| Morphine | 0.1–0.2 mg/kg | | | Over 1 year:<br>0.1–0.3 mg/kg PO or<br>0.1–0.2 mg/kg IV<br>6–12 months:<br>0.1–0.2 mg/kg PO or<br>0.05–0.1 mg/kg IV | PCA: 1 mg dose, 5 min lockout in adults |
| Codeine | 30–60 mg | | 30–60 mg | | Not used in children under 12 yrs |
| Remifentanil | 0.5–1 mcg/kg/min (induction) | 50 mcg/mL (infusion) | 0.05–2 mcg/kg/min (maintenance) | Reduce concentration to 20–25 mcg/mL | Dilute 2 mg in 40 mL 0.9% NaCl |
| Paracetamol | 500–1000 mg | | | 15–20 mg/kg PO (max 80 mg/kg/day)<br>15 mg/kg IV (>3/12 old, max 60 mg/kg/day) | Max 500 mg if <50kg<br>Max daily dose if <3/12 old, 60 mg/kg/day<br>For term neonates (>38/40 – 3/12 old), IV dose 10 mg/kg TDS |
| Ibuprofen | | | 400 mg tds | Over 1 year: 10 mg/kg tds<br>Under 1 year: 5 mg/kg qds | Not to be used if <1 month or <5kg |
| Diclofenac | Max 150 mg/24hr | 25 mg/mL | 75 mg one off IV | 1 mg/kg tds | Not to be used if <6 months |
| Naloxone | 200–400 mcg | | 400 mcg | 4–10 mcg/kg | For opiate reversal; may need repeat doses |

# Local anaesthetics

Calculating concentrations:

1% = 10 mg/ml
0.5% = 5 mg/ml
0.25% = 2.5 mg/ml
0.125% = 1.25 mg/ml

**Table 27.5** Local anaesthetics

| Drug | Maximum dose | Maximum dose with adrenaline | Maximum dose for 70 kg patient | Notes |
|---|---|---|---|---|
| Lidocaine | 3 mg/kg | 6–7 mg/kg | 210 mg/420 mg (with adrenaline) | 1% or 2% concentration. Onset 5–10 min |
| Bupivacaine | 2 mg/kg | 2.5 mg/kg | 140 mg/175 mg (with adrenaline) | 0.125% (usually in epidural infusion); 0.25% or 0.5% concentration. LSCS spinal dose: 2.2–2.7 ml 0.5% heavy bupivacaine |
| Levobupivacaine | 2.5–3 mg/kg | 2.5–3 mg/kg | 210 mg | S-enantiomer of bupivacaine; less cardiotoxic |
| Ropivacaine | 3 mg/kg | 4 mg/kg | 210/280 mg (with adrenaline) | |
| Prilocaine | 6 mg/kg | 9 mg/kg | 420 mg/630 mg (with adrenaline) | 0.5%, 1% or 2% concentration. Onset 5–10 min |
| Cocaine | 3 mg/kg | N/A | 210 mg | Generally reserved for ENT |

Intralipid 20%: 1.5 ml/kg bolus; start IV infusion 15 ml/kg/h. Give up to 2 repeat boluses, increase infusion to 30 ml/kg/h up to maximum 12 ml/kg
For 70 kg patient: give 100 ml bolus, start IV infusion at 1000 ml/h. Give up to 2 further doses of 100 ml, then double rate to 2000 ml/h up to a maximum of 840 ml

# Emergency drugs

**Table 27.6** Emergency drugs

| Drug | Concentration | Average dose 70 kg | Paeds/Other | Notes |
|---|---|---|---|---|
| Adrenaline | 100 mcg/ml (in minijet 1:10 000) | 50–100 mcg boluses = 0.5–1 ml 1:10 000 | 10 mcg/kg (0.1 ml/kg) in paediatric cardiac arrest | IV infusion 2–20 mcg/min (dilute in 5% dextrose) |
| Atropine | 600 mcg/ml | 300–600 mcg | 20 mcg/kg | |
| Ephedrine | 3 mg/ml | 3–60 mg | | Dilute 30 mg in 9 ml 0.9% NaCl |
| Glycopyrrolate | 200 mcg/ml | 200–600 mcg | 4–10 mcg/kg | |
| Metaraminol | 0.5 mg/ml | 0.5–1 mg bolus prn | 10 mcg/kg | Dilute 10 mg in 19 ml 0.9% NaCl |
| Noradrenaline | 80 mcg/ml (4 mg/50 ml) | | | Dilute in 5% dextrose. Starting rate IV infusion = 0.025 mcg/kg/min |
| Phenylephrine | 10 mg/ml | 50–100 mcg bolus | Obs: boluses, or run IV infusion (50 mcg/ml) at 30–40 ml/h | 10 mg in 100 ml 0.9% NaCl = 100 mcg/ml. Use 10–20 ml in syringes as required |

## A note on adrenaline

It is vital to understand the concentration and dilution when using adrenaline.

- 1 ml of 1:1000 = 1 mg
- 1 ml of 1:10 000 = 0.1 mg = 100 mcg
- 1 ml of 1:100 000 = 0.01 mg = 10 mcg
- 1 ml of 1:200 000 = 0.005 mg = 5 mcg

# Antiemetics

**Table 27.7** Antiemetics

| Drug | Dose | Paediatric dose | Notes |
|---|---|---|---|
| Cyclizine | 50 mg | 1 mg/kg | Causes tachycardia |
| Ondansetron | 4 mg | 0.1 mg/kg | Can give up to max 16 mg/24 h in adult |
| Dexamethasone | 4–8 mg (3.3–6.6 mg) | 0.1 mg/kg | |

# Miscellaneous drugs

**Table 27.8** Miscellaneous drugs

| Drug | Dose | Average dose 70 kg | Notes |
|---|---|---|---|
| Aminophylline | 5 mg/kg (loading) | 350 mg | Over 30 min to load, then 0.5 mg/kg/h |
| Amiodarone | 150–300 mg | | Continue 900 mg IVI over 23 h. Paeds: 25 mcg/kg/min for 4 h, then 5–15 mcg/kg/min |
| Clonidine | 1–2 mcg/kg/h | 70–140 mcg/h (infusion 30 mcg/ml) = 2.3–4.6 ml/h | Max 4 mcg/kg/h. May cause rebound hypertension if stopped abruptly. Use in caudal anaesthesia = 1 mcg/kg |
| Dantrolene | 2.5 mg/kg (loading) | 9 vials containing 20 mg for initial bolus | Rpt 1 mg/kg boluses as required up to max 10 mg/kg |
| Esmolol | | 25–100 mg | Paeds 0.5 mg/kg |
| Labetalol | | 5 mg bolus up to 100 mg | 20 mg (over 1 min) for PET, hydralazine 5 mg over 15 min |
| Lorazepam | 4 mg bolus | | Paeds 0.1 mg/kg |
| Magnesium | Varies with indication | In eclampsia: 4 g bolus (8 ml 50% solution) in 32 ml 0.9% NaCl at 160 ml/h | ICU: 5 g = 20 mmol over 60 min for replacement (20 mmol = 10 ml). Asthma: 2 g = 8 mmol over 20–30 min. PET/eclampsia: 4 g/ bolus, IVI 1 g/h (10 ml 50% + 40 ml 0.9% NaCl 10 ml/h), 2 g bolus if further fits (4 ml 50% + 16 ml 0.9% NaCl over 7 min) |
| Mannitol | 0.25–1 g/kg | 0.5 g/kg = 35 g = 350 ml of 10% | 10% = 100 mg/ml; 20% = 200 mg/ml |
| Midazolam | 0.1 mg/kg bolus for agitation | 0.5–5 mg | Maintenance infusion: 0.02–2 mg/kg/h. Paeds: 0.5 mg/kg PO 30 min pre-induction. Reversal: 200 mcg flumazenil |
| Oxytocin | | 5 U postpartum/ERPC | Ergometrine 500 mcg IM (×2 max) (not if hypertensive). Carboprost 250 mcg IM/IU q 15 min (not if asthmatic), max 2 mg |
| Phenytoin | 15 mg/kg over 1 h | 1000 mg loading dose | Dilute to 10 mg/ml in saline |
| Salbutamol | 250 mcg slow IV bolus | 5–20 mcg/min > bolus | Paeds 4 mcg/kg |

# Fluids

**Box 27.1   Quick reference fluid guide**

- Total blood volume = 70 ml/kg
  - Replace with blood if > 20% volume loss (fit, healthy adult)
  - Replace with blood if > 10% volume loss (unwell/elderly/child)
- Paediatric maintenance fluids:
  - (4 ml/kg/h × first 10 kg) + (2 ml/kg/h × second 10 kg) + (1 ml/kg/h × any weight over 20 kg)
  - E.g. 21 kg child would require 61 ml/h
  - Resuscitation requires 10–20 ml/kg as a bolus (10 ml/kg in trauma)
- Paediatric dextrose bolus: 2 ml/kg 10% dextrose
- Paediatric packed red cell transfusion volume = required rise in haemoglobin (g) × weight (kg) × 4 (assuming that Hb of packed cells is 20 g/dl)
- Platelets/Octaplas/Cryoprecipitate = 10 ml/kg

**Chapter**

# 28

# Paediatric physiology and equipment

Emma Plunkett

*Safe paediatric anaesthesia requires meticulous attention to detail, arguably even more so than adult practice. This chapter brings together some of the unique features of paediatric anaesthesia with respect to the differences in physiology and also in the equipment used. Whilst the specialist paediatric anaesthetist is likely to recall all this information relatively easily, if you have not done paediatrics for a while then the tables and list here will help to refresh your memory.*

## Paediatric physiology and equipment[1]

### Airway equipment

The formulae you need to know to calculate sizing of airway equipment are as follows:

$$\text{ETT internal diameter} = \text{Age}/4 + 4$$
$$= \text{Age}/4 + 3.5 \text{ if using a cuffed ETT}$$

$$\text{ETT length (cm)} > 2 \text{ years} = \text{Age}/2 + 12 \text{ (oral)} = \text{Age}/2 + 15 \text{ (nasal) neonates}$$
$$= \text{weight (kg)} + 6 \text{ (oral)}$$

Examples of sizing for paediatric airway equipment are given in Table 28.1. All these sizes are estimations and should not be seen as absolute. We have calculated the weights according to the new APLS formulae and then given examples of tube sizes and depth of insertion so you can look up a starting point easily. Many paediatric drug dosing apps will have this information.

### Breathing

- An Ayre's T-piece (with Jackson Rees modification) can be used up to 20 kg.
  - Fresh gas flow 2–3 × minute volume for spontaneous ventilation.
  - Fresh gas flow 1000 ml + 200 ml × weight for controlled ventilation.
- A Bain circuit can be used from 20 kg.
- A Humphrey ADE system can be used from 10 kg.
- A paediatric circle system can be used from 5 kg.
- An adult ventilator can be used above 20 kg.

*Returning to Work in Anaesthesia*, ed. Emma Plunkett, Emily Johnson and Anna Pierson.
Published by Cambridge University Press. © Cambridge University Press 2016.

**Table 28.1** Paediatric airway equipment

| Age | Approx weight (kg) | Guedel airway size (colour)* | LMA | ETT Size/ depth (oral) |
|---|---|---|---|---|
| 28/40 | 1 | 000 (pink/clear) | Not used | 2.5/7 cm |
| 33/40 | 2 | 000 (pink) | Not used | 3.0/8 cm |
| 38/40 (term) | 3–4 | 00 (blue) | 1 up to 5 kg** | 3.5/9 cm |
| 3 months | 5.5 | 00 (blue) | 1.5** | 4.0/10 cm |
| Use a straight laryngoscope blade (size 0 up to 6 kg) and a curved blade for > 6 kg | | | | |
| 6 months | 7 | 00 (blue) | 1.5** | 4.5/11 cm |
| 1 year | 10 | 0 (black) | 1.5 (up to 10 kg)** | 5.0/12 cm |
| 2 years | 12 | 0 (black) | 2 | 5.5/13 cm |
| 5 years | 18 | 1 (white) | 2 (up to 20 kg) | 6.0/14.5 cm |
| 8 years | 31 | 1 (white) | 2.5 (up to 30 kg) or 3 | 6.5/16 cm |
| 12 years | 43 | 2 (green) | 3 | 7.0/18 cm |
| 16 years | 55 | 2 (green) | 3 (up to 50 kg) or 4 | 7.5/20 cm |

* Guedel colours can change according to the manufacturer, more often seen with adult sizes. Obviously, you should always size it to the patient but we thought it may be useful to include an idea of which one to start with.
** In practice in babies and small infants LMAs often do not sit well and many anaesthetists prefer to intubate (or use a facemask and a regional technique if appropriate).

**Table 28.2** Paediatric ventilation parameters

| Age | Estimated weight (kg) | Respiratory rate | Estimate tidal volume (ml) (7 ml/kg) | Example of ventilator setting |
|---|---|---|---|---|
| Preterm | <2.5 kg | 30–40 | 5–20 | |
| Birth | 3–4 | 30–40 | 25 | Pressure controlled (or regulated) mode |
| 1 year | 10 | 30–40 | 70 | An inspiratory pressure of 16–20 cmH$_2$O |
| 2 years | 12 | 25–30 | 80 | with a PEEP of 4–5 cmH$_2$O is a |
| 5 years | 18 | 20–25 | 125 | reasonable start |
| 8 years | 31 | 15–20 | 200 | |
| 12 years | 43 | 12–20 | 300 | |

PEEP, positive end-expiratory pressure.

- A Newton valve will convert the Nuffield Penlon 200 from a time-cycled flow generator to a pressure generator and is suitable for children up to 20 kg.

Example ventilation parameters are given in Table 28.2.

## Circulation

- A heart rate of less than 60 in a neonate or infant needs CPR.
- Use paediatric defibrillator paddles if under 10 kg.
- Normal neonatal mean arterial pressure = post-conceptional age in weeks.
- Normal haemoglobin at birth is 160–200 g/l at term. In an infant it is 100–120 g/l.
- Preterm infants often have a lower haemoglobin, partly through decreased production and increased consumption but also due to blood lost when sampling.

**Table 28.3** Normal paediatric cardiovascular parameters and emergency cardiovascular drug dosing according to weight

| Age | Approx weight | Heart rate | Systolic blood pressure | Fluid bolus (ml) 10 ml/kg | Adrenaline dose (ml) 0.1 ml/kg 1:10 000 | Atropine dose (mcg) 20 mcg/kg | CPR ratio |
|---|---|---|---|---|---|---|---|
| Estimated blood volume 90 ml/kg for a neonate | | | | | | | |
| Preterm | <3 kg | 120–200 | 50–90 | 5–30* | 0.05–0.3 | 10–60 | 3:1 |
| Birth | 3–4 kg | 100–160 | 70–90 | 30–40 | 0.3–0.4 | 60–80 | |
| Estimated blood volume 85 ml/kg for an infant | | | | | | | |
| 1 year | 10 | 100–160 | 70–90 | 100 | 1 | 200 | 15:2 |
| Estimated blood volume 80 ml/kg for a child | | | | | | | |
| 2 years | 12 | 95–140 | 80–100 | 120 | 1.2 | 240 | 15:2 |
| 5 years | 18 | 80–120 | 90–110 | 180 | 1.8 | 360 | |
| 8 years | 31 | 80–100 | 90–110 | 310 | 3.1 | 600 | |
| 12 years | 43 | 60–100 | 100–120 | 430 | 4.3 | 600 | 30:2** |
| Estimated blood volume 70 ml/kg for an adult | | | | | | | |

\* Particular care needed with volume of drug flushes.
\*\* CPR ratio changes to adult ratio at puberty.

## Blood volume and transfusion

Calculate estimated blood volume at the beginning of the case and transfuse after 15% has been lost (assuming normal starting haemoglobin).

$$\text{Transfusion volume} = \frac{(\text{desired--current haematocrit}) \times \text{estimated blood volume}}{\text{Haematocrit of packed cells (SAG} - M = 0.6; \text{CPD} = 0.65)}$$

## IV access

Peripheral access can be tricky, even for the experienced anaesthetist. The saphenous vein is often used (just anterior to the medial malleolus). Do not forget the intraosseous route in an emergency (see page 141).

Central venous access is by the usual routes with the addition of umbilical catheters in neonates and long lines in all ages. Lines come in many forms but a rough guide would be a 4.5 F gauge for an infant or neonate. Common lengths are 6 cm, 8 cm and 12 cm but this will depend on the site of insertion – it is a good idea to measure before you start).

# References

1.  S. Berg. Paediatric and neonatal anaesthesia. In: K. G. Allman, I. H. Wilson, eds. *Oxford Handbook of Anaesthesia*, 3rd edn. Oxford: Oxford University Press, 2011, pp. 799–860.

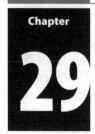

Chapter

# Practical procedures

Laura Tulloch, Laura Fulton and Emily Johnson

*This chapter aims to refresh your memory of the common practical procedures you may be required to undertake in your first few weeks back at work. Whilst you may have your own methods of performing these procedures and these will probably return to you very quickly, the aim here is to pick up on some of the major points and enable you to get back up to speed safely and confidently. In addition to covering some of the common procedures, their indications and complications, the basics of ultrasound, current advice on skin asepsis and the stop before you block campaign are considered.*

## Basic approach to USS

Point-of-care ultrasound has become an important clinical tool for anaesthestists and intensivists. Whether you plan on using USS to perform a peripheral nerve block or to obtain vascular access it is essential that you understand some of the basics of USS.

## Which probe to use?

High frequency probes will give high resolution but limited depth of penetration. Low frequency probes give greater depth of penetration but lower resolution.

High frequency linear array probe (10–15 MHz)
- Best for vascular access and superficial peripheral nerve blockade (e.g. interscalene, supraclavicular and axillary)
- These transducers provide high quality images for superficial structures up to approximately 4 cm.

Low frequency curvilinear probe (2–5 MHz)
- Best for scanning deeper structures such as infraclavicular, popliteal, sciatic regions and abdominal organs
- These transducers penetrate 4–5 cm or more below the skin surface.

## Planes of view

There are two views in which a target vessel or nerve may be imaged:
- Transverse or short axis: the image is a cross section of the structure with the probe held at right angles to the target structure.

*Returning to Work in Anaesthesia*, ed. Emma Plunkett, Emily Johnson and Anna Pierson.
Published by Cambridge University Press. © Cambridge University Press 2016.

- Longitudinal or long axis: the probe and target structure are aligned producing an image of the structure in its longitudinal axis.

## Imaging modes

- 2D: the standard imaging mode.
- M (motion) mode: a 2D image is acquired and a single scan line is placed along the area of interest. The M mode will then show how the structures intersected by that line move toward or away from the probe over time. This mode is used for making measurements of cardiac chambers and valve movements.
- Colour flow Doppler: this is an instrument to characterize blood flow and is useful for differentiating vascular from non-vascular structures. Generally, Blue is blood flowing Away from the transducer, Red is blood flowing Towards (BART)

## Ultrasound appearances of tissues

Artery   Anechoic (black), pulsatile, non-compressible
Vein     Anechoic, non-pulsatile, compressible. Increase in size with Valsalva
Muscle   Hypoechoic (grey) with multiple hyperechoic lines
Tendon   Hyperechoic (white), bright lines longitudinally or bright dots at right angles fibrillary pattern
Nerve    Variable hypo- or hyperechoic
Bone     Hyperechoic

## Needle imaging techniques

It is important to remember that the ultrasound beam is very narrow (1–2 mm wide) and in order for a needle to be seen some part of the needle must be crossing this beam and reflecting waves back to the probe.

### Out-of-plane (short axis)

This technique is commonly used when obtaining vascular access.

With this method, the needle approaches the target perpendicular to the ultrasound beam. The needle will be seen as a bright spot on the image, along with a dark shadow deep to it. Remember that the bright spot denotes the point at which the needle intersects the 2 mm wide ultrasound beam, and may not indicate the needle tip.

When using this method it is important to slide or angulate the probe to check where the needle tip lies. Movement of tissue helps guidance and a steep angle of needle entry is preferred.

The main limitation of this technique is difficulty in visualizing the needle tip.

### In-plane (long axis)

This technique is commonly used for nerve blocks. The advantage is that the whole needle can be visualized, allowing very precise needle positioning and therefore predictable local anaesthetic spread. With in-plane needle imaging, the needle is in the same plane as the ultrasound beam, allowing the entire needle to be seen.

The main limitation of this technique is that maintaining alignment between the needle and the ultrasound beam can be difficult. The best needle images are achieved when the needle is at right angles to the ultrasound beam.

## Tips for maximizing the visibility of the needle

- Use a large gauge ultrasound needle – this offers greater reflection and visibility.
- Angle of approach – for out-of-plane needle insertion – steeper angles (>60°) improve visibility. For in-plane needle insertion, shallow angles of about 30° are best.
- When using the in-plane technique it is also advisable to insert the needle 1–2 cm or so away from the probe in order to allow a shallow-angled approach to the target structure and better visualization of the needle.
- Hydro-dissection – when the needle tip is close to the structure you are targeting, a small amount of saline or local anaesthetic can be injected, which opens up a space that can help identify the tissue planes and needle tip better.

## Improving your image

Depth: adjust the depth so that the target vessel or structure is centred in the image. Reducing the depth will decrease the field of view but will increase the resolution of the relevant structures.

Gain: gain adjusts the acoustic power of the transmitted signals and the amplification of the received signals. Undergaining results in the loss of low level echo signals such as a thrombus. Overgaining results in rescued contrast resolution and increased possibility of artefacts in otherwise 'echo free' areas.

## Central venous catheter insertion

Central venous catheter (CVC) insertion is a core skill for all anaesthetists. It is estimated that 200 000 CVCs are inserted annually in the NHS[1].

## Indications

- Intravenous access (especially if difficult peripheral access)
- Haemodynamic monitoring
- Infusions of irritant substances (e.g. vasoactive drugs, chemotherapy, total parenteral nutrition (TPN))
- Renal replacement therapy
- Transvenous pacing.

## Practicalities of CVC insertion

The principle of CVC insertion is the same regardless of the chosen insertion site; a Seldinger technique is used. The 2002 National Institute for Health and Care Excellence (NICE) guidelines recommend that ultrasound guidance should be used for all elective internal jugular CVC insertions. It is still, however, extremely important to know how to insert CVCs using landmark techniques in case of an emergency or in the event that ultrasound equipment is not readily available.

**Table 29.1** Advantages and disadvantages of CVC insertion sites

| CVC site | Advantages | Disadvantages |
|---|---|---|
| Internal jugular vein (IJV) | Relatively simple to insert<br>Lower risk of pneumothorax than SCV<br>Low infection rates<br>Site of choice in obesity | Less comfortable for patients than SCV |
| Subclavian vein (SCV) | Lowest infection risk<br>Comfortable for patients<br>Useful in trauma or patients with spinal immobilization | Harder to visualize SCV with USS – need to use axillary vein<br>Higher risk of pneumothorax – avoid in severe lung disease<br>Avoid in coagulopathy – unable to compress vessels easily<br>Venous stenosis – avoid in long-term dialysis patients |
| Femoral vein (FV) | Easy insertion, safer for novices to learn<br>Good flow rates for dialysis lines<br>Good choice in the coagulopathic patient<br>No risk of pneumothorax | Higher infection rate<br>Higher thrombosis rate<br>Limits patient mobility |

# Approaches and landmarks

## Internal jugular vein

Identify anatomy: carotid artery, thyroid cartilage, sternocleidomastoid muscle, clavicle

Insertion point:

> *High approach:* medial border of sternal head of sternocleidomastoid, just lateral to the carotid artery at the level of the thyroid cartilage.
> *Middle approach*: apex of triangle formed by the two heads of sternocleidomastoid muscle.
> *Low approach*: posterior border of the sternal head of sternocleidomastoid muscle.

Direct the needle towards the ipsilateral nipple at an angle of 45°. The vein is usually very superficial and only 0.5–2 cm under the skin.

Tips and advice
- Turn head to contralateral side, avoid excessive turning as it changes the relationship of the vein and artery and can collapse the vein.
- If you experience difficulty in cannulating the vein or it keeps collapsing:
  - Make sure you are not compressing the vein too much with the USS probe or your fingers
  - Put the patient more head down
  - Consider giving a fluid bolus
  - Ask the patient to hold their breath or do a Valsalva manoeuver.

## Subclavian vein

Identify anatomy: sternal notch and clavicle

Insertion point: 1 cm below the clavicle, at the junction of the medial third and middle third of the clavicle. Advance needle towards the sternal notch, guiding the needle under the clavicle. Some clinicians advocate identifying the clavicle initially by hitting it with the needle and then 'walking' the needle under the inferior border whilst keeping the needle as horizontal as possible to avoid the dome of the pleura.

Tips and advice
- Turn head to contralateral side.
- Place a rolled up towel or bag of fluids between the scapula to extend the spine.
- It you have difficulty locating the vein, ask an assistant to pull caudally on the ipsilateral arm.
- If you are unable to get beneath the clavicle consider starting more laterally and bending your needle upward slightly.
- If arterial puncture occurs, withdraw the needle and apply firm pressure both above and below the clavicle.
- If a chest drain is already in situ (e.g. following chest trauma) place the CVC on the same side.

### Femoral vein

Identify anatomy: inguinal ligament, femoral artery (the femoral vein lies medial to the artery)

Insertion point: palpate the femoral artery 2 cm below the inguinal ligament and insert the needle 1 cm medial to the pulsation and aim cephalad and slightly medially at an angle of 20–30° to the skin. In adults the vein is usually 2–4 cm below the skin.

Tips and advice
- The patient should be supine with a pillow under the buttocks to elevate the groin. The thigh should be abducted and externally rotated.
- It can be difficult to feel the arterial pulsation especially in obese patients. Get an assistant to retract the abdomen if this is a problem and recheck the landmarks.

## Complications

Early: haematoma; arrhythmia; accidental arterial puncture; pneumothorax; haemothorax; air embolism

Late: infection; thrombosis; vascular erosion

## Catheter tip position

The CVC tip should lie in the superior vena cava at the level of the carina on chest x-ray. If the CVC is within the right atrium it is in too far and should be withdrawn. Ideally the tip of the CVC should not abut the side of the vessel wall as this can lead to erosion of the vein wall.

## Spinal and epidural anaesthesia
### Anatomy (see Figure 29.1)
- The spinal cord terminates at L1–2 in the adult, L3 in children.
- Below this level the lumbar and sacral nerves form the cauda equina.
- The meninges (dura, arachnoid and pia mater) surround the spinal cord from the foramen magnum to S2 level.
- Dural cuffs extend laterally as far as intervertebral foraminae.

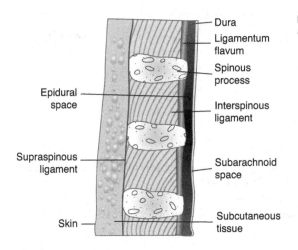

Dura
Ligamentum flavum
Spinous process
Epidural space
Interspinous ligament
Supraspinous ligament
Subarachnoid space
Skin
Subcutaneous tissue

**Figure 29.1** Anatomy of the subarachnoid and epidural space.

- There is a potential space between the dura and arachnoid mater – the subdural space; inadvertent injection into this space is a recognized complication of spinal and epidural injections.
- The epidural (extradural) space lies between the walls of the spinal canal and the spinal dural mater. It is a potential, low pressure space filled with fat, areolar tissue and the internal vertebral venous plexus.
- The ligamentum flavum links the vertebral laminae and is at its thickest in the lumbar region.

# Spinal

Indications
- Wide variety of elective and emergency surgery below the level of the umbilicus (T10).

Approaches and landmarks
- Sitting or lateral position with spine flexed.
- Line between iliac crests (Tuffier's line) passes across L4 and is used to locate L3–4 space, which is most commonly used.
- Midline and paramedian approaches can be used.
- Paramedian – 1–2 cm lateral to upper border of spinous process, insert needle perpendicular to skin and advance to contact bone (lamina), then withdraw and re-angle 15 degrees medially and 30 degrees cephalad to pass over lamina and enter interlaminar space.

Insertion
- Sterilize skin using 0.5% chlorhexidine spray and allow it to dry.
- Drape and use 1% lidocaine to skin if patient awake.
- Insert introducer needle at 90 degrees to skin in midline.
- Spinal needle passes through introducer into supraspinous and interspinous ligaments then the tougher ligamentum flavum and through the dura (see Figure 29.1).
- If bone is contacted withdraw and redirect needle, cephalad in first instance.
- Following dural puncture cerebrospinal fluid (CSF) should flow freely.

**Table 29.2** Volume of hyperbaric bupivacaine 0.5% to achieve desired block height

| Block height | Volume of drug |
|---|---|
| T6–T10 | 2.5–3 ml |
| T11–L1 | 2.5 ml |
| L2–L5 | 2.0 ml |
| S1–S5 | 1–1.5 ml |

Drugs

- Bupivacaine 0.5% heavy or plain. Plain produces a less reliable block and approximately 0.5 ml more volume is required for a similar level block.
- Ropivacaine not licenced for intrathecal use.
- Opioids commonly added are diamorphine 0.25–0.5 mg or fentanyl 10–25 mcg.

Tips and advice

- Position of patient and comfort of operator are key to success, do not be tempted to rush or compromise.
- Accurate identification of L3/4 space is difficult, 70% of clinicians are higher than they think.
- If a second space is attempted go down as level of termination of the conus is variable.
- Sitting position allows easier identification of the midline and gives higher CSF pressure so improves flow.
- Lateral position allows possibility of sedation.

# Epidural

Indications

- Anaesthesia in abdominal and lower limb surgery.
- Acute pain relief post-operatively in thoracic, abdominal or lower limb surgery, labour, trauma and for miscellaneous reasons (e.g. pancreatitis, ischaemic pain).
- Chronic pain states.

Approaches and landmarks

- Position as for spinal.
- Identify the appropriate vertebral space (use landmarks of Tuffier's line indicating spinous process of L4 or tip of scapula is level with T7 and count spaces to correct level).
- Midline/paramedian approaches can be used (as for spinal).

Insertion

- Prepare trolley (see Figure 29.2) and flush the catheter and filter with saline to ensure free passage.
- Clean, drape and infiltrate 1% lidocaine as for spinal. You can use slightly more lidocaine and use the injecting needle to seek the space and infiltrate local into the interspinous ligaments.
- Insert the Tuohy needle in the direction indicated, the higher the level the more cephalad the angle is likely to be. When resistance becomes more obvious remove the trocar.

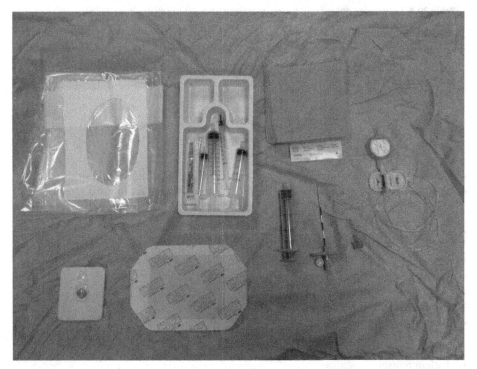

**Figure 29.2** Epidural trolley. Photograph taken by Dr Sam Salib. Reproduced with his kind permission.

- Attach the loss of resistance syringe filled with saline (or air) and carefully advance into ligamentum flavum, constantly checking for loss of resistance as the needle is advanced through the ligament.
- On loss of resistance immobilize the Tuohy and check no blood or CSF flows from the Tuohy needle.
- Note the depth and insert the catheter generously.
- Remove the Tuohy over the catheter and pull back to leave 4–5 cm in the space.
- Check for absence of blood or CSF and look for a meniscal drop.
- Fix the catheter to the skin with a sterile see-through dressing to allow site inspection.
- Fix catheter well up back and over shoulder.

Drugs
- Opioids commonly added are diamorphine 2.5–5 mg or fentanyl 50–100 mcg.

Tips and advice
- Many factors affect spread of epidural solutions; therefore, an understanding of these allow manipulation of the block.
- Drug mass is critical and more important than volume, for a given mass a larger volume will spread more.
- Epidural space increases in volume in a caudal direction so larger volumes are required to achieve the same dermatomal cover the lower the epidural is sited.

**Table 29.3** Dose of local anaesthetic required to achieve either lumbosacral or thoracolumbar block

| Block height (for epidural at L3–4) | Drug | Volume |
|---|---|---|
| Lumbosacral | Lidocaine 2% | 20–25 ml |
| | Bupivacaine 0.5% | 20 ml |
| | Bupivacaine 0.75% | 10–15 ml |
| | Ropivacaine 0.75% | 20–25 ml |
| Thoracolumbar | Lidocaine 2% | 25–30 ml |
| | Bupivacaine 0.5% | 20–25 ml |
| | Bupivacaine 0.75% | 15–20 ml |
| | Ropivacaine 0.75% | 15–25 ml |

- Smaller volumes may be needed in age >40, pregnancy and morbid obesity.
- Position can be used to manipulate the block, sitting will reduce upward spread.

## Contraindications to central neuraxial blockade

Relative

- Aortic stenosis
- History of back surgery
- Systemic sepsis
- Neurological disease

Absolute

- Patient refusal
- Anticoagulation
- Local sepsis.

## Complications of central neuraxial blockade[2,3] (See Chapter 34 for NAP3 summary)

- Hypotension, urinary retention, bradycardia are physiological consequences and should be managed appropriately but if profound lead to nausea and vomiting and faintness.
- Itching is common (1:3–10) with intrathecal opioid.

**Table 29.4** Complications of central neuraxial blockade

| Complication | Incidence |
|---|---|
| Post-dural puncture headache | 1:100 |
| Following dural tap (with 16G Touhy in obstetric population) | 7:10 |
| Failed block | 1:100 |
| Epidural abscess | 1:47 000 |
| Meningitis | 1:200 000 |
| Vertebral canal haematoma | 1:117 000 |
| Transient neurological symptoms | 3:100 |
| Spinal cord damage | 1:100 000 |

# Percutaneous dilatational tracheostomy

Percutaneous dilatational tracheostomy (PDT) has become a well-established procedure on the intensive care unit (ICU) for patients requiring prolonged invasive mechanical ventilation. Tracheostomy offers a number of potential benefits such as increased patient comfort, reduced sedation requirement and a decrease in dead space, all of which may aid the weaning process[4].

## Indications

- To maintain the airway; e.g. reduced level of consciousness, upper airway obstruction, intubation difficulties
- To provide some protection to the airway; e.g. bulbar palsy
- For bronchial toilet; e.g. excessive secretions/inadequate cough
- For weaning from IPPV; e.g. patient comfort, reduction of sedation.

## Landmarks

The tracheostomy is usually inserted at the level of the second and third tracheal rings, which can usually be found at the midway point between the cricoid cartilage and the sternal notch. Many operators will perform the tracheal puncture under bronchoscopic guidance to ensure adequate positioning and to avoid puncture of the posterior tracheal wall.

## Percutaneous tracheostomy kits

The method for PDT insertion involves using a Seldinger-based technique first described by Ciaglia in 1985[5]. A needle is inserted through the neck into the trachea followed by a guide-wire through the needle. The needle is removed and a white plastic sheath is positioned over the wire to act as a guide for the dilators and prevent the guide-wire becoming kinked. A series of dilators are used until the stoma is sufficiently dilated to pass a tracheostomy tube loaded onto a dilator into the trachea. The correct placement of the tracheostomy tube should be confirmed with EtCO$_2$ and/or bronchoscopy.

In the UK, a modification of the Ciaglia technique using a single tapered dilator is the most commonly used technique[6] (see Figure 29.3). A newer method called the balloon dilation technique involves similar steps to the serial dilation technique but instead of a curved dilator a pressurized balloon is used to dilate the trachea to allow passage of the tracheostomy tube (see Figure 29.3).

## Types of tracheostomy

Cuffed or uncuffed: cuffed tubes are necessary when positive-pressure ventilation is required or the airway needs protecting from aspiration from oral or gastric secretions.

Fenestrated or unfenestrated: fenestrated tubes have an opening on the outer cannula, which allows air to pass through the patient's oral/nasal pharynx. Fenestrated tubes allow the patient to speak and cough more effectively.

Adjustable flange: may be used in obese patients or patients with large necks where an extended proximal length of the tracheostomy tube is required to get enough of the tube inside the airway.

Patient Name .........................................

D.O.B ..................................................

Hospital Number ...................................

(Attach Addressograph label)

University Hospital NHS
of South Manchester
NHS Foundation Trust

| AICU Percutaneous Tracheostomy Insertion | | Airway | Dr |
| --- | --- | --- | --- |
| | | Tracheostomy | Dr |

| Indication for tracheostomy | |
| --- | --- |
| Discussion with patient / relatives | |
| USS neck | |

| Clotting / Anticoagulants checked | | LA + 1:200,000 adrenaline | |
| --- | --- | --- | --- |
| NG feed off / aspirated | | Aseptic technique | |
| Difficult upper airway? | | Bronchoscopy guided | |
| FiO₂ | | ETCO₂ present | |
| PEEP | | Tracheostomy sutured | |
| Pinsp | | Inner tube replaced | |

| Tracheal ring level and position of tracheostomy insertion | |
| --- | --- |

Additional documentation and complications here and on reverse
.................................................................................................................
.................................................................................................................
.................................................................................................................
.................................................................................................................

| CXR required? | Result: |
| --- | --- |

| Tracheostomy size | |
| --- | --- |
| Emergency bed head sign complete | |

| Signature | |
| --- | --- |
| Print | |
| Designation | |
| Date | |

Attach Bronchoscope sterilisation sticker here

**Figure 29.3** University Hospital of South Manchester Percutaneous Tracheostomy Insertion Checklist. Reproduced with kind permission from the Intensive Care Society.

Inner tube/no inner tube: the Intensive Care Society recommends the use of tracheostomies with inner tubes where possible owing to the reduction in problems with tube obstruction[7].The disadvantage of tracheostomies with inner tubes is the reduced internal diameter and its implications for air flow.

The Manchester Tracheostomy Checklist (Figure 29.3) is a useful aide memoire for the procedure[8]. It is included in the Intensive Care Society tracheostomy standards document 2014.

# Skin antisepsis for central neuraxial blockade (CNB)[9]

Guidance was issued in 2014 following case reports that implicated chlorhexidine in the causation of permanent neurological injury and a survey that demonstrated a wide variation in practice. An expert Working Party consisting of members of the Association of Anaesthetists of Great Britain and Ireland (AAGBI) with representatives from the Obstetric Anaesthetists' Association (OAA), Regional Anaesthesia UK (RAUK) and the Association of Paediatric Anaesthetists of Great Britain and Ireland (APAGBI) reviewed the evidence on the commonly available solutions and made consensus recommendations specifically relating to skin asepsis for CNB.

**Key points from the guideline are as follows:**

Recommended aseptic technique for CNB includes:
- Thorough hand washing with surgical scrub
- Wearing cap, mask, gown and gloves
- Use of a large sterile drape
- 0.5% chlorhexidine in alcohol.

Why 0.5% chlorhexidine in alcohol?

Studies have shown it is more effective than povidone iodine in terms of speed of onset (faster) and duration of action (longer). It also remains effective in the presence of blood and is associated with fewer skin reactions. Chlorhexidine in alcohol has superior antibacterial action than the aqueous preparation. There is lack of evidence that 2% chlorhexidine is more effective than 0.5%, but there is evidence that it is more neurotoxic. Therefore it should not be used.

How to use it safely
Measures must be taken to prevent chlorhexidine reaching the CSF. These include:
- Keeping it away from drugs and equipment
- Not pouring into containers near the same surface as equipment
- Covering equipment while it is applied by swab, applicator or spray
- Allowing solution to dry before starting the procedure (which includes palpating the surface anatomy)
- Gloves should be checked and changed if contaminated.

Use in paediatrics
The minimum volume necessary to ensure antisepsis should be used in children under 2 months.

# STOP before you block

## Notice for anaesthetists and anaesthetic assistants

- A STOP moment must take place immediately before inserting the block needle

- The anaesthetist and anaesthetic assistant must double-check:
    - the surgical site marking
    - the site and side of the block

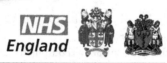

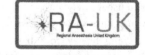

SAFE ANAESTHESIA LIAISON GROUP

Nottingham University Hospitals NHS NHS Trust

**Figure 29.4** Stop before you block poster. Reproduced here with permission from The Safe Anaesthesia Liaison Group and P. Townsley, J. Maybin, J. French, N. Bhandal, N. Bedforth of Nottingham University Hospitals NHS Trust (http://www.respond2articles.com/ANA/forums/post/851.aspx).

The working party acknowledged the three commonly used methods of application: solution with gallipot and sponges, pre-soaked applicator sponges and multiuse spray. They discussed the potential for crossover error and contamination of equipment and did not make any specific recommendation. They noted that pre-soaked applicator sponges are currently only available containing 2% chlorhexidine solution and acknowledged work that demonstrated that a single spray achieved skin sterilization.

## Stop before you block

Inadvertent wrong-sided peripheral nerve blocks were highlighted by the Safe Anaesthesia Liaison Group (SALG) in an alert in 2010[10]. Although not classified as a 'Never Event' by the National Patient Safety Agency they have potentially serious consequences. Review of experience demonstrated that wrong-sided blocks were occurring even with appropriate marking of the surgical site and adherence to the World Health Organization sign-in procedure.

SALG and RAUK introduced the Stop Before You Block campaign in 2011. Based on an initiative from Nottingham University Hospitals this national campaign is endorsed by The Royal College of Anaesthetists and the AAGBI.

The Stop Before You Block process[11]:

1. Perform **WHO 'sign-in'** as usual.
2. **Vigilance** when:
   - There are distractions in the anaesthetic room
   - There is delay between 'Sign in' and performance of the block
   - After turning the patient, the block site will have 'moved' relative to the anaesthetist
   - Lower limb blocks are performed as surgical marking may not be visible
   - Operator does not regularly perform regional anaesthesia.
3. A **'STOP' moment occurs IMMEDIATELY before insertion of the nerve block needle.** Initiated by any member of the team, the anaesthetist and anaesthetic assistant double-check the surgical site marking and the side of the block by:
   - Visualizing the surgical arrow indicating site of surgery
   - Asking the conscious patient to confirm side of surgery or in the unconscious patient, checking the consent form for operative side.

The campaign promotes a standardized poster for display, and encourages local additions to the process and audit of uptake. This is shown in Figure 29.4.

## References

1. The National Institute for Clinical Excellence (NICE). Guidance on the use of ultrasound locating devices for placing central venous catheters (NICE technology appraisal No. 49). London: NICE, 2002.
2. http://www.labourpains.com/assets/_managed/cms/files/InfoforMothers/REGIONAL-ANAESTHESIA/Feb%2015%20Regional%20Anaesthesia%20for%20CS%20English-1.pdf (accessed 2 January 2016).
3. M. C. Dale, M. R. Checketts. Complications of regional anaesthesia. *Anaesth Intensive Care Med* 2014; 14(4): 142–5.
4. http://ceaccp.oxfordjournals.org/content/early/2014/01/02/bjaceaccp.mkt068.full#T3 (accessed 11 September 2015).

5. P. Ciaglia, R. Firsching, C. Syniec. Elective percutaneous dilatational tracheostomy. A new and simple bedside procedure; preliminary report. *Chest* 1985; 87: 715–19.

6. T. Veenith, S. Ganeshamoorthy, T. Standley, J. Carter, P. Young. Intensive care unit tracheostomy: a snapshot of UK practice. *Int Arch Med* 2008; 1: 21–7.

7. A. Bodenham, D. Bell, S. Bonner, et al. Standards for the care of adult patients with a temporary tracheostomy; standards and guidelines. London: Intensive Care Society Standards, 2014. Available at http://www.ics.ac.uk/ics-homepage/guidelines-and-standards/ (accessed 28 February 2015)

8. G. Rajendran, S. Hutchinson. Checklist for percutaneous tracheostomy in critical care. *Crit Care* 2014; 18(2): 425.

9. Association of Anaesthetists of Great Britain and Ireland. Safety guideline: skin asepsis for central neuraxial blockade. *Anaesthesia* 2014; 69(11): 1279–86. doi: 10.1111/anae.12844.

10. Safe Anaesthesia Liason Group. Wrong Site Blocks During Surgery. London: National Patient Safety Agency, 2011. Available at http://www.aagbi.org/sites/default/files/SALG_statement_WSB_10_11_10.pdf (accessed 29 March 2015).

11. Royal College of Anaesthetists http://www.rcoa.ac.uk/sites/default/files/SBYB-SupportingInfo .pdf (accessed 29 March 2015).

**Chapter**

# 30

# Resuscitation algorithms

Emily Johnson and Anna Pierson

*Anaesthetists are often called to be involved in resuscitation attempts. It is therefore essential you are familiar with the most recent resuscitation guidelines prior to returning to work. Many may choose to attend resuscitation courses in order to prepare for this responsibility; however, this represents a significant time and expense commitment making it unfeasible for all, in which case running through the guidelines below should help your preparations.*

## Adult advanced life support

As anaesthetists it is both required and expected of us that we are able to manage life-threatening situations either in those patients who are peri-arrest, or those in whom cardiac arrest has already occurred. Anaesthetists make a considerable contribution to resuscitation services within a hospital and are heavily involved in the assessment and management of critically ill patients, with the aim of preventing cardiac arrest[1]. Having an advanced life support (ALS) qualification is mandatory, therefore even if your certification is valid, it is worth revising the main algorithms before you return to work. Although the principles will obviously be familiar, a reminder of the flowsheet will help to guide you. On occasion, we may be required to lead the resuscitation attempt and, at the very least, are in a good position to view the situation as a whole.

The UK Resuscitation Council makes regular updates to ALS material, and guidelines change every few years. Notably, the most recent change was made in October 2015. The main adaptations are highlighted in the algorithms in Figures 30.1 to 30.4. Latest updates and additions can be found at www.resus.org.uk[2].

## Paediatric advanced life support

It is a rare and stressful occasion when anaesthetists are required to administer paediatric life support. However, it is valuable to refresh your knowledge of the paediatric life support guidelines prior to a return to work. A paediatric list may be something you feel apprehensive about on your return, and any steps you can take to make this experience more comfortable will have a positive impact on your confidence and most likely on the patient's and parents' experience too.

*Returning to Work in Anaesthesia*, ed. Emma Plunkett, Emily Johnson and Anna Pierson.
Published by Cambridge University Press. © Cambridge University Press 2016.

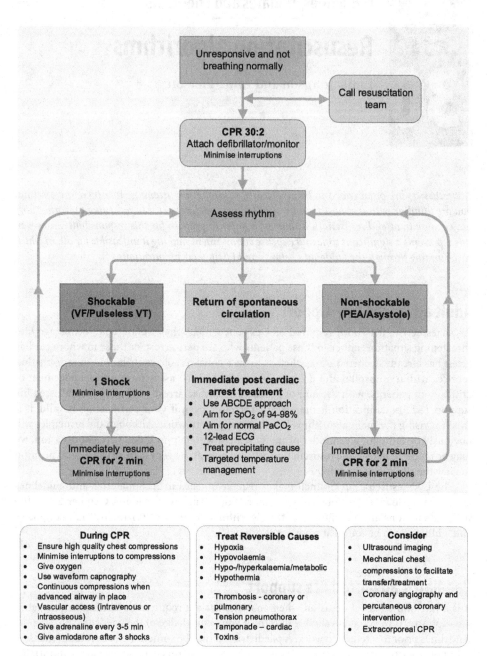

**Figure 30.1** Adult Advance Life Support algorithm. Reproduced with the kind permission of the Resuscitation Council (UK).

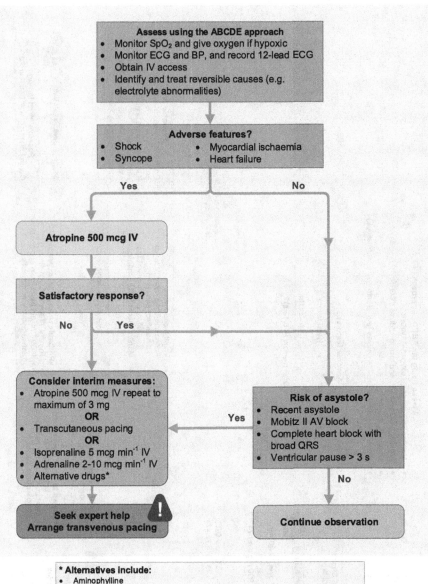

**Figure 30.2** Adult Bradycardia Algorithm. Reproduced with the kind permission of the Resuscitation Council (UK).

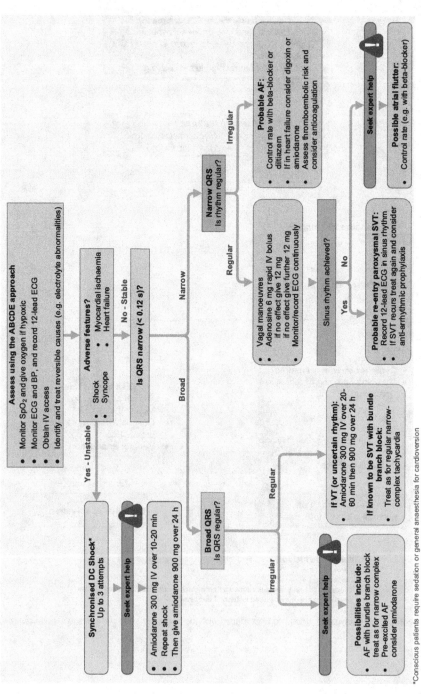

**Assess using the ABCDE approach**
- Monitor SpO₂ and give oxygen if hypoxic
- Monitor ECG and BP, and record 12-lead ECG
- Obtain IV access
- Identify and treat reversible causes (e.g. electrolyte abnormalities)

**Adverse features?**
- Shock
- Syncope
- Myocardial ischaemia
- Heart failure

**Yes - Unstable**

**Synchronised DC Shock***
Up to 3 attempts

Seek expert help

- Amiodarone 300 mg IV over 10-20 min
- Repeat shock
- Then give amiodarone 900 mg over 24 h

**No - Stable**

**Is QRS narrow (< 0.12 s)?**

**Broad**

**Narrow**

**Broad QRS**
Is QRS regular?

**Irregular**

Seek expert help

**Possibilities include:**
- AF with bundle branch block treat as for narrow complex
- Pre-excited AF consider amiodarone

**Regular**

**If VT (or uncertain rhythm):**
- Amiodarone 300 mg IV over 20-60 min then 900 mg over 24 h

**If known to be SVT with bundle branch block:**
- Treat as for regular narrow-complex tachycardia

**Narrow QRS**
Is rhythm regular?

**Regular**

**Vagal manoeuvres**
- Adenosine 6 mg rapid IV bolus if no effect give 12 mg if no effect give further 12 mg
- Monitor/record ECG continuously

**Sinus rhythm achieved?**

**Yes**

**No**

**Probable re-entry paroxysmal SVT:**
- Record 12-lead ECG in sinus rhythm
- If SVT recurs treat again and consider anti-arrhythmic prophylaxis

**Irregular**

**Probable AF:**
- Control rate with beta-blocker or diltiazem
- If in heart failure consider digoxin or amiodarone
- Assess thromboembolic risk and consider anticoagulation

Seek expert help

**Possible atrial flutter:**
- Control rate (e.g. with beta-blocker)

*Conscious patients require sedation or general anaesthesia for cardioversion

**Figure 30.3** Adult Tachycardia Algorithm. Reproduced with the kind permission of the Resuscitation Council (UK).

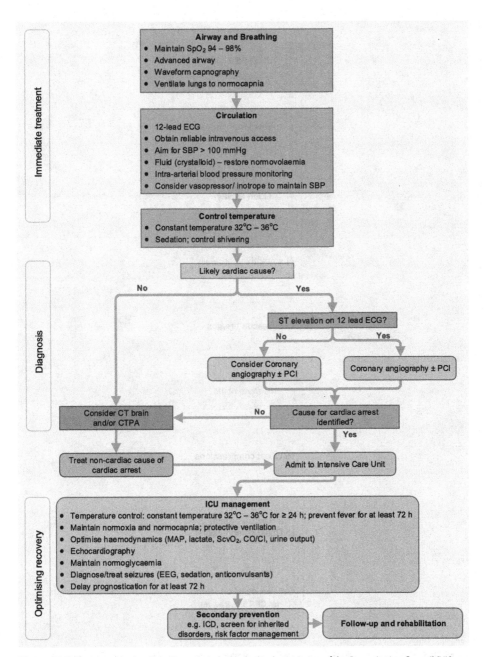

**Immediate treatment**

**Airway and Breathing**
- Maintain $SpO_2$ 94 – 98%
- Advanced airway
- Waveform capnography
- Ventilate lungs to normocapnia

**Circulation**
- 12-lead ECG
- Obtain reliable intravenous access
- Aim for SBP > 100 mmHg
- Fluid (crystalloid) – restore normovolaemia
- Intra-arterial blood pressure monitoring
- Consider vasopressor/ inotrope to maintain SBP

**Control temperature**
- Constant temperature 32°C – 36°C
- Sedation; control shivering

**Diagnosis**

Likely cardiac cause?

No / Yes

ST elevation on 12 lead ECG?

No → Consider Coronary angiography ± PCI

Yes → Coronary angiography ± PCI

Consider CT brain and/or CTPA ← No ← Cause for cardiac arrest identified?

Yes

Treat non-cardiac cause of cardiac arrest → Admit to Intensive Care Unit

**Optimising recovery**

**ICU management**
- Temperature control: constant temperature 32°C – 36°C for ≥ 24 h; prevent fever for at least 72 h
- Maintain normoxia and normocapnia; protective ventilation
- Optimise haemodynamics (MAP, lactate, $ScvO_2$, CO/CI, urine output)
- Echocardiography
- Maintain normoglycaemia
- Diagnose/treat seizures (EEG, sedation, anticonvulsants)
- Delay prognostication for at least 72 h

**Secondary prevention**
e.g. ICD, screen for inherited disorders, risk factor management → **Follow-up and rehabilitation**

**Figure 30.4** Post-resuscitation Care. Reproduced with the kind permission of the Resuscitation Council (UK).

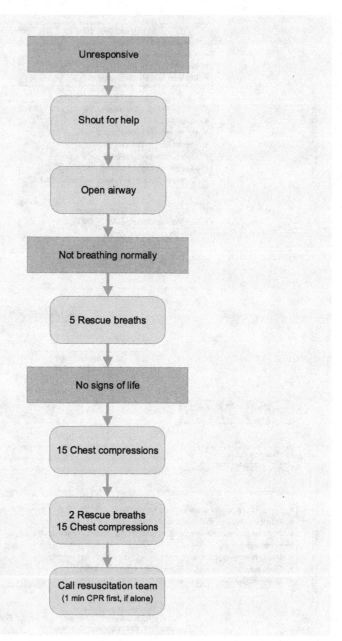

**Figure 30.5** Paediatric Basic Life Support algorithm. Reproduced with the kind permission of the Resuscitation Council (UK).

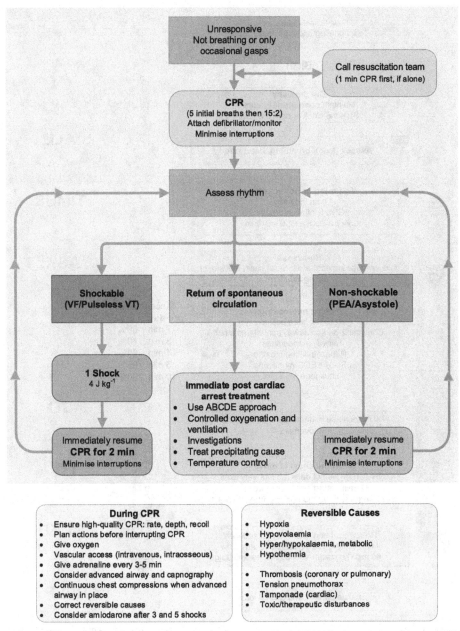

**Figure 30.6** Paediatric Advanced Life Support algorithm. Reproduced with the kind permission of the Resuscitation Council (UK).

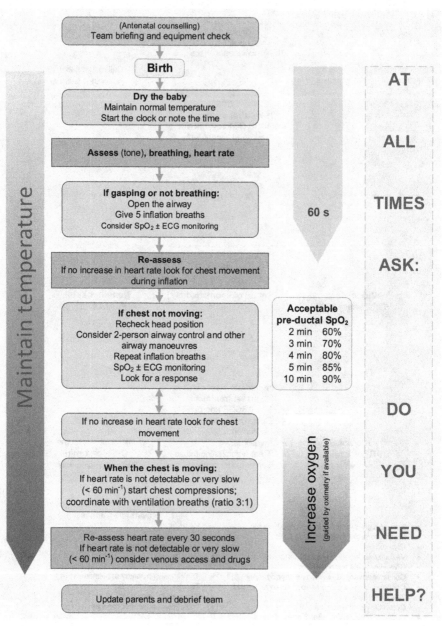

**Figure 30.7** Newborn Life Support algorithm. Reproduced with the kind permission of the Resuscitation Council (UK).

**Table 30.1** WETFLAG mnemonic

| WETFLAG | Doses | Example for a 1 year old 10 kg child |
|---|---|---|
| Weight*<br>Birth<br>1–12 months<br>1–5 yr<br>5–12 yr | 3–3.5 kg<br>(age in months/2)+4<br>(age in years×2)+8<br>(age in years×3)+7 | <br><br>10 kg<br>10 kg<br> |
| Energy for defibrillation | 4 J/kg | 40 J |
| Tracheal tube size:<br>Internal diameter<br>Length (oral) | <br>Age/4+4<br>Age/2+12 | <br>4 mm uncuffed<br>12 cm at lips |
| Fluid bolus (crystalloid) | 10–20 ml/kg | 100–200 ml |
| Lorazepam dose for seizures** | 0.1 mg/kg | 1 mg |
| Adrenaline dose for CPR iv/io | 0.01 mg/kg | 0.1 mg |
| Glucose 10% dose iv/io | 2 ml/kg | 20 ml |

\* Resuscitation council guidelines suggest (age in years + 4) x2 from age 1 upwards.
\*\* Some versions miss this out, using "FL" for fluids.

For the infrequent paediatric anaesthetist, or even the experienced paediatric anaesthetist returning to work after a break, it is worth considering some emergency calculations for every case undertaken. The WETFAG mnemonic is a well-accepted method of doing this and is also frequently used in A&E departments when a paediatric admission is expected. This is shown in Table 30.1.

The paediatric basic and advanced life support algorithms are shown in Figures 30.5 to 30.7. In addition the newborn life support algorithm is included as it is sometimes required of the anaesthetist to assist with a newborn resuscitation, especially in cases where intubation is proving difficult. Although there will generally be a paediatrician present leading the resuscitation it is useful to revise the principles.

# References

1. J. Nolan, J. Soar. ACSA References: Guidelines for the Provision of Anaesthetic Services; Anaesthesia services for resuscitation 2015 (Chapter 8). Available at https://www.rcoa.ac.uk/system/files/GPAS-2015-08-RESUSCIT.pdf (accessed 1 August 2015).
2. Resuscitation guidelines. London: Resuscitation Council, 2015. www.resus.org.uk/resuscitation-guidelines/ (accessed 4 January 2016).

# Intensive care guidelines

Laura Tulloch and Emily Johnson

*The aim of this chapter is to group together some of the intensive care guidelines you may need to refer to in your first few weeks back at work. It is made up of useful, recent or well-recognized guidelines including the surviving sepsis guidelines and those for emergency intubation outside theatre. In addition there is information on paediatric retrieval services, management of traumatic brain injury and safe tracheostomy management. This should allow quick reference or more in-depth consideration in conjunction with other related sections of the book.*

## Surviving Sepsis Campaign guidelines

The Surviving Sepsis Campaign (SSC) is a collaboration of international critical care societies committed to reducing mortality from severe sepsis and septic shock. The SSC produced their 3rd edition of the SSC guidelines in 2012[1]. A recent study has shown that compliance with the SSC care bundles is associated with a 25% relative risk reduction in mortality[2].

The SSC guidelines are summarized below:

Initial resuscitation
*Within 3 hours*

- Measure lactate level
- Take blood cultures
- Give broad-spectrum antibiotics
- Consider whether there is adequate source control
- Give a fluid challenge (up to 30 ml/kg) crystalloid if hypotensive or lactate >4

*Within 6 hours*
In non-fluid responders – initiate goal-directed therapy (Grade 1C)

- Mean arterial pressure (MAP) > 65 mmHg
- Central venous pressure (CVP) 8–12 mmHg
- Aim for central venous or mixed venous saturation 70% or 65% respectively
- Urine output >0.5 ml/kg/h

Haemodynamic support and adjunctive therapy
**Fluid therapy**

- Crystalloid is the initial fluid choice (Grade 1B)
- Avoid use of hydroxyethyl starches (Grade 1B)
- Consider using albumin when substantial amounts of crystalloids used (Grade 2C)

*Returning to Work in Anaesthesia*, ed. Emma Plunkett, Emily Johnson and Anna Pierson.
Published by Cambridge University Press. © Cambridge University Press 2016.

## Vasopressors

- Noradrenaline first-line agent (Grade 1C)
- Consider adding in adrenaline or vasopressin if required (Grade 2B)
- Low dose dopamine should not be used for renal protection (Grade 1A)

## Inotropic therapy

- Use dobutamine if evidence of low cardiac output state/hypoperfusion despite adequate MAP (Grade 1C)

## Corticosteroids

- Only use steroids if fluid resuscitation and vasopressor therapy are unable to restore haemodynamic stability (Grade 2C)

## Other supportive therapy

## Blood products

- Transfusion trigger of Hb < 70 g/l in the absence of extenuating circumstances (myocardial ischaemia, acute haemorrhage, ischaemic heart disease) (Grade 1B)
- Maintain platelets $>10 \times 10^9$/l in the absence of bleeding (Grade 2D)

## Immunoglobulins

- Not recommended (Grade 2B)

## Selenium

- Not recommended (Grade 2C)

## Mechanical ventilation in sepsis-induced acute respiratory distress syndrome (ARDS)

- Low tidal volume (6 ml/kg) (Grade 1A)
- High positive end-expiratory pressure (PEEP) strategy (Grade 1B)
- 30–45 degree head up to prevent ventilator-associated pneumonia (Grade 1B)
- Consider prone position if $PaO_2/FiO_2 < 100$ (Grade 2B)
- Conservative fluid strategy rather than liberal in patients with no evidence of tissue hypoperfusion (Grade 1C)

## Sedation, analgesia and paralysis

- Short course of non-depolarizing muscle relaxants of no greater than 48 hours for patients with early ARDS and $PaO_2/FiO_2 < 150$ mmHg (Grade 2C)

## Glucose control

- Start an insulin sliding scale if two measurements of blood glucose >10 mmol/l (Grade 1A)

## Deep vein thrombosis prophylaxis

- If there are no contraindications patients should receive low molecular weight heparin (LMWH) and pneumatic compression devices wherever possible (Grade 2C)

## Stress ulcer prophylaxis/nutrition

- Use $H_2$ blocker or proton pump inhibitor in those with bleeding risk factors (Grade 1B)
- Administer oral/enteral feed as tolerated within the first 48 hours (Grade 2C).

## The Sepsis Six

Survive Sepsis is a UK Sepsis Trust initiative that has produced a set of interventions which can be delivered by any junior doctor within 1 hour – the Sepsis Six[3]. The principle of this initiative is doing simple things to make a big difference:

1. **Administer high-flow oxygen**
2. **Take blood cultures**
3. **Give broad-spectrum antibiotics**
4. **Give intravenous fluid challenges**
5. **Measure serum lactate and haemoglobin**
6. **Measure accurate hourly urine output.**

# Emergency intubation outside theatre

Emergency intubation in the emergency department (ED) or on ICU can be a life-saving intervention. It is well recognized that emergency intubation outside of the theatre environment can be more technically difficult and have a higher rate of complications. In the 4th National Audit Project (NAP4) audit, nearly 20% of all of the airway incidents occurred in the ICU[4]. Another study found that 28% of patients undergoing emergency intubation suffered life-threatening complications such as hypotension or hypoxaemia[5].

There are obvious technical differences between intubating a starved, elective, ASA 1 patient and intubating a critically unwell trauma victim with unstable physiology and facial fractures; however, it is often how you manage the non-technical factors that can make the biggest impact. Non-technical factors such as situational awareness, equipment issues, having less experienced assistance and an unfamiliar environment can make a difficult situation much worse. For this reason you should find out where the difficult intubation trolley and emergency drugs (including sugammadex) are kept in the ED/ICU when starting a new job and familiarize yourself with the equipment.

One of the key recommendations from the NAP4 audit was the implementation of a checklist for all ICU/ED intubations. This is not a new concept; a pre-intubation checklist has been used successfully in pre-hospital care and in settings where non-anaesthetists routinely intubate in ED/ICU.

An example of a pre-intubation checklist which has been developed by the Safer Intubation Project[6] is shown in Figure 31.1.

# Paediatric intensive care retrieval services

Whether you are a career paediatric anaesthetist or not, if you work in a centre without an on-site paediatric intensive care unit (PICU) it is likely that you will be called to assist if a critically ill child presents to your hospital.

Anaesthetic involvement is usually required to help stabilize critically ill babies and children and initiate intensive care prior to their transfer to a PICU. This can be a daunting task, especially if several years have passed since your last paediatric attachment, or your exposure to very sick children has been limited.

In general, paediatric intensive care transfer teams will undertake transfer of critically ill children to specialist centres. There will be an expectation, however, that you should start stabilizing the child prior to the transfer team's arrival. Often the transfer team can offer excellent clinical advice and support prior to their arrival; many have websites that contain

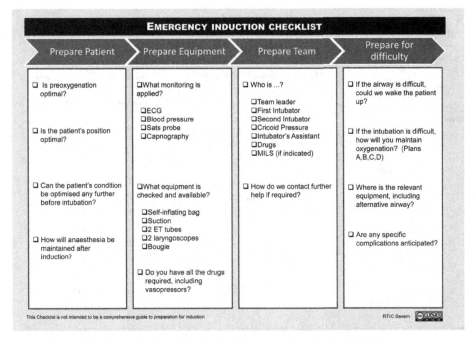

**Figure 31.1** Safer Intubation Checklist. Reproduced with permission from Tim Bowles, RTIC.

useful resources such as clinical guidelines, drug calculators, checklists and even apps that you can download that may prove invaluable.

An example of a checklist developed by the KIDS retrieval service for a ventilated child is shown in Figure 31.2[7].

## Useful resources/websites

| | |
|---|---|
| www.kids.bch.nhs.uk | Kids Intensive Care and Decision Support |
| | Birmingham Children's Hospital |
| www.cats.nhs.uk | Children's Acute Transfer Service |
| | Great Ormond Street Hospital |
| http://www.strs.nhs.uk | South Thames Retrieval Service |
| | Evelina Children's Hospital, located at St Thomas' Hospital |
| http://www.sort.nhs.uk | Southampton Oxford Retrieval Team |
| | Southampton General Hospital and the Radcliffe Hospital |
| http://www.nwts.nhs.uk | North West & North Wales Paediatric Transport Service |
| | Royal Manchester Children's Hospital and Alder Hey Children's Hospital |
| http://www.sheffieldchildrens.nhs.uk | Embrace transfer service for Yorkshire and the Humber |
| | Sheffield Children's Hospital |

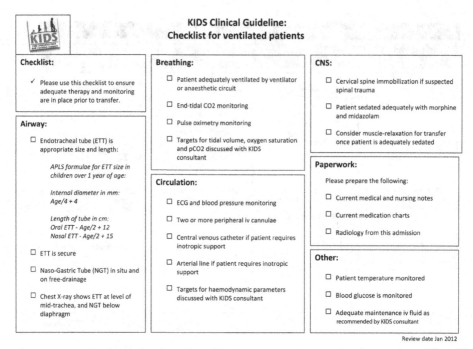

**Figure 31.2** Checklist for ventilated patients. Reproduced with permission from Kids Intensive Care and Decision Support, Birmingham Children's Hospital.

# Management of patients with traumatic brain injury

The principles of management of traumatic brain injury are important to all anaesthetists and have been covered in questions included in Chapters 7 and 16. A useful algorithm has been developed by St George's neurocritical care unit[8] and is shown in Figure 31.3. This should aid management of patients with head injuries.

# National Tracheostomy Safety Project Guidelines

Patients with tracheostomies are not only commonplace in the ICU, but many are now managed in the ward environment. The NAP4 audit found that tracheostomy complications were attributable to half of all airway-related deaths and cases of brain damage in critical care.

The National Confidential Enquiry into Patient Outcome and Death (NCEPOD) published a report (On the Right Trach?) in 2014 which reviewed care received by patients who underwent tracheostomy insertion. One of the principal recommendations was that bedside staff caring for tracheostomy patients must be competent in recognizing and managing common airway complications, including tube obstruction or displacement[9].

The National Tracheostomy Safety Project (NTSP) is a UK-based group that was developed to improve the management and care of patients with tracheostomies. The NTSP have developed educational resources and emergency guidelines for all healthcare professionals to follow in the event of an airway problem in both laryngectomy patients and those with tracheostomies[10].

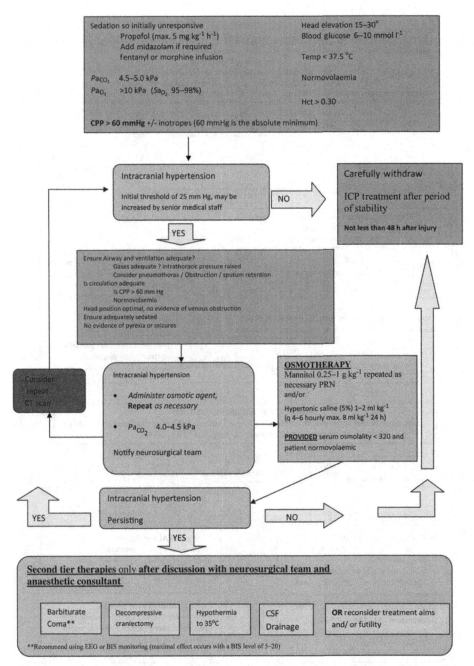

**Figure 31.3** Management algorithm for patients with severe traumatic brain injury. Reproduced with permission from Oxford University Press and Dr Judith Dinsmore.

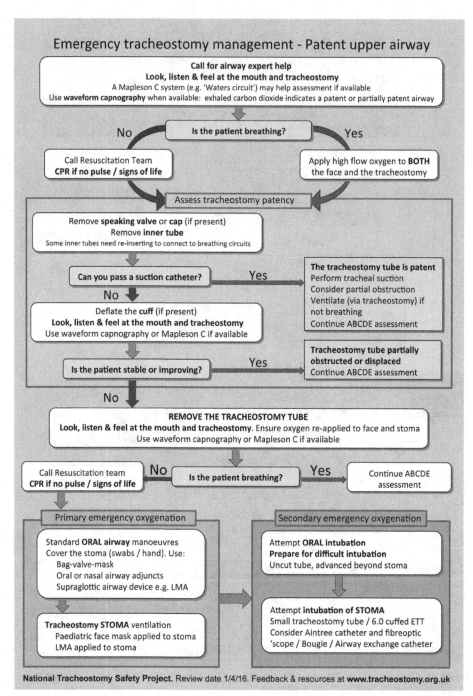

**Figure 31.4** Emergency tracheostomy management. Reproduced from McGrath B. A., Bates L., Atkinson D., Moore J. A. Multidisciplinary guidelines for the management of tracheostomy and laryngectomy airway emergencies. *Anaesthesia.* 2012 Jun 26. doi: 10.1111/j.1365–2044.2012.07217, with permission from the Association of Anaesthetists of Great Britain & Ireland/Blackwell Publishing Ltd.

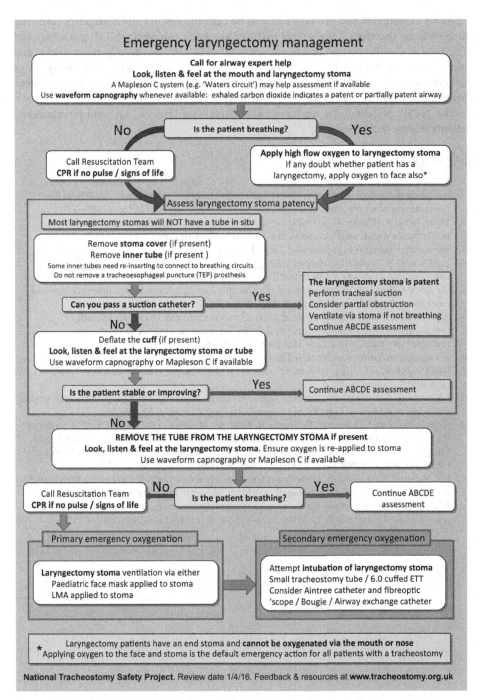

**Figure 31.5** Laryngectomy algorithm. Reproduced from McGrath B. A., Bates L., Atkinson D., Moore J. A. Multidisciplinary guidelines for the management of tracheostomy and laryngectomy airway emergencies. *Anaesthesia*. 2012 Jun 26. doi: 10.1111/j.1365–2044.2012.07217, with permission from the Association of Anaesthetists of Great Britain & Ireland/Blackwell Publishing Ltd.

As an anaesthetist you are very likely to be called to help at any emergency involving these patients, therefore it is essential that you know the emergency NTSP guidelines and are able to deal with common problems such as tube blockage and dislodgement quickly and safely. The guidelines highlight early use of oxygen on the stoma and the face, early use of capnography and connection to a Mapleson C circuit. This may be obvious, but remember that it is impossible to orally intubate a patient with a laryngectomy.

The NTSP guidelines for tracheostomy emergencies (Figure 31.4) and laryngectomy patients (Figure 31.5) are shown[11].

## References

1. R. P. Dellinger, M. M. Levy, A. Rhodes et al. Surviving Sepsis Campaign Guidelines Committee including the Pediatric Subgroup. Surviving sepsis campaign: international guidelines for management of severe sepsis and septic shock: 2012. *Crit Care Med* 2013; 41: 580–637.
2. M. M. Levy, A. Rhodes, G. S. Phillips et al. Surviving sepsis campaign: association between performance metrics and outcomes in a 7.5-year study. *Crit Care Med* 2015; 43(1): 3–12.
3. www.survivingsepsis.org/ (accessed 2 March 2015).
4. T. M. Cook, N. Woodall, J. Harper, J. Benger. Fourth National Audit Project. Major complications of airway management in the UK: results of the Fourth National Audit Project of the Royal College of Anaesthetists and the Difficult Airway Society. Part 2: intensive care and emergency departments. *Br J Anaesth* 2011; 106: 632–42.
5. S. Jaber, J. Amraoui, J. Y. Lefrant et al. Clinical practice and risk factors for immediate complications of endotracheal intubation in the intensive care unit: a prospective, multiple-center study. *Crit Care Med* 2006; 34: 2355–61.
6. www.saferintubation.com (accessed 28 February 2015).
7. http://kids.bch.nhs.uk/wp-content/uploads/2015/12/KIDS-pre-transfer-checklist-Dec-2015.pdf (accessed 9 January 2016).
8. J. Dinsmore. St George's neurocritical care unit management algorithm for patients with severe traumatic brain injury. *Contin Educ Anaesth Crit Care Pain* 2013; 13: 189–95.
9. K. A. Wilkinson, I. C. Martin, H. Freeth, K. Kelly, M. Mason. On the Right Trach? A review of the care received by patients who underwent a tracheostomy. London: National Confidential Enquiry into Patient Outcome and Death, 2014. www.ncepod.org.uk/2014report1/downloads/On%20the%20Right%20Trach_FullReport.pdf (accessed 2 March 2015).
10. UK National Tracheostomy Safety Project. www.tracheostomy.org.uk (accessed 2 March 2015).
11. B. A. McGrath, L. Bates, D. Atkinson, J. A. Moore. National Tracheostomy Safety Project. Multidisciplinary guidelines for the management of tracheostomy and laryngectomy airway emergencies. *Anaesthesia* 2012; 67(9): 1025–41. doi: 10.1111/j.1365-2044.2012.07217.

**Chapter**

# Analgesic ladders

Alifia Tameem

*Pain management is a key role of all anaesthetists. This chapter provides a recap of the World Health Organization (WHO) analgesic ladder and the adapter ladder for acute, chronic and cancer pain.*

## Analgesic ladders

In 1986, the World Health Organization (WHO) proposed a 3-step guideline for management of patients with cancer pain. This came to be recognized as the 'Pain Ladder' or 'Analgesic Ladder', and has gradually extended to treating non-malignant pain. The ladder proposed a 3-step approach using simple, over-the-counter drugs initially, moving up to strong opioids for severe pain (Figure 32.1). Prior to the advent of the analgesic ladder, clinicians were reluctant to prescribe strong opioids for fears of addiction and misuse, but these guidelines transformed prescribing practices and legitimized opioids for certain conditions[1].

The WHO ladder was updated in 1996 and the five main recommendations were [2,3]:

1) *'By mouth'* – administer analgesics orally whenever possible. Alternative routes should be reserved for patients who have gastrointestinal problems.
2) *'By the clock'* – they should be given on a regular basis rather than on an 'as needed' basis. Analgesics given at fixed time intervals based on the duration of action of the drug result in better pain management. The subsequent dose should ideally be administered before the previous one has worn off. The dose of the drug is titrated to effect/side effects and some patients may need rescue analgesia for breakthrough and incident pain.
3) *'By the ladder'* – pain is subjective and patients should be treated with analgesics as per 'their' intensity of pain. Patients' pain should be evaluated using simple pain evaluation scales and treated accordingly. Use only one drug from the respective group and if ineffective, use stronger drugs from the group rather than replacing it by a similarly efficacious drug.
4) *'For the individual'* – pain doses should be specifically tailored to individuals as they demonstrate variable response to drugs. Apart from strong opioids, most analgesic drugs have a standard dosing regime with a maximum allowable safe dose. Strong opioids on the other hand are titrated to effect in individual patients; i.e. optimum pain relief with tolerable side effect profile.

*Returning to Work in Anaesthesia*, ed. Emma Plunkett, Emily Johnson and Anna Pierson.
Published by Cambridge University Press. © Cambridge University Press 2016.

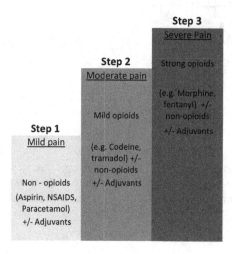

**Figure 32.1** WHO analgesic ladder – 3-step approach.

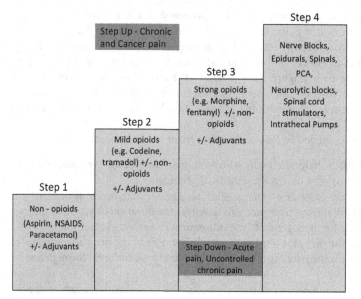

**Figure 32.2** Adapted analgesic ladder for acute, chronic and cancer pain.

5) *'Attention to detail'* – in order to achieve adequate pain relief, regular, individualized administration of painkillers is vital. The patients and their family should be provided with a documented personal plan once the drug dose and timing are established.

Since its initiation in 1986, there have been several iterations of the WHO analgesic ladder. Its use has been extended to encompass acute and chronic non-cancer pain. One of the new adaptations includes a fourth step wherein nerve blocking/modulation procedures can be contemplated (Figure 32.2). The important difference is that patients can be commenced on treatment directly at the stage they present rather than starting at step 1 and then gradually progressing upwards. For example, severe pain can be treated directly with step 3 medications. Additionally, there is consideration for rapid step-down treatment once pain is adequately controlled.

Simple analgesics for mild pain can include paracetamol and non-steroidal anti-inflammatory drugs, such as ibuprofen or naproxen. For moderate pain, the regime can be escalated to include weak opioids such as codeine and tramadol, along with the drugs from step 1. Strong opioids such as morphine, oxycodone, methadone or fentanyl should be considered for severe pain, along with alternative routes of administration. Transdermal opioid is one such choice, which helps to minimize systemic side effects common to this class of drug. Sublingual and buccal preparations provide good, rapid analgesia, hence are suitable for incident pain. Antineuropathic drugs play an important role in managing neuropathic pain; these include antidepressants (amitriptyline), anticonvulsants (gabapentin, pregabalin), N-methyl-D-aspartate (NMDA) receptor drugs (ketamine), steroids and anxiolytics.

Though the WHO analgesic ladder has been criticized for lacking strong evidence of effectiveness, it definitely provides a robust framework enabling us to manage analgesia in patients in a structured manner.

## References

1.  G. Vargas-Schaffer. Is the WHO analgesic ladder still valid? Twenty-four years of experience. *Can Fam Physician* 2010; 56(6): 514–17.
2.  Reid C., Davies A. The World Health Organization three-step analgesic ladder comes of age. *Palliat Med* 2004; 18: 175–6.
3.  *Cancer Pain Relief: With a Guide to Opioid Availability*, 2nd edn. Geneva: World Health Organization, 1996

Chapter

# 33

# Difficult Airway Society (DAS) guidelines

Emily Johnson and Emma Plunkett

*In this chapter airway management guidelines are considered and key points highlighted. This includes the DAS adult, paediatric and obstetric guidelines and the introduction of the Vortex Approach. The importance of planning and team working in airway management cannot be over emphasized. Careful consideration of the DAS guidelines will help refresh your knowledge and aid appropriate airway management planning on your return to work.*

## The DAS adult intubation guidelines

The four plans, A, B, C and D, remain, but have been updated and adapted after consideration of emergency evidence and option. The following points were highlighted by the DAS Guidelines group as particularly new or emerging themes[1]:

- The importance of planning, team working and human factors is recognized.
- New techniques for pre-oxygenation and maintenance of oxygenation are included.
- Facemask ventilation after induction is supported in a rapid sequence induction (RSI) as well as elective induction.
- Videolaryngoscopy is part of plan A.
- It is recommended that cricoid pressure should be removed if there is any difficulty with laryngoscopy or intubation and it should remain off for insertion of a supraglottic airway device (SAD) in plan B (see Figure 33.3a).
- Plan B focusses on oxygenation using SAD (preferably second generation), rather than intubation through SAD although this is still an option. (The intubating laryngeal mask airway (ILMA) is not explicitly recommended.)
- Consideration of the degree of neuromuscular blockade is highlighted as important if intubation fails.
- Standardization of plan D is recommended with surgical cricothyroidotomy as the default. (Cannula techniques remain as an alternative if the anaesthetist is trained and skilled in the particular technique but jet ventilation should be reserved for experts.)

## The DAS extubation guidelines

Extubation is a high-risk phase of anaesthesia and complications are common and may result in significant morbidity and mortality. Despite this it has not received the same level of attention as intubation. Several international airway guidelines recognized the need for a management strategy for extubation without any detailed discussion, except specifically for

*Returning to Work in Anaesthesia*, ed. Emma Plunkett, Emily Johnson and Anna Pierson.
Published by Cambridge University Press. © Cambridge University Press 2016.

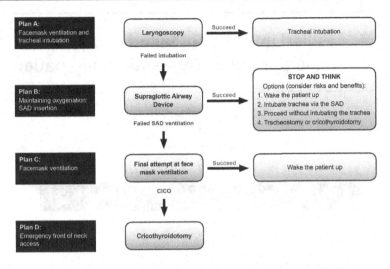

This flowchart forms part of the DAS Guidelines for unanticipated difficult intubation in adults 2015 and should be used in conjunction with the text.

**Figure 33.1** Basic Structure of DAS Guidelines flow chart. Reproduced from Difficult Airway Society 2015 guidelines for unanticipated difficult intubation in adults. C. Frerk, V. S. Mitchell, A. F. McNarry, C. Mendonca, R. Bhagrath, A. Patel, E. P. O'Sullivan, N. M. Woodall and I. Ahmad, Difficult Airway Society intubation guidelines working group. *British Journal of Anaesthesia*, 115(6): 827–48 (2015) doi: 10.1093/bja/aev371.

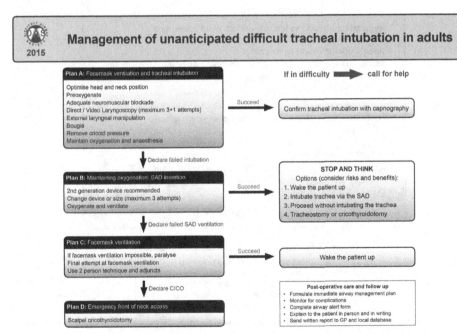

This flowchart forms part of the DAS Guidelines for unanticipated difficult intubation in adults 2015 and should be used in conjunction with the text.

**Figure 33.2** DAS Management of unanticipated difficult intubation in adult patient. Reproduced from Difficult Airway Society 2015 guidelines for unanticipated difficult intubation in adults. C. Frerk, V. S. Mitchell, A. F. McNarry, C. Mendonca, R. Bhagrath, A. Patel, E. P. O'Sullivan, N. M. Woodall and I. Ahmad, Difficult Airway Society intubation guidelines working group. *British Journal of Anaesthesia*, 115(6): 827–48 (2015) doi: 10.1093/bja/aev371.

# Failed intubation, failed oxygenation in the paralysed, anaesthetised patient

**2015**

## CALL FOR HELP

Continue 100% O₂
Declare CICO

**Plan D:** Emergency front of neck access

Continue to give oxygen via upper airway
Ensure neuromuscular blockade
Position patient to extend neck

### Scalpel cricothyroidotomy

**Equipment:** 1. Scalpel (number 10 blade)
2. Bougie
3. Tube (cuffed 6.0mm ID)

**Laryngeal handshake to identify cricothyroid membrane**

**Palpable cricothyroid membrane**
Transverse stab incision through cricothyroid membrane
Turn blade through 90° (sharp edge caudally)
Slide coude tip of bougie along blade into trachea
Railroad lubricated 6.0mm cuffed tracheal tube into trachea
Ventilate, inflate cuff and confirm position with capnography
Secure tube

**Impalpable cricothyroid membrane**
Make an 8-10cm vertical skin incision, caudad to cephalad
Use blunt dissection with fingers of both hands to separate tissues
Identify and stabilise the larynx
Proceed with technique for palpable cricothyroid membrane as above

**Post-operative care and follow up**
- Postpone surgery unless immediately life threatening
- Urgent surgical review of cricothyroidotomy site
- Document and follow up as in main flow chart

This flowchart forms part of the DAS Guidelines for unanticipated difficult intubation in adults 2015 and should be used in conjunction with the text.

**Figure 33.3** DAS Failed intubation, failed oxygenation in the paralysed, anaesthetised patient. Reproduced from Difficult Airway Society 2015 guidelines for unanticipated difficult intubation in adults. C. Frerk, V. S. Mitchell, A. F. McNarry, C. Mendonca, R. Bhagrath, A. Patel, E. P. O'Sullivan, N. M. Woodall and I. Ahmad, Difficult Airway Society intubation guidelines working group. *British Journal of Anaesthesia*, 115(6): 827–48 (2015) doi: 10.1093/bja/aev371.

# FIBREOPTIC GUIDED TRACHEAL INTUBATION THROUGH SUPRAGLOTTIC AIRWAY DEVICE (SAD) USING AINTREE INTUBATION CATHETER

NHS
Lanarkshire

Please ensure the SAD is in place; give 100% oxygen;
confirm adequate sedation/anaesthesia, ventilation & paralysis

### Aintree catheter

- 56cm long hollow catheter
- 6.5mm outer diameter; 4.7mm inner diameter
- Easily preloaded onto an appropriately sized intubating fibroscope (maximum insertion cord diameter - 4.2mm)
- Flexible enough for loading over fibroscope
- Stiff enough to facilitate railroading of tracheal tube
- Comes with 2 rapifit adaptors (please refer to manufacturer's guidelines)
- Used for SAD assisted orotracheal fibreoptic intubation

**4**
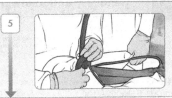

Note depth of AIC. With assistant immobilising SAD and the operator maintaining the position of AIC, the FS alone is withdrawn after removal of securing tape.

**1**
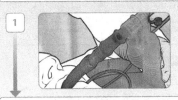

Having prepared the fibrescope (FS) and camera system, lubricate the outer surfaces of both the Aintree Intubation Catheter (AIC) and FS. Preload AIC onto FS and secure with tape. Attach a 15mm bronchoscopic swivel connector (with port) to SAD and attach the anaesthetic circuit to the swivel connector. Confirm adequate anaesthesia, muscle relaxation and assisted ventilation.

**5**
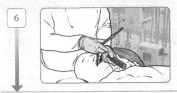

Briefly disconnect SAD (along with swivel connector) from anaesthetic circuit, deflate cuff (if present) and start withdrawing SAD (along with swivel connector), applying counter pressure on AIC to prevent movement. Once the SAD cuff becomes visible, grasp AIC in the mouth and fully remove SAD with the swivel connector. The process should be done with care. Again note the depth of AIC at the lips, ensuring that it **never exceeds 26cm**.

**2**
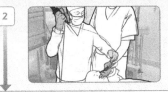

The SAD should be immobilised by an assistant. Introduce FS with loaded AIC through top port of swivel connector into the SAD lumen.

**6**
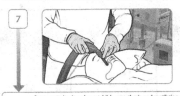

Using a laryngoscope, railroad the tracheal tube (ETT) over AIC ensuring a 'tip anterior' orientation.
Use a conventional ETT - minimum size is 7.0 and pre cut to appropriate length.

**3**
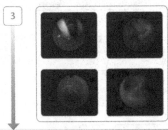

Sequentially visualise SAD aperture bars (if present), glottis, tracheal rings and finally carina as the FS passes caudally. **Never advance beyond carina.**

**7**

Reconnect circuit and re-establish anaesthesia and ventilation.
Confirm end-tidal $CO_2$. Consider FS confirmation of ETT position.

Permission for use granted by Cook Medical Incorporated, Bloomington, Indiana.
Authors: Dr. Rajinuhan Padmanabhan, Consultant Anaesthetist, NHS Lanarkshire
Dr. Barry McGuire, Consultant Anaesthetist, NHS Tayside
Illustrations produced by Andy Morris, Medical Illustration Department, NHS Lanarkshire. 26/01/2011

The AIC was invented in Liverpool, UK;
Reference: Anaesthesia,1996, volume 51, pages 1123-1126.

- This is not an airway rescue technique
- It should be performed in a controlled stepwise process
- The process is designed to provide continued ventilation/oxygenation via the SAD and swivel connector until the SAD is removed and tracheal tube is railroaded in place
- Oxygen can be delivered via the AIC in situations where railroading of tracheal tube is prolonged; assisting ventilation via this route is often suboptimal (narrow diameter/lack of cuff) - Refer to manufacturer's guidelines for methods of oxygen delivery.

**Recommendations**
1. Consider a second anaesthetist in addition to a trained assistant.
2. Use a camera system for fibrescope.

**Caution**
The aintree catheter is not recommended with the LMA Supreme.

**Figure 33.3a** (cont.)

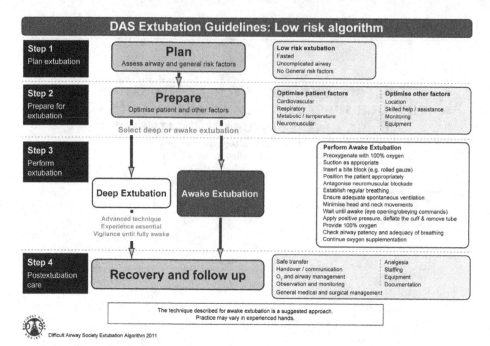

**Figure 33.4** DAS Extubation Guidelines: Low risk algorithm. Reproduced from Popat M., Mitchell V., Dravid R., Patel A., Swampillai C., Higgs A. Difficult Airway Society Guidelines for the management of tracheal extubation. *Anaesthesia* 2012; 67: 318–40, with permission from the Association of Anaesthetists of Great Britain & Ireland/Blackwell Publishing Ltd.

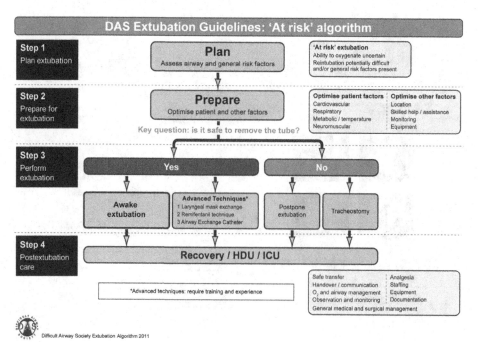

**Figure 33.5** DAS Extubation Guidelines: High risk algorithm. Reproduced from Popat M., Mitchell V., Dravid R., Patel A., Swampillai C., Higgs A. Difficult Airway Society Guidelines for the management of tracheal extubation. *Anaesthesia* 2012; 67: 318–40, with permission from the Association of Anaesthetists of Great Britain & Ireland/ Blackwell Publishing Ltd.

the management of the difficult airway. Following up on this in 2012, the DAS developed guidelines for the management of extubation in perioperative practice. The guidelines discuss the problems arising during extubation and recovery and promote a strategic, step-wise approach to extubation. They emphasize the importance of planning and preparation, and include practical techniques for use in clinical practice and recommendations for post-extubation care[2]. Figures 33.4 and 33.5 show the low-risk and high-risk algorithms, respectively. The basic algorithm is also available on the DAS website.

## The APA and DAS paediatric guidelines

The DAS paediatric difficult intubation guidelines relate to management of the unanticipated difficult airway in children 1 to 8 years old. The following three guidelines are available on the DAS website:

1. Difficult mask ventilation during routine induction of anaesthesia in a child aged 1 to 8 years
2. Unanticipated difficult tracheal intubation during routine induction of anaesthesia in a child aged 1 to 8 years
3. Cannot intubate and cannot ventilate (CICV) in a paralysed anaesthetised child aged 1 to 8 years.

It was identified that most paediatric airway management strategies were developed from adult practice. Therefore, following extensive literature review, external review and a con-sultation period the APA and DAS have developed these guidelines jointly (Figures 33.6 to

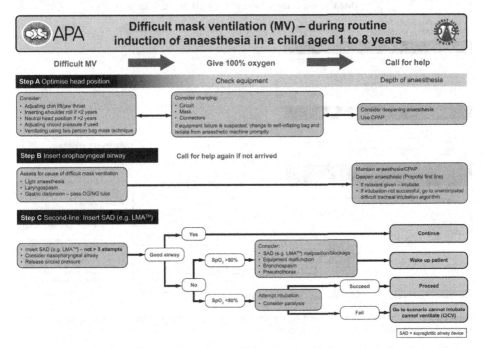

**Figure 33.6** APA and DAS Difficult mask ventilation guideline. Reproduced with permission from Dr Ann Black, Chair, Paediatric Airway Guidelines Group and Paediatric Anaesthesia.

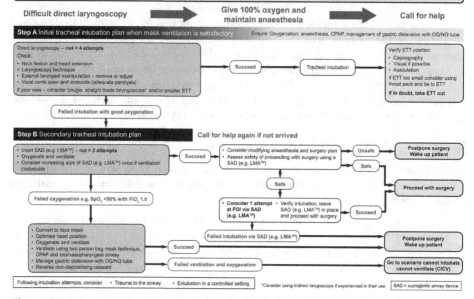

**Figure 33.7** APA and DAS Unanticipated difficult tracheal intubation guideline. Reproduced with permission from Dr Ann Black, Chair, Paediatric Airway Guidelines Group and Paediatric Anaesthesia.

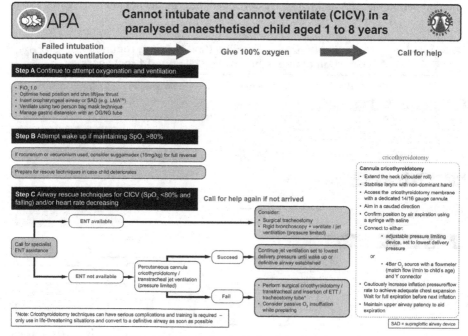

**Figure 33.8** APA and DAS CICV Guideline. Reproduced with permission from Dr Ann Black, Chair, Paediatric Airway Guidelines Group and Paediatric Anaesthesia.

33.8). It is noted there is very little grade 1 evidence to support practice in paediatric airway management.

## The OAA and DAS obstetric difficult intubation guidelines

The development of difficult airway guidelines specific to obstetric anaesthesia is a new endeavour. A public consultation was performed in 2014 regarding the proposed four algorithms and two tables.

Algorithms:

1. Safe obstetric general anaesthesia
2. Obstetric failed intubation
3. Can't intubate, can't oxygenate
4. A combination of 1–3

Tables:

1. Criteria to be used in the decision to wake or proceed following failed intubation
2. Management after a failed intubation: How to wake or proceed and what to do after waking.

The guidelines have been designed around the principles of simplicity, safety (multiple attempts at intubation can be dangerous), a review of practice (anaesthesia is usually continued after failed intubation), familiarity and human factors. We have included algorithm 4 (Figure 33.9) and the two tables (Figures 33.10 and 33.11). The other algorithms can be found on the OAA and DAS websites. We would like to highlight a few key points that the authors mention, many of which are similar themes to those in the updated general adult guidelines.

- Attention to detail in planning and preparation is vital. This can be difficult in practice in category 1 Caesarean sections.
- Mask ventilation may be considered post induction.
- Early reduction or release of cricoid should be considered if there is any difficulty obtaining a view.
- Abandoning intubation attempts sooner rather than later to avoid trauma.
- Early insertion of a second generation SAD is suggested if intubation fails and do not remove this even if it is not possible to ventilate.
- If difficult to ventilate, exclude laryngeal spasm and consider further neuromuscular antagonists.
- Many of the factors that will help determine whether to wake or proceed with surgery are known preoperatively and these can be considered in advance planning.
- The two new factors are the airway device in situ and the presence of any airway pathology. Difficult airway maintenance or airway abnormality will indicate an increased risk of further deterioration.
- The second table gives useful practical guidance of how to manage the situation after a failed intubation.

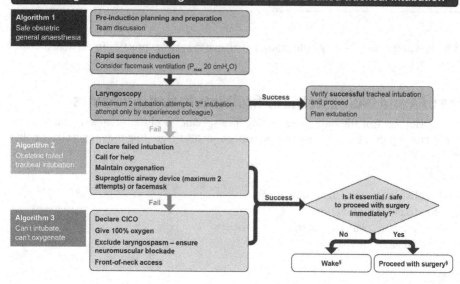

**Master algorithm – obstetric general anaesthesia and failed tracheal intubation**

**Algorithm 1**
Safe obstetric general anaesthesia

Pre-induction planning and preparation
Team discussion

→

Rapid sequence induction
Consider facemask ventilation ($P_{max}$ 20 $cmH_2O$)

→

Laryngoscopy
(maximum 2 intubation attempts; 3rd intubation attempt only by experienced colleague)

— Success → Verify **successful** tracheal intubation and proceed
Plan extubation

Fail ↓

**Algorithm 2**
Obstetric failed tracheal intubation

Declare failed intubation
Call for help
Maintain oxygenation
Supraglottic airway device (maximum 2 attempts) or facemask

— Success →

Fail ↓

**Algorithm 3**
Can't intubate, can't oxygenate

Declare CICO
Give 100% oxygen
Exclude laryngospasm – ensure neuromuscular blockade
Front-of-neck access

Is it essential / safe to proceed with surgery immediately?*

No → Wake§    Yes → Proceed with surgery§

*See Table 1, §See Table 2
© Obstetric Anaesthetists' Association / Difficult Airway Society (2015)

**Figure 33.9** Joint OAA and DAS Obstetric Difficult Intubation Guideline (Algorithm 4). Reproduced from Mushambi M. C., Kinsella S. M., Popat M., Swales H., Ramaswamy K. K., Winton A. L., Quinn A. C. Obstetric Anaesthetists' Association and Difficult Airway Society guidelines for the management of difficult and failed tracheal intubation in obstetrics. *Anaesthesia* 2015; 70: 1286–306, with permission from Obstetric Anaesthetists' Association/ Difficult Airway Society.

## Table 1 – proceed with surgery?

| Factors to consider | | WAKE | ← → | | PROCEED |
|---|---|---|---|---|---|
| **Before induction** | Maternal condition | • No compromise | • Mild acute compromise | • Haemorrhage responsive to resuscitation | • Hypovolaemia requiring corrective surgery<br>• Critical cardiac or respiratory compromise, cardiac arrest |
| | Fetal condition | • No compromise | • Compromise corrected with intrauterine resuscitation, pH < 7.2 but > 7.15 | • Continuing fetal heart rate abnormality despite intrauterine resuscitation, pH < 7.15 | • Sustained bradycardia<br>• Fetal haemorrhage<br>• Suspected uterine rupture |
| | Anaesthetist | • Novice | • Junior trainee | • Senior trainee | • Consultant / specialist |
| | Obesity | • Supermorbid | • Morbid | • Obese | • Normal |
| | Surgical factors | • Complex surgery or major haemorrhage anticipated | • Multiple uterine scars<br>• Some surgical difficulties expected | • Single uterine scar | • No risk factors |
| | Aspiration risk | • Recent food | • No recent food<br>• In labour<br>• Opioids given<br>• Antacids not given | • No recent food<br>• In labour<br>• Opioids not given<br>• Antacids given | • Fasted<br>• Not in labour<br>• Antacids given |
| | Alternative anaesthesia<br>• regional<br>• securing airway awake | • No anticipated difficulty | • Predicted difficulty | • Relatively contraindicated | • Absolutely contraindicated or has failed<br>• Surgery started |
| **After failed intubation** | Airway device / ventilation | • Difficult facemask ventilation<br>• Front-of-neck | • Adequate facemask ventilation | • First generation supraglottic airway device | • Second generation supraglottic airway device |
| | Airway hazards | • Laryngeal oedema<br>• Stridor | • Bleeding<br>• Trauma | • Secretions | • None evident |

Criteria to be used in the decision to wake or proceed following failed tracheal intubation. In any individual patient, some factors may suggest waking and others proceeding. The final decision will depend on the anaesthetist's clinical judgement.
© Obstetric Anaesthetists' Association / Difficult Airway Society (2015)

**Figure 33.10** Criteria to be used in the decision to wake or proceed following failed intubation (Table 1). Reproduced from Mushambi M. C., Kinsella S. M., Popat M., Swales H., Ramaswamy K. K., Winton A. L., Quinn A. C. Obstetric Anaesthetists' Association and Difficult Airway Society guidelines for the management of difficult and failed tracheal intubation in obstetrics. *Anaesthesia* 2015; 70: 1286–306, with permission from Obstetric Anaesthetists' Association/Difficult Airway Society.

## Table 2 – management after failed tracheal intubation

| Wake | Proceed with surgery |
|---|---|
| • Maintain oxygenation<br>• Maintain cricoid pressure if not impeding ventilation<br>• Either maintain head-up position or turn left lateral recumbent<br>• If rocuronium used, reverse with sugammadex<br>• Assess neuromuscular blockade and manage awareness if paralysis is prolonged<br>• Anticipate laryngospasm / can't intubate, can't oxygenate | • Maintain anaesthesia<br>• Maintain ventilation - consider merits of:<br>  ◦ controlled or spontaneous ventilation<br>  ◦ paralysis with rocuronium if sugammadex available<br>• Anticipate laryngospasm / can't intubate, can't oxygenate<br>• Minimise aspiration risk:<br>  ◦ maintain cricoid pressure until delivery (if not impeding ventilation)<br>  ◦ after delivery maintain vigilance and reapply cricoid pressure if signs of regurgitation<br>  ◦ empty stomach with gastric drain tube if using second-generation supraglottic airway device<br>  ◦ minimise fundal pressure<br>  ◦ administer $H_2$ receptor blocker i.v. if not already given<br>• Senior obstetrician to operate<br>• Inform neonatal team about failed intubation<br>• Consider total intravenous anaesthesia |

### After waking

• Review urgency of surgery with obstetric team
• Intrauterine fetal resuscitation as appropriate
• For repeat anaesthesia, manage with two anaesthetists
• Anaesthetic options:
  ◦ Regional anaesthesia preferably inserted in lateral position
  ◦ Secure airway awake before repeat general anaesthesia

© Obstetric Anaesthetists' Association / Difficult Airway Society (2015)

**Figure 33.11** Management after a failed intubation (Table 2). Reproduced from Mushambi M. C., Kinsella S. M., Popat M., Swales H., Ramaswamy K. K., Winton A. L., Quinn A. C. Obstetric Anaesthetists' Association and Difficult Airway Society guidelines for the management of difficult and failed tracheal intubation in obstetrics. *Anaesthesia* 2015; 70: 1286–306, with permission from Obstetric Anaesthetists' Association/Difficult Airway Society.

### The Vortex

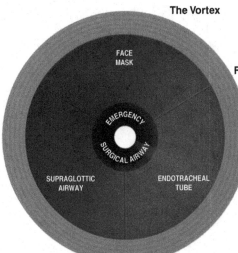

**For Each NSA Technique Consider:**

1. Manipulations:
  ▪ Head & Neck
  ▪ Larynx
  ▪ Device

2. Adjuncts
3. Size/Type
4. Suction/$O_2$ Flow
5. Muscle Tone

MAXIMUM THREE TRIES AT EACH NON-SURGICAL AIRWAY TECHNIQUE
AT LEAST ONE TRY SHOULD BE HAD BY MOST EXPERIENCED AVAILABLE CLINICIAN

vortexapproach.org
© Copyright Nicholas Chrimes & Peter Fritz, 2013

**Figure 33.12** The Vortex Approach. Reproduced from The Vortex Approach by Dr Nicholas Chrimes and Dr Peter Fritz.

# The Vortex Approach

The Vortex Approach has been developed by Dr Chrimes and Dr Fritz in Melbourne, Australia[3,4]. They feel the existing algorithms for management of difficult airways are too complex to use under stress and have therefore designed a more simple approach with the aim of creating a universal template for airway management similar to that for cardiac arrest training. The idea of the Vortex is that it can be applied across disciplines in advanced airway management as a 'high stakes cognitive aid' to focus decision making. It emphasizes the importance of oxygen delivery and can be used regardless of the airway management strategy that was chosen initially[5]. The tool (see Figure 33.12) is presented as a funnel in three segments. Each segment represents a non-surgical airway management technique – face mask, supraglottic airway and endotracheal tube. After an optimal attempt at each has been made (allowing up to three attempts) the operator moves onto the next at the same time conceptually sliding down the funnel towards the surgical airway.

## References

1. http://www.das.uk.com/content/update_on_new_das_guidelines_2015_3 (accessed 4 January 2016).
2. Membership of the Difficult Airway Society ExtubationGuidelines Group. Difficult Airway Society Guidelines for the management of tracheal extubation. *Anaesthesia* 2012; 67(3): 318–40.
3. http://vortexapproach.com (accessed 4 January 2016).
4. N. C. Chrimes. The Vortex: striving for simplicity, context independence and teamwork in an airway cognitive tool. *Anaesthesia* 2015; 115(1): 148–9.
5. A. Sille'n. Cognitive tool for dealing with unexpected difficult airway. *Br J Anaesth* 2014; 112(4): 773–4.

Chapter

# National Audit Project (NAP) summaries

## 34

Fran Haigh and Anna Pierson

To date there have been five National Audit Projects (NAPs) completed, with a sixth on Peri-operative Anaphylaxis currently under development. The Health Services Research Centre is responsible for the management of the NAPs and is overseen by the Royal College of Anaes-thetists (RCoA) Council. NAP1 looked at the supervisory role of consultant anaesthetists and NAP2 the place of mortality and morbidity review meetings. Since these first two projects the NAPs have been used to study an important anaesthesia-related topic of low incidence. This chapter considers NAPs 3, 4 and 5 in more detail, providing a summary of their key findings, and concludes with an outline of the awaited NAP6.

## NAP3: Major Complications of Central Neuraxial Block in the United Kingdom (reported 2009)

### Introduction

Historically it has been difficult to obtain genuinely informed consent from patients to whom we are offering central neuraxial block because the incidence of serious complications was not known; figures quoted have varied from as high as 1 in 1000 to 1 in 100 000. NAP3 was designed to inform this consent process by answering three key questions:

1. What types of central neuraxial blocks (CNBs) are used in the UK and how often?
2. How often are they associated with complications leading to major harm?
3. What happens to the patients experiencing these complications?

### The project

First an assessment of the number of CNBs performed annually in the UK National Health Service (NHS) was made (for denominator information). Then the major complications of CNBs performed over 12 months were audited (for numerator information).

CNBs were classified as epidurals, spinals, combined spinal epidurals (CSE) and caudals. They included those performed perioperatively for both adults and children, all CNBs on the labour ward and, in the chronic pain setting, whether they were administered by an anaes-thetist or non-anaesthetist. Major complications were classified as permanent injury, death or paraplegia.

The project sought to review all patients with a potentially life-changing complication for 6 months in order to assess outcome as well as incidence. As well as neurological

*Returning to Work in Anaesthesia*, ed. Emma Plunkett, Emily Johnson and Anna Pierson.
Published by Cambridge University Press. © Cambridge University Press 2016.

complications it also looked at harm resulting from wrong route error or cardiovascular collapse. However, the report does not provide any information on the incidence of minor complications or major complications without permanent harm.

## The results at a glance

In the UK NHS, over 700 000 CNBs are performed per year: 46% spinals and 41% epidurals, with 45% for obstetric indications and 44% perioperative.

There were 84 major complications reported with 52 meeting all the inclusion criteria. The data were interpreted both 'pessimistically', giving 30 permanent injuries, and 'optimistically', giving 14. Therefore, the figures which we can now confidently quote to our patients are:

Pessimistically, 1 in 24 000 for permanent injury after CNB and 1 in 50 000 for paraplegia/death.

Optimistically, 1 in 54 000 for permanent injury after CNB and 1 in 140 000 for paraplegia/death.

In the 30 patients with permanent harm, 60% occurred after epidural block, 23% after spinal and 13% after CSE. Given the relative numbers of each performed, the incidence of complications of CSE was at least twice those of spinals and epidurals.

These incidences are lower than those of similar (but smaller) historic studies and therefore reassuring to clinicians and patients. Also reassuring is the finding that two-thirds of patients with complications initially judged to be severe made a full recovery. Patients for whom prognosis was poor were those with vertebral canal haematoma and spinal cord ischaemia.

Most complications leading to harm occurred in the perioperative setting as opposed to the obstetric or pain settings and with the majority occurring after epidurals. Perioperative epidurals represent approximately 1 in 7 of all CNBs but accounted for more than half of all the complications leading to harm. In contrast, wrong route errors were more common in obstetric practice than other clinical areas.

Incidences for the different patient populations are shown in Table 34.1.

**Table 34.1** Incidences of permanent harm with CNB

| Indications | Pessimistic | Optimistic |
| --- | --- | --- |
| Overall | 1 in 23 500 | 1 in 50 500 |
| Paraplegia and death | 1 in 54 500 | 1 in 141 500 |
| Overall death | <1 in 100 000 | <1 in 200 000 |
| Perioperative overall | 1 in 12 500 | 1 in 24 000 |
| Obstetric | 1 in 80 000 | 1 in 300 000 |
| Chronic pain | 1 in 40 000 | Had full recovery |
| Paediatrics | No permanent harm | No permanent harm |

## Avoidable harm

Several cases reported to the NAP3 study suggest that failure to identify and understand the relevance of inappropriately weak legs after CNB led to avoidable harm. Contributing factors to delays in diagnosis and intervention were: failure to monitor, poor understanding of abnormal findings (by nurses and doctors), poor interdepartmental referral processes, scanning equipment being unavailable out of hours and a lack of availability of beds in tertiary referral centres for patients requiring specialized emergency surgery.

In response to the NAP3 findings some hospitals have developed algorithms for the management of leg weakness with epidural analgesia. An example of these can be found in Appendix 3 of the full NAP3 report[1].

## NAP3 application

Following the NAP3 project an application (app) has been developed for use with smartphones. Its main feature is a calculator into which the user inputs three variables:

The patient population: perioperative, obstetric, chronic pain or paediatric.

The type of block: spinal, epidural, CSE or caudal.

The statistic sought: permanent harm and death, paraplegia and death, or death.

The app then displays the calculated incidence of complications both 'pessimistically' and 'optimistically', enabling the practitioner to have an informed discussion with the patient about the risks and benefits of the proposed procedure.

The full NAP3 report is freely available online[1].

# NAP4: Major Complications of Airway Management in the United Kingdom (reported 2011)

## Introduction

NAP4 was a collaboration between the Royal College of Anaesthetists (RCoA) and the Difficult Airway Society. The audit was designed to answer the following questions:

1. What types of airway device are used during anaesthesia and how often?
2. How often do major complications, leading to serious harm, occur in association with airway management in anaesthesia both in intensive care units (ICUs) and in emergency departments (EDs) in the UK?
3. What is the nature of these events and what can we learn from them, in order to reduce their frequency and consequences?

## The project

First an assessment was made of the number of general anaesthetics (GAs) performed and the airway devices used annually in the UK NHS (for denominator information). Then the major complications of GAs performed over 12 months was audited (for numerator information).

Major complications were classified as death, brain damage, the need for an emergency surgical airway, unanticipated ICU admission or prolongation of ICU stay.

Data on complications was collected from all areas of the hospital in which GAs are performed including operating theatres, ICUs and EDs.

## The results at a glance

- In the UK NHS, approximately three million patients receive a GA each year.
- 56% of these are managed with a supraglottic airway, 38% with an endotracheal tube (including tracheostomy tubes) and 5% with a face mask.

- Over the 1-year audit period there were 184 cases of major airway complications including 38 deaths.
- A disproportionate number of events reported to NAP4 occurred either in ICU or the ED and the outcome of these events was more likely to lead to permanent harm or death than events in the operating theatre.
- In the theatre environment NAP4 suggests we see a rate of one major airway complication per 22 000 GAs and one death per 180 000 GAs.

The results showed that a minority of hospitals accounted for disproportionately high percentages of reported cases. Because of this anomaly, further statistical analysis was conducted which suggested that as few as 25% of relevant incidents may have been reported. These rates of complications must therefore be seen as an indication of the lower limit of incidence.

## Emergency airways

- An emergency airway was attempted in 80 (43%) of the 184 cases.
- Approximately 60% of the time emergency cannula cricothyroidotomy failed, whereas a surgical technique was almost universally successful. Equipment, training, insertion technique and ventilation technique were all factors in failed attempts.
- In the operating theatre there were 58 emergency airways attempted with 51 (88%) making a full recovery from the incident. Half were tracheostomies and half were cricothyroidotomies. These were performed by a surgeon in 33 cases and by an anaesthetist in 25.
- Of the 29 cricothyroidotomies attempted, 19 were with a narrow-bore (<2 mm) cannula, seven with a wide-bore cannula and three with a surgical approach. The three first choice surgical cricothyroidotomies were all successful whereas 58% of all the other attempts failed.
- In ICU, there were 12 emergency airways attempted; three out of five attempts at needle cricothyroidotomy failed. All other emergency airway attempts were successful.
- In ED, there were 10 emergency airways attempted. All three needle cricothyroidotomies failed but were rescued by a surgical or percutaneous approach.

## The causes of major airway complications

Poor judgement was identified as the commonest cause of the events reported to NAP4. For example, there were many cases where awake fibre-optic intubation was indicated but not used or where there was a clear indication for a rapid sequence induction but this was not performed. Aspiration was the single commonest cause of death in anaesthesia events.

Lack of education and training was also a key element in many cases seen. Poor or incomplete airway assessment or failure to act on its findings led to poor airway outcomes. In addition, a failure to plan or lack of clear strategy for dealing with a difficult or failed intubation or impossible mask ventilation were factors in the NAP4 events. It was also observed that multiple repeat attempts at intubation were tried rather than changing approach.

Many cases of aspiration were seen when supraglottic airway devices (SADs) were inappropriately used in obese patients (defined as BMI $> 30$ kg/m$^2$) or those with multiple risk factors for aspiration.

Airway management was only considered to be good in 19% of cases and elements of care were judged to be poor in three-quarters.

Anaesthesia for head and neck surgery and for obese patients featured frequently in the case reports. Particular complications in obese patients included an increased frequency of aspiration and other complications during the use of SADs and difficulty at tracheal intubation and airway obstruction during emergence or recovery. When rescue techniques were necessary in obese patients they failed more often than in the non-obese.

In ICU, failure to use capnography in ventilated patients was a likely contributor to more than 70% of deaths. The incorrect interpretation of capnograph traces also led to several major complications. In cardiac arrest it must be remembered that cardiopulmonary resuscitation leads to an attenuated but visible expired carbon dioxide trace.

Displaced tracheostomy, and to a lesser extent displaced tracheal tubes, was the most frequent cause of major morbidity and mortality in ICU. The NAP4 report gives an example of an algorithm for management of tracheostomy and endotracheal tube displacement on ICU[2].

One-third of events occurred during emergence or recovery and obstruction was the common cause in these events. This finding of the NAP4 project led the Difficult Airway Society to develop a set of Extubation Guidelines[3].

## Recommendations

Every patient to be anaesthetized should undergo a thorough airway assessment and have a complete plan made for the management of their airway. This should include a plan for failure, i.e. a strategy (logical sequence of plans) to deal with a difficult or failed intubation/ventilation scenario.

At-risk patients must be identified and appropriately managed. The safest technique may not be the most familiar to the anaesthetist but they should seek assistance from colleagues and always ensure the appropriate level of equipment and support is immediately available in case of difficulty.

Capnography must be used and correctly interpreted in every case of GA including in ICU and ED and rapid sequence induction outside of the operating theatre should be treated the same as in theatre with equivalent levels of equipment and support.

Anaesthetists should be trained in both the technique of needle cricothyroidotomy and the surgical airway. NAP4 does not conclude that we should perform one rather than the other technique but it does indicate the possibility that needle cricothyroidotomy is intrinsically inferior to a surgical technique.

Anaesthetists should be educated in how to deal with a displaced tracheostomy and all patients on ICU should have an emergency re-intubation plan.

The full NAP4 report can be found on the RCoA website[2].

# NAP5: Accidental Awareness during General Anaesthesia in the United Kingdom and Ireland (reported 2014)

## Introduction

Being aware during general anaesthesia is something patients cite as their most significant fear and it is an event which all anaesthetists seek to avoid. Previous indicators of how frequently awareness occurs have been based on interview studies where patients are repeatedly interviewed during the days after their operation for signs of awareness. NAP5 differs in that it investigated spontaneous reports of accidental awareness from patients. It sought to address the following questions:

1. How many patients spontaneously report accidental awareness under general anaesthesia (AAGA)?
2. How do these patients present: when, to whom and in what manner?
3. To what extent can risk factors be identified?
4. Is specific depth of anaesthesia monitoring used and does it alter the incidence of AAGA?

## The project

NAP5 was the largest yet of the National Audit Projects as for the first time it involved reporting from all hospitals in Ireland as well as the UK. Over the period of a year all new patient reports of AAGA were reported anonymously to a central, secure, online database. All new reports were considered even if the event had happened years previously; as long as this was the first time the patient had reported the case of AAGA then it was included for analysis. Information was collected on the anaesthetic and surgical techniques and any sequelae. These were then assessed by a multidisciplinary panel and categorized as certain/probable/possible/unlikely episodes of AAGA.

## The results at a glance

Three hundred reports were reviewed in full and, out of these, 141 were classified as certain or probable cases of AAGA. Delay in patient reporting ranged from none up to 62 years after the event. Half of all cases occurred during induction. One-third occurred during maintenance (when pain was more likely to be experienced) and one-fifth on emergence.

The estimated incidence varied widely depending on the surgical specialty and whether neuromuscular blockade (NMB) was used. Overall the incidence of patient reports of AAGA is approximately 1:19 000 anaesthetics but this rises to 1:8000 when NMB is used, 1:136 000 when it is not.

As seen with previous studies about awareness the high-risk surgical specialties were cardiothoracic (1:8600) and obstetrics, i.e. Caesarean section (1:670).

Most reports described events lasting less than 5 minutes with a wide range in the type of experience described; some very trivial, others hugely distressing describing feelings of torture or dying. This was particularly apparent when NMB was used.

The results showed that between 75% and 95% of cases of AAGA were deemed to be preventable.

## Risk factors for AAGA

- Drug factors: NMB, thiopentone, total intravenous anaesthesia (TIVA) techniques
- Patient factors: female gender, age (25–45 years), obesity, previous AAGA and possibly difficult airway management
- Subspecialties: obstetric, cardiac, thoracic, neurosurgical
- Organizational factors: emergencies, out-of-hours operating, junior anaesthetists.
- ASA grade was not found to be a risk factor for AAGA.

## Neuromuscular blockade (NMB)

This is a highly significant risk factor for AAGA. NMB is used in fewer than half of UK GAs; however, 93% of reports to NAP5 concerned patients who had received NMB. They were more likely to experience the most distressing sensations of paralysis and therefore had more long-term psychological sequelae. There were 17 cases of awake paralysis due to drug error. Residual paralysis was experienced by a number of cases of AAGA on emergence. This was due to mistiming the switch-off of anaesthesia; with the failure to use a nerve stimulator being a key factor.

## TIVA

AAGA was twice as likely during TIVA as during volatile anaesthesia. However, in the operating theatre most TIVA was administered using target-controlled infusion (TCI) and AAGA occurred after failure to deliver the intended dose, i.e. disconnection, tissued cannula, etc. Most cases of AAGA during TIVA occurred when non-TCI techniques were used, which was more common outside the operating theatre, e.g. manual infusion, intermittent boluses for the transfer of paralysed patients. Three-quarters of cases were considered preventable. Approximately 20% of reports to NAP5 involved AAGA after sedation rather than general anaesthesia. This represents a failure of communication between anaesthetists and patients.

## Depth of anaesthesia monitoring

Specific depth of anaesthesia (DOA) monitors are still rarely used during general anaesthesia (processed EEG in 2.8% of GAs). It appears to be used in a targeted fashion, in approximately 1% of cases where a volatile agent is given without NMB, but in up to 23% of cases of TIVA with NMB. There was only one report of AAGA with adverse psychological sequelae when DOA was used and overall NAP5 findings are supportive of its use.

## Obstetrics

Obstetrics was significantly over-represented in NAP5 (approximately 10% of all reports, whereas obstetric GAs represent only 0.8% of the total GAs given). Almost all cases occurred after Caesarean section and at induction or early on in surgery. The obstetric population do have many of the risk factors for AAGA as listed above. It is possible that the high number of obstetric cases may explain why 'female gender' appears to be a risk factor for AAGA.

## 'Mind the gap'

Half of all cases occurred during induction. These were likely due to transfer of patient from anaesthetic room to theatre with interruption in anaesthetic delivery, either because of omission of enough drug during transfer or forgetting to turn on the vapour on arrival in the operating theatre. Anaesthetists should be mindful of awareness occurring during this gap; an observation which contributes to the argument for anaesthetic rooms to be dispensed with.

In 25% of cases of AAGA during maintenance anaesthesia no cause could be determined. It is suggested that resistance to anaesthetic drugs may be a plausible explanation.

## Long-term effects of AAGA

Moderate or severe long-term sequelae were experienced by 41% of patients reporting AAGA. They were more likely to occur if the patient had experienced the sensation of paralysis or if there was unsympathetic early management and denial of events by clinicians. Conversely, a good understanding of what had happened seemed to mitigate immediate and longer-term psychological distress. The NAP5 team have developed an Awareness Support Pathway for managing patients who report AAGA[4].

## Recommendations

The NAP5 report includes 64 recommendations. Some key ones are outlined below:

1. Nerve stimulators should be considered as essential in monitoring guidelines whenever NMB drugs are used.
2. All anaesthetists should be adequately trained in the use of TIVA.
3. Anaesthetists should be familiar with the principle, use and interpretation of specific DOA monitoring techniques which should be considered in circumstances where patients undergoing TIVA may be at higher risk of AAGA. These include use of neuromuscular blockade, at conversion of volatile anaesthesia to TIVA and during use of TIVA for transfer of patients.
4. If AAGA is suspected, immediate verbal reassurance should be given to the patient during the episode to minimize adverse consequences, as well as additional anaesthetic to limit the duration of the experience.
5. All reports of AAGA should be treated seriously and all anaesthetic departments should have a policy to manage reports of AAGA. The NAP5 Awareness Support Pathway, or similar, should be instituted[4].
6. Patients should be provided with information about the risks of AAGA as part of the consent process for GA and there should be documentation of this discussion. This is particularly important for obstetric patients undergoing Caesarean section who should be regarded as being at increased risk of AAGA.
7. Patients undergoing elective procedures under sedation should have clear written information provided to them. This should emphasize that during sedation the patient is likely to be aware, and may have recall, but that the intention is to improve comfort and reduce anxiety. It should be stressed that sedation is not general anaesthesia.

The full NAP5 report can be found on the RCoA website[5].

# NAP6: Perioperative Anaphylaxis

The Sixth National Audit Project of the Royal College of Anaesthetists (NAP6), supported by the Health Services Research Centre of the National Institute of Academic Anaesthesia (NIAA) will examine perioperative anaphylaxis[6]. Following the success of recent NAP reports, it is hoped that the awareness raised by the previous projects will facilitate the collection of useful, clinically relevant data. All UK NHS hospitals will be encouraged to participate, with data collection commencing in November 2015. An Allergen survey will then be carried out in spring 2016.

As with all NAPs, the decision to focus on perioperative anaphylaxis underwent a rigorous selection process; a background to NAP6 and plans for the project are summarized by Professor Tim Cook, College Advisor for NAPs, in the November 2013 edition of the Bulletin[7].

So, why look at anaphylaxis? Perioperative anaphylaxis is a relatively rare occurrence within anaesthesia; however, it often results in serious and potentially life-threatening complications, not forgetting the impact of morbidity and mortality on the patient. The incidence of anaesthesia-associated anaphylaxis is thought to be between 1 in 3000 and 1 in 20 000; these figures are predominantly obtained from non-UK studies. It can occur in any patient and in response to all manner of allergens. These include drugs, anaesthetic drugs (of which a few are known to be the more common culprits), colloids, materials used in operative procedures (e.g. surgical dyes, bone cement, haemostatic agents), antibiotics and solutions used for surgical preparation (e.g. betadine, chlorhexidine).

Despite ever-evolving knowledge on the pathophysiology of anaphylaxis, the epidemiology and clinical impact within anaesthesia are less clear. Little is known about the natural history of the condition, but it is thought that over the course of a year, one or two patients are admitted to ICU in every hospital as a result of anaesthesia-associated anaphylaxis. NAP6 hopes to collect extensive information concerning perioperative anaphylactic events, thus enabling clinicians to ultimately improve patient care.

Guidelines are widely available which inform clinical management of such events (Resuscitation Council UK, Association of Anaesthetists of Great Britain and Ireland, British Society of Allergists and Clinical Immunologists) – these may provide standards against which the findings of NAP6 may be audited. Ultimately, any suspected anaesthesia-associated anaphylaxis requires investigation and the UK has approximately 30 clinics set up to do this.

A NAP studying anaphylaxis will provide ample opportunity for (and indeed, in order to succeed in its aims, will require) multispecialty collaboration. Although the precise logistics are not as yet available, the questions NAP6 aims to address may include:

- How frequently do serious anaphylactic reactions occur?
- What is the epidemiology of the condition?
- What is the outcome of such events in the immediate and longer term?
- What are the causative agents?

# References

1.  http://www.rcoa.ac.uk/system/files/CSQ-NAP3-Full_1.pdf (accessed 4 January 2016).
2.  http://www.rcoa.ac.uk/system/files/CSQ-NAP4-Full.pdf (accessed 4 January 2016).
3.  http://www.das.uk.com/content/das-extubation-guidelines (accessed 4 January 2016).
4.  http://nap5.org.uk/NAP5-Anaesthesia-Awareness-Pathway (accessed 4 January 2016).
5.  http://nap5.org.uk/NAP5report#pt (accessed 4 January 2016).
6.  http://www.nationalauditprojects.org.uk/NAP6home (accessed 6 September 2015).
7.  T. Cook. NAP6 Anaphylaxis: what and why? Royal College of Anaesthetists Bulletin 82 November 2013, 42–3. Available at https://www.rcoa.ac.uk/document-store/bulletin-82-november-2013 (accessed 4 January 2016).

# National Institute for Health and Care Excellence (NICE) guidance

Laura Fulton

*Adherence to NICE guidelines may be used to measure clinical effectiveness of an organization and guidelines ultimately exist in order to improve patient care. This chapter summarizes some of the recent publications relevant to anaesthetic practice.*

## NICE guidance

### Guidance on the use of ultrasound locating devices for placing central venous catheters[1]

Literature suggests that the failure rate for initial insertion of central venous catheters (CVCs) is as high as 35%. Complications such as inadvertent arterial puncture and pneumothorax are well described, becoming more likely in the obese patient or in those with distorted anatomy. The potential advantage of ultrasound (US) guidance is the reduction in incidence of complications associated with initial venous puncture. NICE reviewed 20 clinical trials and an economic analysis model to conclude that evidence supports the clinical and cost-effectiveness of the use of US.

Guidance summary:

- 2D US guidance is the preferred method for cannulating the internal jugular vein. It should be considered for all CVC insertions in both adults and children, whether elective or emergency.
- Operators should have training in US-guided technique.
- Doppler US is not recommended.
- Landmark method should be taught alongside US technique. Operators should maintain their ability to use landmark method in case of emergency situations when US is not available.

### Inadvertent perioperative hypothermia[2]

This guideline applies to surgical patients undergoing elective or emergency surgery under general, regional or combined anaesthesia. It does not cover procedures under local anaesthesia, pregnant women, patients <18 years, patients undergoing therapeutic hypothermia or head injured patients with impaired temperature regulation. It outlines steps to be taken in the perioperative period to prevent and treat hypothermia.

*Returning to Work in Anaesthesia*, ed. Emma Plunkett, Emily Johnson and Anna Pierson.
Published by Cambridge University Press. © Cambridge University Press 2016.

Key guidance applicable to the anaesthetist:

- Patients should be managed as higher risk if: ASA II–V, preoperative temperature <36.0 °C, undergoing combined general and regional anaesthesia, major or intermediate surgery, at risk of cardiovascular complications or have received premedication.
- Temperature should be measured on arrival in the anaesthetic room and every 30 minutes until end of surgery.
- Critical incident reporting should be considered if temperature is <36.0 °C on arrival in the anaesthetic room and induction of anaesthesia should not begin until temperature is >36.0 °C unless dictated by clinical urgency.
- Ambient temperature in theatre should be 21.0 °C whilst the patient is exposed and may be reduced once forced air warming is established.
- Patients should be covered and only exposed for surgical preparation.
- IV fluids >500 ml and blood products should be warmed to 37.0 °C using a fluid warming device.
- High-risk patients having surgery <30 minutes and all patients having surgery >30 minutes should be warmed from induction using a forced warm air device.
- Forced warm air devices should be set at maximum and adjusted to maintain temperature of at least 36.5 °C.
- Irrigation fluids should be warmed to 38–40 °C.
- Temperature should be recorded and documented on admission to recovery and every 15 minutes. Patient should not be discharged unless temperature is >36.0 °C. If temperature is <36.0 °C patients should be actively warmed using forced air warming until discharge or until temperature is 36.5–37.5 °C.

# CardioQ-ODM oesophageal Doppler monitor[3]

Guidance summary:

- The CardioQ oesophageal Doppler (CardioQ) is a relatively simple method of monitoring cardiac output by placement of a single-use US probe into the oesophagus to determine flow velocity. From this, values such as stroke volume and cardiac output can be derived, thus monitoring response to fluid therapy. CardioQ should be considered for use in patients undergoing major or high-risk procedures and in surgical patients in whom a clinician would consider using invasive cardiovascular monitoring.
- Clinical studies reviewed included patients undergoing bowel, cardiac, gynaecological, general, urological surgery and surgery for fractured neck of femur. The evidence supported a reduction in perioperative complications and length of hospital stay when fluid management was guided by CardioQ in combination with central venous pressure (CVP) monitoring versus CVP monitoring alone. NICE concluded that clinical evidence demonstrates that the use of CardioQ reduces perioperative complications, the use of central lines and reduces length of hospital stay.
- Reviewing the financial evidence NICE concluded that it demonstrates potential cost savings when CardioQ is used in place of CVP monitoring and when CardioQ is used in

conjunction with CVP monitoring. There was insufficient evidence to support the use of CardioQ in preference to other cardiac output monitoring technology in the critical care setting.

- NICE highlights that this recommendation is not intended to limit the use of other technologies that may offer similar advantages.

## Intravenous fluid therapy in adults in hospital[4]

NICE gives recognition to the complexity of fluid balance. It acknowledges delegation to junior members of the team, error and monitoring as issues. The guidance offers evidence-based advice on IV fluid therapy and includes an outline of physiology, indications for IV therapy and choice of fluids. This guidance does not apply to patients who are <16, in pregnancy, patients with severe liver or kidney disease, traumatic brain injuries, diabetes or burns. It does not apply to patients needing inotropes or those on intensive monitoring. NICE states that it is therefore less relevant in critical care and during anaesthesia.

Key recommendations:

- IV therapy should be administered as part of a protocol that addresses resuscitation, routine maintenance, replacement, redistribution and reassessment. The NICE protocol can be viewed in the full guidance.
- Patients should have an IV fluid management plan that includes a fluid prescription over 24 hours and a plan for assessment and monitoring.
- Assessment should include history, examination, monitoring and investigations and should initially be at least once daily.
- Complications of fluid management should be reported as critical incidents.
- A 500 ml bolus of crystalloid containing sodium in the range 130–154 mmol/l over less than 15 minutes should be used for resuscitation.
- Initial prescription for IV fluid for routine maintenance should be:

   25–30 ml/kg/day water and approximately 1 mmol/kg/day of sodium/potassium and chloride and approximately 50–100 g/day glucose to limit ketosis as a result of starvation.

- Hospitals should have an IV fluid lead responsible for training and governance.

## References

1.  National Institute for Health and Care Excellence (NICE). TA49. Guidance on the use of ultrasound locating devices for placing central venous catheters. London: NICE, 2002. Available at https://www.nice.org.uk/guidance/ta49/resources/guidance-on-the-use-of-ultrasound-locating-devices-for-placing-central-venous-catheters-2294585518021 (accessed 9 January, 2016)
2.  National Institute for Health and Care Excellence (NICE). CG65. Inadvertent perioperative hypothermia. Hypothermia: prevention and management in adults having surgery. London: NICE, 2008. Available at https://www.nice.org.uk/guidance/cg65/resources/hypothermia-prevention-and-management-in-adults-having-surgery-975569636293 (accessed 9 January, 2016)

3. National Institute for Health and Care Excellence (NICE). MTG3. CardioQ-ODM oesophageal doppler monitor. London: NICE, 2011. Available at https://www.nice.org.uk/guidance/mtg3/resources/cardioqodm-oesophageal-doppler-monitor-1788110750149 (accessed 9 January 2016).

4. National Institute for Health and Care Excellence (NICE). CG174. Intravenous fluid therapy in adults in hospital. London: NICE, 2013. Available at https://www.nice.org.uk/guidance/cg174/resources/intravenous-fluid-therapy-in-over-16s-in-hospital-35109752233669 (accessed 9 January 2016).

# Index